THE MOUTH
Diagnosis and Treatment

THE MOUTH
Diagnosis and Treatment

DRORE EISEN, M.D., D.D.S.
Dermatology Associates of Cincinnati
Cincinnati, Ohio

DENIS P. LYNCH, D.D.S., Ph.D.
Professor, Department of Biologic and Diagnostic Sciences
College of Dentistry
Professor, Department of Medicine, Division of Dermatology
College of Medicine, The University of Tennessee, Memphis
Memphis, Tennessee

*with **318** color illustrations*

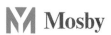 Mosby

St. Louis Baltimore Boston Carlsbad Chicago Minneapolis New York Philadelphia Portland
London Milan Sydney Tokyo Toronto

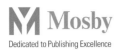

Mosby
Dedicated to Publishing Excellence

A Times Mirror
Company

Vice President and Publisher: Anne S. Patterson
Editor: Susie Baxter
Developmental Editor: Ellen Baker Geisel
Project Manager: Patricia Tannian
Project Specialist: Suzanne C. Fannin
Book Design Manager: Gail Morey Hudson
Manufacturing Manager: Karen Lewis
Cover Designer: Teresa Breckwoldt

Printed in the United States of America
Composition by Accu-color, Inc.
Lithography/color Film by Accu-color, Inc.
Printing/binding by Von Hoffmann Press

Mosby–Year Book, Inc.
11830 Westline Industrial Drive
St. Louis, Missouri 63146

Library of Congress Cataloging in Publication Data

Eisen, Drore.
    The mouth: diagnosis and treatment / Drore Eisen, Denis P. Lynch.
        p. cm.
    Includes index.
    ISBN 0-8151-3105-4 (alk. paper)
    1. Mouth--Diseases. I. Lynch, Denis P. II. Title.
    [DNLM: 1. Mouth--Diseases--diagnosis. 2. Mouth Diseases--therapy.
WU 140 E36m 1998]
RC815.E37 1997
616.3' 1--dc21
DNLM/DLC
for Library of Congress   97-4386
                                                                    CIP

97 98 99 00 01 / 9 8 7 6 5 4 3 2 1

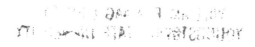

This book is dedicated to the women in our lives

Jane, Sara, Natalie, Monica, Sydney, and Shannon

They encourage us in our professions,
sustain us in our scholarly efforts, and continue to be there when we need them the most.
Husbands and fathers cannot ask for more love and support than that.

Foreword

It is essential that clinicians have a high degree of competence in and are well-educated about oral medicine. Skillful examination of the mouth plays an ever-increasing role in the evaluation and treatment of patients with diverse health problems. The educated eye of the conscientious clinician may recognize subtle evidence of important systemic diseases or infections, the initial manifestations of cutaneous disorders, or significant local problems. Timely recognition allows for the prompt institution of appropriate therapy for disorders such as human immunodeficiency virus (HIV) infection, mucocutaneous blistering diseases, and premalignant and malignant tumors.

Diseases of the skin appear mysterious to many physicians, and those of the mouth may be even more confusing and often overlooked. Although a complete understanding of the etiology and pathophysiology of many oral disorders remains unclear, accurate diagnosis may be made and treatment of great value to patients may be instituted, provided the disorders are detected.

The Mouth: Diagnosis and Treatment is important to clinicians in various disciplines—both primary care physicians and many specialists in medicine and dentistry. This book discusses all aspects of mucosal disease including neoplasia; oral manifestations of systemic, genetic, and dermatologic diseases; and the oral manifestations of infections, including HIV disease. Entire chapters are devoted to the technique of accurate oral examination and the treatment of oral disease. Hundreds of color photographs of oral diseases will aid the clinician in accurate diagnosis and thus lead to appropriate therapy. The book will be of great benefit as a clinical and therapeutic guide and reference.

Drs. Eisen and Lynch are uniquely qualified to author this text. Dr. Eisen holds both D.D.S. and M.D. degrees. Following a medical internship, he trained in dermatology and has continued his interest in oral medicine. He is the author of many articles and chapters on this topic and is a frequently invited speaker, both nationally and internationally. Dr. Lynch is an oral and maxillofacial pathologist with extensive training in oral medicine and has a Ph.D. in experimental pathology. As professor in both the College of Dentistry and College of Medicine at the University of Tennessee, Memphis, he is the author of numerous journal publications and book chapters and has been a featured speaker at numerous professional meetings and symposia. I commend this book with enthusiasm to colleagues in both medicine and dentistry as an excellent resource for use in the diagnosis and treatment of oral disease.

Kenneth A. Arndt, M.D.

Dermatologist-in-chief
Beth Israel Hopital
Professor of Dermatology
Harvard Medical School
Boston, Massachusetts

Preface

The concept of *The Mouth: Diagnosis and Treatment* was born of a desire to provide clinical direction to physicians and dentists who, in the course of practice, encounter oral abnormalities. Its intended use is as a guidebook, providing practical information about diagnoses and treatments. Both gross and microscopic features of oral entities are presented to aid the clinician in understanding the pathophysiology of the underlying condition. Because the oral cavity is a reflection of patients' general health, the importance of identifying oral abnormalities as they relate to systemic, dermatologic, and genetic disorders has been emphasized. Recently, the advent of increased usage of immunosuppressive therapies and the prevalence of the human immunodeficiency virus in the general population have resulted in a reemergence of serious, life-threatening oral infections of various etiologies. Recognizing their impact on oral structures, several chapters have been devoted to infectious diseases that practitioners of multiple disciplines may encounter. Because the therapeutic modalities for oral disorders are scattered among the dental and medical archives, this information has been consolidated and an entire chapter has been devoted to current therapy. It represents a compilation of these sources integrated with a unique emphasis on methods derived from our own extensive clinical experience.

As a dually trained dentist and dermatologist and dentist and oral and maxillofacial pathologist, we are familiar with the educational process in medical and dental schools. Traditionally, medical training deemphasizes the oral cavity, and, consequently, physicians may feel less than familiar with normal and abnormal oral features. Therefore we have incorporated chapters on normal oral anatomy and basic methods of diagnosis, including examination and biopsy techniques. Dentists, although expertly prepared for the recognition of normal and abnormal oral anatomy, may be unfamiliar with underlying systemic entities and the medical treatments required to alleviate oral disorders. It is hoped that the use of this book will encourage a multidisciplinary approach toward recognition and treatment of the numerous diseases that affect the oral cavity. Our ultimate goal in presentation of this work is to enrich our colleagues with a unified resource that will enhance their effectiveness as healers, especially of patients afflicted with oral disease.

We wish to gratefully acknowledge our medical and dental colleagues who supported our effort by contributing material from their personal collections: Jane Anne Blankenship, Timothy M. Johnson, Michael A. Kahn, Anne W. Lucky, Kenneth H. Neldner, J. Robert Newland, C. Mark Nichols, Barry R. Rittman, and Harry K. Sharp.

Drore Eisen
Denis P. Lynch

Contents

Detailed Contents

CHAPTER 1

Normal Oral Anatomy

The oral cavity is the site of many neoplasms, reactive processes, infections, and manifestations of systemic disease. The detection of these abnormalities can be achieved only by those who recognize normal oral structures and their anatomic variations. For most practitioners, this goal can best be accomplished by repeatedly performing oral cavity examinations in all patients, including those without oral complaints.

LIPS

The lips, normally vividly pinkish-red (vermilion), surround the entrance to the oral cavity. The vermilion border of the lips represents the line of demarcation between the oral mucosa and the cutaneous surface (Fig. 1-1). The surface of the vermilion borders is thin and slightly wrinkled in the anteroposterior axis. Although the vermilion borders exhibit hyperparakeratosis microscopically, they do not exhibit clinical evidence of keratinization, such as scale or leukoplakia.

The mucosal surfaces of the lips are normally smooth and glistening because of the presence of saliva. When labial mucosa is palpated, underlying minor salivary glands can be detected, most prominently in the lower lip. If the lips are everted, dried, and observed for a period of time, mucous saliva can be observed as secretions from numerous orifices of the minor salivary glands (Fig. 1-2). Occasionally, the lingual branch of the mental nerve can be noted as a pale, whitish arborizing structure immediately beneath the mucosal surface, lateral to the midline. Both the maxillary and mandibular labial mucosa are attached to the gingiva and alveolar bone by a midline frenum. This weblike attachment normally extends to the height of the junction between the alveolar mucosa and the attached gingiva (Fig. 1-3).

BUCCAL MUCOSA

The buccal mucosa, like the labial mucosa, contains minor salivary glands and normally exhibits a glistening, saliva-coated surface. The linea alba can often be detected as a bilaterally symmetric, white, elevated ridge coursing in an anteroposterior direction at the level of interdigitation of the teeth, which conforms to the space between the teeth at rest. Over three fourths of individuals will also exhibit Fordyce's granules in the oral mucosa. These whitish-yellow papules, normally measuring less than 2 mm, can occur as solitary entities or coalescing plaques. Although most prevalent on the buccal mucosa opposite the posterior maxillary teeth, Fordyce's granules commonly develop on the vestibular and labial mucosa and less frequently on other oral surfaces (Fig. 1-4). The lesions histologically consist of ectopic sebaceous glands and should be considered a normal variant (Fig. 1-5). Stensen's papillae represent the site of drainage of the parotid gland into the oral cavity and are found on the posterosuperior aspect of the buccal mucosa adjacent to the maxillary molars. Serous saliva can be expressed from Stensen's duct when the parotid gland is massaged externally. Another normal variation observed on the buccal mucosa is leukoedema, which results from excess hydration of the mucosal epithelium. The mucosa appears opalescent, whitish-gray, and wrinkled (Fig. 1-6). Although at first glance the lesion may resemble leukoplakia, when the involved mucosa

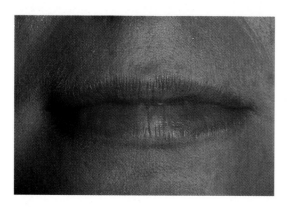

FIG. 1-1   The vermilion borders of the lips are normally pinkish-red and slightly wrinkled. Pigment is commonly seen in nonwhite persons and, when present, is bilateral and evenly distributed. Although the vermilion border is microscopically keratinized, clinical leukoplakia should not be evident.

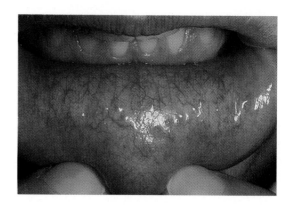

FIG. 1-2   Minor salivary glands of the lower lip, although palpable, are not normally apparent clinically. Punctate salivary secretions are visible, however, if the lower labial mucosa is dried and salivary flow is stimulated.

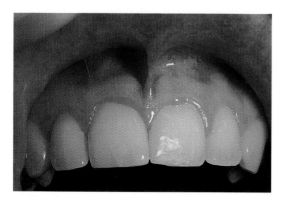

FIG. 1-3   The labial frenula attach the lips to the gingiva and underlying alveolar bone.

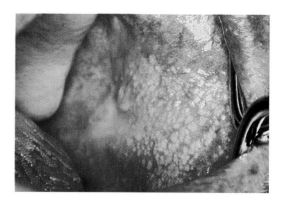

FIG. 1-4   Fordyce's granules are present in the majority of the population and represent ectopic sebaceous glands. They may be isolated or widespread and involve the buccal, vestibular, and labial mucosa and, occasionally, the vermilion borders of the lips.

FIG. 1-5   Fordyce's granules are normal sebaceous glands that are trapped within oral mucosa during embryonic development of the oral cavity.

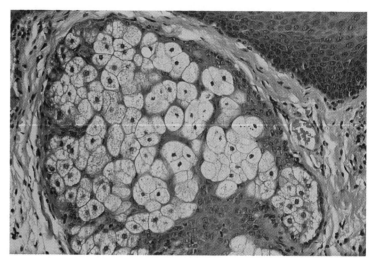

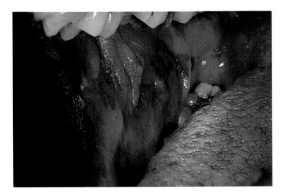

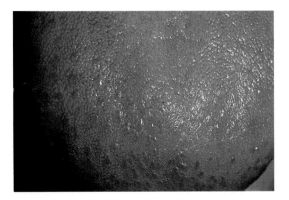

FIG. 1-6   Leukoedema is most commonly found on the buccal mucosa in non-Caucasian persons. It is distinguished clinically from leukoplakia by its disappearance when the cheek is stretched.

FIG. 1-7   The fungiform papillae near the anterior tip of the tongue are interspersed among the more numerous filiform papillae on the dorsal surface of the tongue.

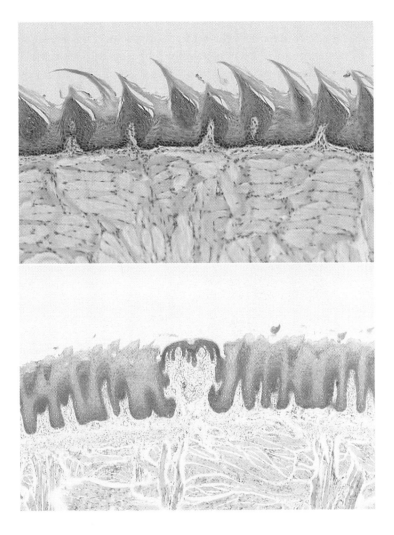

FIG. 1-8   The filiform papillae *(top)* are short, hairlike projections that cover the dorsal surface of the tongue. The fungiform papillae *(bottom)* are larger, pedunculated structures located primarily on the anterior, dorsal, and lateral surfaces of the tongue (×44).

is distended and stretched, the white cast completely disappears. Leukoedema is more prominent in dark-skinned individuals.

TONGUE

The tongue is comprised primarily of voluntary muscle and is covered by highly specialized, keratinized mucosa that contains taste buds. The dorsal surface of the tongue is normally pink and covered by abundant papillae of various types, which have been adapted for taste and mastication. The filiform papillae are most numerous and appear clinically as short, hairlike projections that are evenly distributed over the entire dorsal surface of the tongue. Interspersed among the filiform papillae are larger, red, pedunculated, mushroom-shaped fungiform papillae that are concentrated near the anterior tip and lateral surfaces of the tongue (Figs. 1-7 and 1-8). At the junction of the anterior two thirds and posterior one third of the tongue lie the circumvallate papillae. Approximately 6 to 10 of these papillae are arranged in an inverted V-shaped pattern, each surrounded by a small depression (Fig. 1-9). These are the largest of the lingual papillae and may occasionally be mistakenly identified by patients as abnormal growths. Taste buds are most prevalent in the circumvallate papillae; there are an average of 250 taste buds in each papilla compared with fungiform papillae, which have no more than 20 taste buds in each.

The lateral surface of the tongue is also salmon-pink and is frequently fissured in the superoinferior axis, especially in the posterior segments. In addition, the lingual tonsils are commonly present on the lateral borders of the posterior third of the tongue. These irregularly shaped, soft lobules are comprised of accessory lymphoid tissue (Figs. 1-10 and 1-11). These lymphoid aggregates may become enlarged and inflamed secondary to mechanical irritation by sharp teeth cusps, fractured teeth, or chronic infection.

Sublingual veins are prominent on the ventral surface of the tongue. They are very superficial and tortuous, making them readily adaptable to tongue movements. In addition, small fronds of mucosa, the plicae sublingualis, hang from the undersurface of the tongue. The ventral surface of the tongue is attached to the floor of the mouth by the lingual frenum. This attachment is variable in length and inserts in the midline of the ventral tongue (Fig. 1-12).

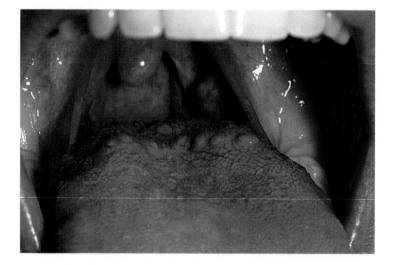

FIG. 1-9   The circumvallate papillae define the junction of the anterior two thirds and posterior one third of the tongue and are surrounded by high concentrations of taste buds.

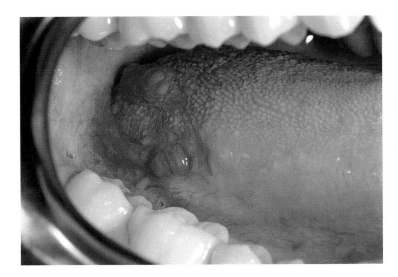

FIG. 1-10   Accessory lymphoid tissue, or lingual tonsil, is normally found in healthy individuals. The tissue may become enlarged and tender secondary to mechanical trauma or local infection.

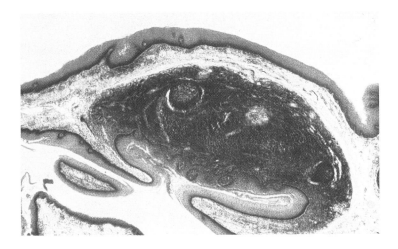

FIG. 1-11   Normal lymphoid tissue is readily identified in lingual tonsils. Germinal centers may be noted, especially in the presence of inflammatory stimuli ($\times$27.5).

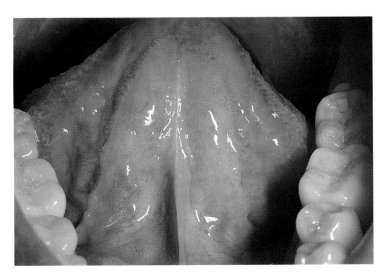

FIG. 1-12   The sublingual vasculature is long and tortuous to allow for the extraordinary mobility of the tongue. Superficial veins are often prominent, especially in geriatric individuals. The plicae sublingualis are found bilaterally on the ventral surface of the tongue, equidistant from the sublingual frenum and the lateral border. The lingual frenum originates in the midline of the ventral tongue and inserts into the floor of the mouth.

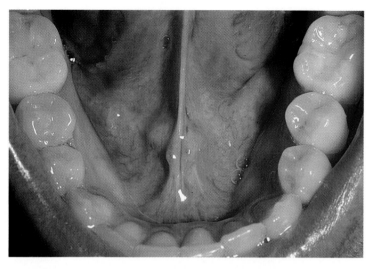

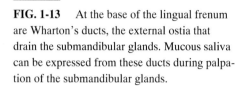

FIG. 1-13 At the base of the lingual frenum are Wharton's ducts, the external ostia that drain the submandibular glands. Mucous saliva can be expressed from these ducts during palpation of the submandibular glands.

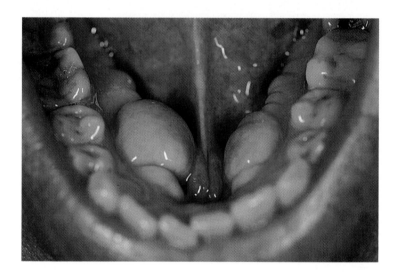

FIG. 1-14 Although often prominent, mandibular tori rarely cause functional impairment. They may require removal before the construction of a mandibular denture.

FLOOR OF THE MOUTH

The floor of the mouth, like the buccal and labial mucosa, is salmon-pink, smooth, and glistening. On either side of the base of the lingual frenum are two punctate papillae. These represent the ostia of Wharton's ducts, which drain saliva from the submandibular glands (Fig. 1-13). The submandibular glands may be palpated in the posterior floor of the mouth and appear as firm masses lateral and inferior to the tongue. The patency of these ducts may be demonstrated by drying the floor of the mouth, massaging the submandibular glands with bimanual palpation, and visualizing expressed saliva. The submandibular saliva is thicker than that produced by the parotid glands because of the higher percentage of mucous acini in the submandibular gland. The sublingual glands are more difficult to palpate because they lie further posteriorly than the submandibular glands.

Mandibular tori are otherwise normal exostoses that may be observed when examining the floor of the mouth (Fig. 1-14). These bony protuberances are generally bilateral and occur in approximately 5% to 10% of the population; however, one fifth of mandibular tori is unilateral. The growths, which may be smooth or lobular, arise on the lingual surface of the mandible at the level of the roots of the premolar teeth. The lesions require surgical removal only when they cause functional impairment or interfere with construction of a dental prosthesis.

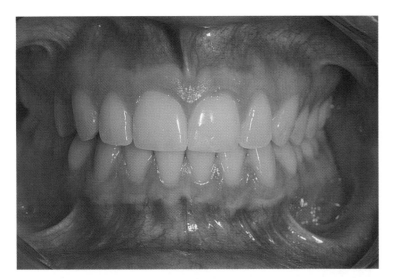

FIG. 1-15   The attached gingiva adjacent to the teeth is keratinized and lighter in color than the nonkeratinized, vascular alveolar mucosa.

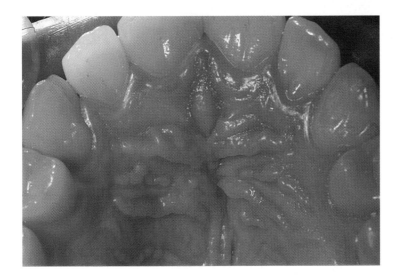

FIG. 1-16   The palatal rugae consist of fibrous connective tissue covered by keratinized mucosa. Immediately posterior to the central incisor teeth is the incisive papilla, which marks the exit of the nasopalatine neurovascular bundle.

HARD PALATE

The hard palate and attached gingiva adjacent to the teeth are areas of the oral cavity that are covered by masticatory or parakeratinized epithelium, and these areas are subject to the greatest mechanical stimulation during mastication and other oral functions. Masticatory mucosa is lighter pink compared with the darker pink or red mucosa found in other oral sites because of a thick layer of keratin and a less vascular lamina propria. The lining or nonkeratinized mucosa that is found on the maxillary and mandibular alveoli, vestibules, cheeks, lips, floor of the mouth, ventral tongue, and soft palate is pinker because of the rich and extensive capillary network beneath a semitransparent epithelium (Fig. 1-15).

The anterior portion of the hard palate is covered by the palatal rugae, which are apparent clinically as firm, fibrous folds of soft tissue. Posterior to the maxillary central incisors is the incisive papilla, which overlies the incisive foramen, representing the inferior ostia of the nasopalatine duct. The neurovascular bundle, which supplies the anterior hard palate and the nasopalatine artery, vein, and nerve, is contained within this duct (Fig. 1-16). A small midline indentation, the palatine raphe, can often be noted in the palatal vault and represents the embryologic fusion of the palatal shelves (Fig. 1-17).

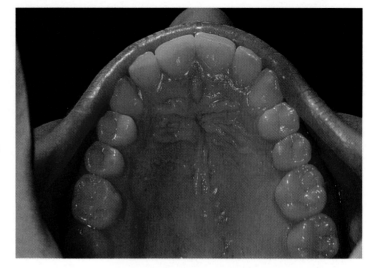

FIG. 1-17   The palatine raphe, which represents the site of fusion of the palatal shelves, presents as a shallow, midline depression of the palate.

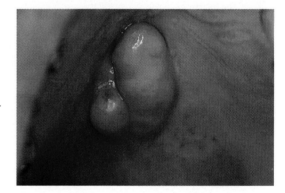

FIG. 1-18   Palatal tori, although capable of attaining significant size, rarely cause problems with oral function, and patients are often unaware of their presence. Preprosthetic surgical removal may be required to achieve adequate biomechanical retention of a maxillary denture.

Palatal tori, like mandibular tori, are bony exostoses that are observed in more than 20% of the population, twice as frequently in females as in males. They occur in the midline of the palate and present clinically in a great variety of shapes and sizes (Fig. 1-18). Palatal tori are generally discovered during early adulthood and may become ulcerated secondary to mechanical trauma. No treatment is indicated unless the tori interfere with function.

SOFT PALATE

The junction of the hard and soft palates occurs at approximately the area of the maxillary second molars. At this location the fovea palatinae, representing the orifices of aggregates of mucous glands, can occasionally be seen on either side of the palatine raphe. The soft palate, lacking osseous support, is highly mobile and, during speech and swallowing, extends posteriorly closing the nasopharynx. The hamular process is an osseous palpable projection immediately posterior to the junction of the hard and soft palates, which functions as an attachment site for several muscles essential for deglutition and mandibular movement. The uvula, a freely movable midline extension of the soft palate, may occasionally be noted to be bifid, although this should be considered to be a normal variant. As with other mucosal surfaces in the mouth, both the hard and soft palates contain minor salivary glands. Although these structures are not palpable, drying of the palate followed by observation reveals the presence of mucous saliva at the glandular ostia (Fig. 1-19).

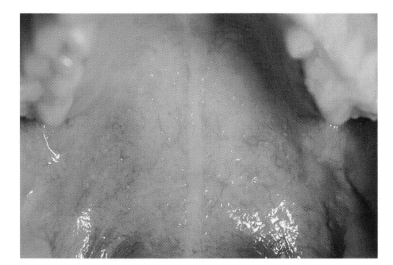

FIG. 1-19   The fovea palatinae are small depressions located lateral to the median palatal raphe at the junction of the hard and soft palates and represent aggregates of minor salivary glands. Additional minor salivary glands are present throughout the hard and soft palates.

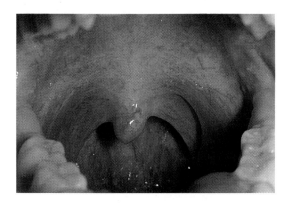

FIG. 1-20   Besides the oral pharyngeal tonsils, additional accessory lymphoid tissue is present on the posterior oral pharynx (Passavant's pad). Such tissue is of normal color and only becomes prominent when inflamed by chronic irritation or infection. It plays a significant role in phonation and deglutition.

OROPHARYNX

The most prominent structures in the oropharynx are the tonsils. In the absence of inflammation, they are salmon-pink with a bosselated surface architecture. The posterior wall of the oropharynx also contains accessory lymphoid tissue (Passavant's pad or adenoids), which appears as slightly elevated mucosal-colored papules (Fig. 1-20). The accessory lymphoid tissue at the posterolateral borders of the tongue (lingual tonsils), palatine tonsils, and Passavant's pad comprises Waldeyer's throat ring.

GINGIVA

The gingiva and alveolar mucosa comprise clinically visible periodontal structures. They are divided into several distinct anatomic regions. The marginal gingiva, immediately adjacent to the crowns of the teeth, is 1 to 2 mm in height and forms the superior edge of the gingival sulcus. In the absence of inflammation, the coronal edge of the marginal gingiva is knife-edged in appearance. The attached gingiva, like the masticatory mucosa of the hard palate, is parakeratinized and firmly bound to the underlying bone. The surface is characteristically stippled in health; however, in the presence of inflammation, it becomes smooth and edematous. The interdental papillae completely fill the space between teeth and contain a subtle depression (Fig. 1-21). Both the marginal gingiva and interdental papillae lack stippling. The mucogingival junction demarcates attached gingiva from alveolar mu-

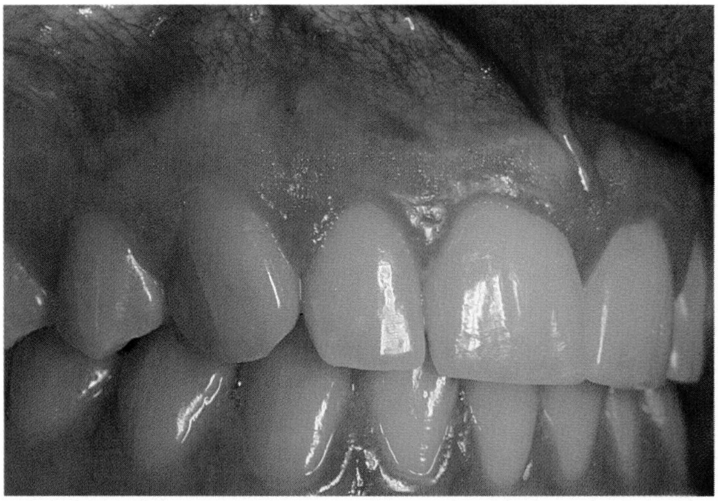

FIG. 1-21   The marginal gingiva has a knife-edged border. The attached gingiva, which is keratinized, is lighter in color than the adjacent alveolar mucosa. In the absence of inflammation, the surface is stippled, resembling an orange peel. The interdental papillae are not stippled and normally fill the entire interdental space.

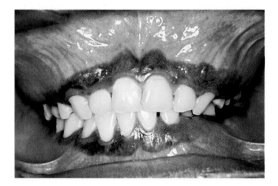

FIG. 1-22   Ethnic pigmentation of the gingiva may be intense but can be differentiated from disorders of pigmentation by its uniform distribution and historical presence.

cosa and is easily visualized. Alveolar mucosa is nonkeratinized and therefore redder than attached gingiva and, unlike the rough and stippled attached gingiva, is smooth.

ORAL PIGMENTATION

Pigmentation is commonly observed in the oral cavity of nonwhite persons. Diffuse patches of pigmentation in various configurations and sizes have their onset in infancy or puberty, and the incidence of such findings increases through early adulthood. The pigmentation is most prevalent on the gingiva and is distinctly absent from the alveolar mucosa (Fig. 1-22). Other sites are also frequently involved, such as the buccal mucosa, palate, and dorsal tongue (Fig. 1-23).

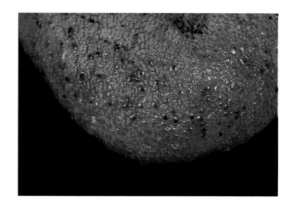

FIG. 1-23   Pigmentation of the fungiform papillae may be found in non-Caucasian persons, usually in association with other physiologic pigmentation of the oral mucosa.

Table 1-1   Timetable of Normal Development Pattern of Teeth

TOOTH	FORMATION	ERUPTION
DECIDUOUS MAXILLARY		
Central incisor	4 months in utero	7.5 months
Lateral incisor	4.5 months in utero	9 months
Cuspid	5 months in utero	18 months
First molar	5 months in utero	14 months
Second molar	6 months in utero	24 months
DECIDUOUS MANDIBULAR		
Central incisor	4.5 months in utero	6 months
Lateral incisor	4.5 months in utero	7 months
Cuspid	5 months in utero	16 months
First molar	5 months in utero	12 months
Second molar	6 months in utero	20 months
PERMANENT MAXILLARY		
Central incisor*	3-4 months	7-8 years
Lateral incisor*	10-12 months	8-9 years
Cuspid*	4-5 months	11-12 years
First premolar*	18-21 months	10-11 years
Second premolar*	24-30 months	10-12 years
First molar	At birth	6-7 years
Second molar	30-36 months	12-13 years
Third molar	7-9 months	17-21 years
PERMANENT MANDIBULAR		
Central incisor*	3-4 months	6-7 years
Lateral incisor*	3-4 months	7-8 years
Cuspid*	4-5 months	9-10 years
First premolar*	21-24 months	10-12 years
Second premolar*	27-30 months	11-12 years
First molar	At birth	6-7 years
Second molar	30-36 months	11-13 years
Third molar	8-10 months	17-21 years

*Succedaneous tooth that replaces an exfoliated primary tooth.

DENTITION

The primary dentition begins to develop at approximately 6 months in utero with the eruption of the first primary teeth, usually the central incisors, occurring at approximately 6 to 9 months of age. There are 20 primary or deciduous teeth, each arch containing four incisors, two cuspids, and four molars. All primary teeth are normally fully erupted by the age of 3 years. Calcification of the permanent dentition begins with the mandibular first molar around the time of birth. There are 32 teeth in the permanent dentition comprised of four incisors, two cuspids, four premolars, and six molars per arch. Twenty of these teeth (the incisors, cuspids, and premolars) are succedaneous teeth, replacing exfoliated primary teeth in the dental arch. Exfoliation of primary teeth begins by the age of 6 years. By the age of 14 years, all of the primary teeth have exfoliated and all of the permanent teeth, with the exception of third molars (wisdom teeth), have erupted. Third molars do not normally erupt until the end of the second or beginning of the third decade of life and, in many instances, remain unerupted. The schedule of eruption of the primary and permanent dentitions is outlined in Table 1-1.

SUGGESTED READINGS

General

Avery JK: *Oral development and histology,* ed 2, New York, 1994, Thieme Medical.

Carranza FA, Newman MG: *Clinical periodontology,* ed 8, Philadelphia, 1996, WB Saunders.

Getchell TV et al: *Smell and taste in health and disease,* New York, 1991, Raven Press.

Meyer J, Squier CA, Gerson SJ: *The structure and function of oral mucosa,* New York, 1984, Pergamon Press.

Rice DH, Becker TS: *The salivary glands,* New York, 1994, Thieme Medical.

Ten Cate AR: *Oral histology: development, structure, and function,* ed 4, St Louis, 1994, Mosby.

Specific

Archard HO, Carlson KP, Stanley HR: Leukoedema of the human oral mucosa, *Oral Surg Oral Med Oral Pathol* 25:717, 1968.

Durocher RT, Thalman R, Fiore-Donno G: Leukoedema of the oral mucosa, *J Am Dent Assoc* 85:1105, 1972.

English WR et al: Individuality of human palatal rugae, *J Forensic Sci* 33:718, 1988.

Ettinger RL, Manderson RD: A clinical study of sublingual varices, *Oral Surg Oral Med Oral Pathol* 38:540, 1974.

Friend GW et al: Oral anomalies in the neonate, by race and gender, in an urban setting, *Pediatr Dent* 2:157, 1990.

Halperin V et al: The occurrence of Fordyce spots, benign migratory glossitis, median rhomboid glossitis, and fissured tongue in 2,478 dental patients, *Oral Surg Oral Med Oral Pathol* 6:1072, 1953.

Kleinman HZ: Lingual varicosities, *Oral Surg Oral Med Oral Pathol* 23:546, 1967.

Kolas S et al: The occurrence of torus palatinus and torus mandibularis in 2,478 patients, *Oral Surg Oral Med Oral Pathol* 6:1134, 1953.

Martin JL: Leukoedema: a review of the literature, *J Natl Med Assoc* 84:938, 1992.

Martin JL, Crump EP: Leukoedema of the buccal mucosa in Negro children and youth, *Oral Surg Oral Med Oral Pathol* 34:49, 1972.

Seah YH: Torus palatinus and torus mandibularis: a review of the literature, *Aust Dent J* 40:318, 1995.

Sewerin I: The sebaceous gland in the vermilion border of the lips and in the oral mucosa in man, *Acta Odontol Scand* 33:13, 1975.

Waitzer S, Fisher BK: Oral leukoedema, *Arch Dermatol* 120:264, 1984.

CHAPTER 2

Diagnosis of Oral Diseases

The primary objectives of an oral cavity examination are to distinguish between health and disease and to recognize normal anatomic structures and their variations. Therefore knowledge of the structure and function of normal oral mucous membranes is crucial to the recognition of oral diseases. This is best accomplished by a careful and methodic inspection of all of the oral structures, complemented by a complete medical and dental history. Because the great majority of lesions in the oral cavity represent reactive processes to either trauma or infections rather than neoplasms, the precise etiology can often be uncovered by a meticulous history and clinical examination.

Because medications often result in oral side effects, a detailed drug history should be routinely obtained. Oral habits and use of dentifrices and mouthwashes should also be recorded because these may also precipitate oral mucosal reactions.

When the diagnosis of an oral abnormality cannot be confirmed on the basis of clinical features, the examination may be supplemented by an excisional or incisional biopsy of the oral mucosa. The microscopic findings correlated with the clinical examination are usually sufficient to confirm the diagnosis.

Clinicians should be encouraged to use photography to document oral diseases and to monitor progress during therapy. Most 35-mm, single-lens reflex cameras can be easily adapted for intraoral use. In fact, several photographic systems have been designed exclusively for intraoral use.

EXTRAORAL EXAMINATION

The initial clinical evaluation of a patient with an oral complaint should begin with an extraoral head and neck examination, which may reveal additional pertinent data. The skin should be inspected for the presence of neoplasms. For example, in patients with multiple hamartoma syndrome, the recognition of cutaneous tricholemmomas on the face is necessary to establish the diagnosis because histopathologic examination of the oral mucosal papillomatosis does not reveal any distinctive histologic properties that would indicate the presence of the syndrome. Changes in color of the facial skin may result from medications such as minocycline or systemic conditions such as Addison's disease, both of which may produce similar changes in the oral mucosa.

All facial structures should be palpated for the presence of masses. Parotid gland tumors may cause intraoral abnormalities, but they are best detected by palpation of the skin overlying the preauricular region. All of the lymph nodes of the neck should be routinely palpated, especially the anterior cervical chain. Lymphadenopathy may result secondary to intraoral infection or from metastatic oral malignancies. Inflammatory lymphadenopathy is characteristically tender on palpation, whereas metastatic disease is normally asymptomatic and results in lymph nodes that are firm and fixed to the underlying tissue. Palpation of the submandibular glands may reveal firmness or tenderness indicative of either neoplasia or infection. The tips of the small digits should be placed in the external auditory canal as patients open their mouth and move the mandible laterally. Frequently, asymptomatic crepitance, clicking, and popping of the temporomandibular joint may be detected and confirmed by auscultation.

The lips should be inspected for color and surface abnormalities, which may indicate actinic damage. Healthy lips are smooth and pliable and do not demonstrate any areas of induration. Maceration or fissuring at the commissures may be a consequence of an underlying nutritional disorder, infections caused by various fungal and bacterial organisms, or decreased vertical dimension secondary to loss of tooth structure or overclosure of the jaws in edentulous patients.

INTRAORAL EXAMINATION

As with any general physical examination, the oral cavity should be examined in a consistent pattern. The examination of the oral cavity is an acquired skill that improves with repetition. Adequate lighting is an invaluable aid that is essential for maximum intraoral visualization. Although present in dental offices, bright overhead lighting is usually absent in medical offices. For those practitioners who do not normally use a fixed or head-mounted examination light, a hand-held flashlight or pen light may be sufficient to supplement ambient room lighting.

The color of all oral mucous membranes should be evaluated because it varies greatly among ethnic groups. Changes in the color of the oral mucosa may be indicative of a systemic disease or may simply represent a variation in the pigmentation of normal mucosa. This awareness may greatly aid in identifying early oral manifestations of systemic diseases and lead to prompt treatment of infections and neoplasms.

The lips should be everted and the labial mucosa inspected. Healthy labial mucosa is smooth, soft, and well lubricated by the numerous minor salivary glands. These glands may be palpated, especially in the lower lip. Self-inflicted and other minor trauma to the lower labial mucosa is common and may result in the formation of a mucocele, which arises most frequently in this location. The buccal mucosa should be examined with the mouth partially opened and the anterior corners of the mouth everted. Normal variations that are commonly noted include diffuse patches of racial or ethnic pigmentation; yellow ectopic sebaceous glands (Fordyce's granules); the linea alba, characterized by a white, hyperkeratotic ridge traversing the buccal mucosa at the level of tooth occlusion; and, in nonwhite persons, leukoedema. Stensen's duct, the orifice of the parotid gland, is visible as a small, punctate, soft-tissue mass opposite the maxillary first (6-year) molars. Saliva may be expressed and visualized after the buccal mucosa is dried with gauze and the cheek is massaged extraorally. The parotid saliva should be clear, thin, and watery; and the procedure should not result in any discomfort to the patient. The buccal mucosa should be well lubricated with saliva but may feel granular because of the presence of minor salivary and sebaceous glands. Almost all of the vesiculoerosive diseases manifest with erythema, blisters, and erosive lesions involving the buccal mucosa.

The dorsal surface of the tongue may be easily visualized by having the patient protrude the tongue and attempt to touch the tip of the chin. The filiform papillae should uniformly cover the dorsal surface. A large number of nutritional deficiencies may result in atrophy of the papillae with associated taste alterations. The lateral borders of the tongue can be visualized after grasping the tongue with gauze and gently pulling and rotating the tongue laterally. In contrast to the dorsal surface, the lateral surface of the tongue is smoother and more erythematous. Normal fissuring in the superoinferior axis may be noted, as well as accessory lymphoid tissue, especially in the posterior lateral tongue, which appears as mucosal-colored, bosselated enlargements. Various pathologic processes manifest on the lateral tongue because this location is subjected to trauma during normal masticatory function.

The ventral surface of the tongue can be inspected as the patient touches the palatal vault with the tip of the tongue. The sublingual mucosa should be smooth and glistening. The prominent sublingual vasculature may impart a blue color to the overlying mucosa. Intraoral squamous cell carcinomas arise most frequently in the ventrolateral tongue. These areas should be meticulously examined for the presence of premalignant and malignant lesions, which frequently present initially as subtle white or red plaques. In the absence of strong clinical evidence and history of the origin of lesions on the tongue, obvious masses or chronic ulcerations should always be biopsied.

Examination of the floor of the mouth should reveal mucosa that is salmon-pink, soft, and freely movable. The ostia of Wharton's ducts, which drain the submandibular glands, are evident at the base of the sublingual frenum on either side of the midline. Pooled saliva can be removed with gauze, and bimanual palpation of the submandibular glands should result in the expression of clear, slightly mucoid saliva.

Direct visual inspection of the hard palate is difficult and is aided by the use of an intraoral mirror. The mucous membrane covering the hard palate is keratinized, accounting for its paler pink color compared with most other oral mucosal surfaces. Recurrent intraoral herpes simplex infections are found on the hard palate in addition to on the attached gingivae. The abundant supply of mucous salivary glands also results in a high incidence of minor salivary gland neoplasms in this location. The incisive papilla appears as a small, firm, sessile, oval nodule immediately posterior to the maxillary central incisors. The anterior hard palate is covered by a series of fibrous ridges or rugae. The soft palate is nonkeratinized, salmon-pink, and relatively vascular. It is most easily inspected when patients are instructed to say "Ahhh." Deviation of the soft palate to one side may be indicative of a neurologic problem or an occult neoplasm.

Examination of the oral pharynx may be difficult in patients with an active gag reflex, although, in the majority of patients, inspection can be accomplished without suppressing the gag reflex with topical anesthetics. The tonsillar pillars are visualized using either a tongue blade or intraoral mirror to depress the posterior tongue and move it laterally. The surface of the tonsils comprises multiple crypts that are highly vascular and more erythematous than surrounding tissues. Accessory lymphoid tissue or adenoids, appearing as irregular, pale, mucosal papules, can be noted on the oral pharyngeal walls. This tissue may enlarge considerably in the presence of infection. Almost all of the primary viral infections that affect the oral cavity, including herpangina and hand-foot-and-mouth disease, involve the oropharynx and result in pharyngeal ulcerations.

The gingivae should be examined with the mouth partially closed and the lips retracted. Like the hard palate, the gingiva is keratinized, pink, and firmly attached to the underlying bone. In contrast, the alveolar mucosa is smooth, red, vascular, and well demarcated from the attached gingivae. In addition to the hard palate, recurrent intraoral herpes simplex infections also affect the keratinized, attached gingivae. In contrast, aphthous stomatitis generally develops on the nonkeratinized mucosal surfaces such as the alveolar, buccal, and labial mucosa. The presence of gingival pigmentation varies greatly and is common in nonwhite persons. In contrast, alveolar mucosa is not normally pigmented, even in dark-skinned individuals. Gingival disease may also be an indicator of a diverse group of underlying systemic disorders, including human immunodeficiency virus infection. Because the gingivae are frequently subjected to chronic trauma and irritation from accumulated plaque and calculus, a great number of reactive lesions and eruptions arise on these oral surfaces. Most important, the health of the gingiva is a reflection of the patient's personal oral hygiene. Failure to maintain adequate oral hygiene will result in significant gingival inflammation, bleeding, and loss of underlying periodontal support of the teeth.

The teeth should be examined last. Gross decay between the teeth or on the occlusal surfaces may indicate poor oral hygiene. Decay at the gingival margins may be the first manifestation of severe xerostomia, as is seen in Sjögren's syndrome. Root surface caries is commonly noted in geriatric patients with gingival recession. A significant number of local and systemic disturbances may result in teeth abnormalities, influencing their size, shape, and number. Evidence of malformed teeth frequently provides clues for identifying a specific congenital abnormality or genetic syndrome. Hypodontia, the congenital absence of one or more teeth, is a common anomaly that most often involves the third molars and maxillary lateral incisors, although it may be associated with inherited disorders. Hyperdontia, or supernumerary teeth, is less common and more frequently associated with several genetic disorders including Gardner's syndrome and oral-facial-digital syndrome.

DIAGNOSTIC TESTS

After a thorough patient history and examination, the diagnosis of an oral condition may remain uncertain. Diagnostic tests provide supplemental information that may be invaluable in establishing a definitive diagnosis. The selection of a diagnostic test or procedure should be based on its value in confirming or excluding a disease process or condition, the attendant risks involved (e.g., morbidity), and the relative expense to the patient.

ORAL BIOPSY

Accurate diagnosis of oral disease is often delayed or postponed because of a hesitation to perform intraoral biopsies. Consequently, treatment of oral diseases is often delayed, resulting in less desirable outcomes. Provided that the clinician is familiar with the normal anatomy of the biopsy site and the basic tenets of good surgical technique, intraoral biopsies can be accomplished with great success.

Several generalizations can be made when performing minor oral surgical procedures and biopsies. Prophylactic antibiotics should be administered before invasive procedures in patients with valvular heart disease and other conditions that predispose them to infective endocarditis, as well as patients with endoprostheses (e.g., prosthetic hip and knee replacements). The local anesthetic should preferably contain a vasoconstrictor, such as epinephrine, to minimize bleeding and retard the vascular diffusion of the anesthetic agent. Topical lidocaine applied to the oral mucosa before the local anesthetic can be used to reduce the initial discomfort of needle insertion.

Vascular-rich areas of the oral cavity requiring biopsy, including the floor of the mouth, Stensen's duct, retromolar trigone, and palate, require extra precautions. Because arteries, veins, and lymphatics tend to course in a posteroanterior direction, incisions should be made parallel to these structures. In general, the biopsy site should be selected from the most representative area of the lesion. Often an additional biopsy specimen is taken from the periphery of a lesion adjacent to normal tissue. When a gingival lesion is biopsied, the specimen should preferentially be obtained from the attached gingiva adjacent to the alveolar mucosa and not from the marginal gingiva to prevent a permanent cosmetic gingival defect. The specimen should be handled gently to preserve cellular detail and should be immediately immersed into an appropriate fixative after removal.

Commonly used surgical modalities include scalpel excision with the use of a chalazion clamp. The clamp is most useful on mobile mucosa such as the lip, tongue, and buccal mucosa. When tightened until it is securely positioned, the clamp provides stability and a relatively bloodless field of operation. Another simple and safe ambulatory technique involves the use of a biopsy punch. Disposable punches may be obtained in graduated sizes ranging from 2 to 6 mm. For biopsies of the lips and buccal mucosa, the free hand of the operator should maintain opposing pressure on the patient's skin during the procedure. Because the majority of oral lesions extend no deeper than the superficial submucosa, punch biopsies may be kept relatively superficial. When a margin of surrounding normal tissue is required, the small size of the punch biopsy may make it difficult to obtain an adequate sampling of tissue. In such cases a larger biopsy punch can be used, or, alternatively, a wedge incision can be made with a scalpel. Oral mucosal specimens, especially those obtained from small punches, should be placed epithelium-side down on a piece of cardboard or other stiff paper before placement in fixative to permit proper orientation of the specimen in the laboratory for sectioning. Deep tissue sampling for lesions that require it should be performed by scalpel incision. Punch biopsies of the oral cavity do not normally require sutured closure and heal adequately within several weeks by secondary intention. Postsurgical hemostasis can be obtained by digital pressure with gauze, aluminum chloride, or silver nitrate; electrodesiccation is infrequently required.

IMMUNOFLUORESCENCE TESTS

The deposition of immunoglobulins and complement components in the oral mucosa is a common feature of autoimmune and other immunologically mediated diseases and conditions. The presence of such substances is ascertained by direct immunofluorescence staining of appropriately fixed biopsy specimens. The most commonly used transport medium for biopsy specimens is Michel's solution. This solution consists of a mixture of buffering salts that preserve the cellular architecture of biopsied tissues and prevent the denaturation of immunoglobulin and complement proteins in the specimen. Biopsy specimens ultimately undergo frozen sectioning; however, specimens may be kept in Michel's solution for months without any appreciable negative effects. Formalin-fixed specimens are inadequate for direct immunofluorescence because the tissue-bound immunoglobulin proteins are denatured by the formalin and become unreactive with antiimmunoglobulin antibody.

When biopsy specimens for direct immunofluorescence studies are obtained, intact perilesional tissue should be selected and ulcerated mucosa should be avoided. When multiple mucosal sites are involved, the selection of an appropriate biopsy site should be governed by the level of disease present and the ease of procuring an appropriate tissue sample.

Examples of immunofluorescence findings of diagnostic value include intercellular deposition of IgG and C3 in pemphigus vulgaris, basement membrane zone deposition of IgG and C3 in cicatricial pemphigoid, shaggy pattern of fibrinogen deposition at the basement membrane zone in lichen planus, and linear IgA deposits along the basement membrane zone, usually without C3, in linear IgA disease. None of these findings is exclusively diagnostic for the conditions listed. All immunofluorescence findings require careful correlation with routine histopathologic and clinical features. Immunoelectron microscopy and immunoblotting may occasionally be necessary to differentiate the oral vesiculoerosive diseases from one another, especially cicatricial pemphigoid, epidermolysis bullosa acquisita, and linear IgA disease.

Indirect immunofluorescence, a method of detecting circulating antibodies by reacting patients' sera with an appropriate mucosal substrate, is an invaluable method used not only for diagnosing vesiculoerosive disorders, but also for monitoring patients' response to therapy. Indirect immunofluorescence has its greatest use in the diagnosis and management of pemphigus vulgaris and paraneoplastic pemphigus.

VIRAL DIAGNOSTIC TESTS

The Tzanck test is a simple and practical diagnostic procedure for oral eruptions suspected of being viral, as well as for other noninfectious acantholytic processes such as pemphigus vulgaris. When the test is performed on a vesicle in the oral cavity, the roof of the lesion should be removed and a sample of the base of the lesion should be obtained by gently scraping it with a scalpel. Generally, oral vesicles rupture shortly after they appear, and the base of an ulceration may be tested with generally reliable results. The material should be transferred to a slide; treated with Wright's, Giemsa's, or another appropriate histochemical stain; and examined for the presence of acantholytic epithelial cell aggregates (Tzanck cells), characteristic giant cells, and other cytopathic effects observed in herpesvirus infections.

The most reliable diagnostic procedure for confirming a suspected viral infection of the oral cavity is viral culturing. After they are rubbed on the base of a lesion, multiple swabs from different anatomic sites may be inserted into one culture vial. Samples should be obtained from intact vesicles or recent ulcerations because such sites yield the highest percentage of positive results. Viral culturing is not equally effective for all oral viral infections. Cultures of herpes simplex infections become positive usually within 3 days, whereas varicella zoster virus is difficult to isolate from oral lesions.

Immunologic and immunohistochemical testing for the presence of specific viral antigens can be accomplished by a variety of mechanisms including immunofluorescence, immunoperoxidase, *in situ* hybridization, specific molecular probes, and polymerase chain reaction–based techniques. All of these mechanisms require an appropriately submitted biopsy specimen. Although these diagnostic technique tests were once used exclusively for investigational purposes, they have in recent years become commercially available.

FUNGAL DIAGNOSTIC TESTS

With the exception of dental caries and periodontal disease, oral candidiasis remains the most common infection of the oral cavity. Accurate diagnosis of the infection is essential for the timely institution of appropriate therapy.

The classic method of diagnosing oral candidiasis involves potassium hydroxide digestion of a mucosal smear. The remaining fungal organisms that resist such digestion can be viewed by dark-field or phase contrast microscopy. Such smears may also be examined by light microscopy after Gram's staining, staining with periodic Schiff's reagent, or using a silver-containing histochemical stain such as Gomori's methenamine silver. Oral candidiasis may also be diagnosed with fluorescent microscopy using calcofluor white (an industrial whitening substance used in the paper industry), which binds to fungal cell walls and fluoresces when exposed to the appropriate excitatory wavelength of light. Although this method is extremely rapid, it requires the use of a fluorescent microscope, which is not routinely found in medical and dental offices.

Traditional culturing of suspected oral candidiasis can be performed by swabbing the infected area and inoculating culture tubes or plates containing appropriate growth media such as Nickerson's or Sabouraud's agar. Culturettes are also available for in-office use that contain appropriate growth media. Unfortunately, *Candida* organisms grow more slowly than most bacteria, and growth may not be detected for several days.

Rapid diagnosis of oral candidiasis can be achieved inexpensively through the use of latex agglutination. Several diagnostic kits are commercially available, although all have been developed exclusively for use in the diagnosis of vulvovaginal candidiasis. The method requires little technical expertise, is relatively inexpensive and highly accurate, and yields results within 2 minutes.

SUGGESTED READINGS

General

Bates B: *A guide to physical examination and history taking,* ed 5, New York, 1995, JB Lippincott.

Bengel W et al: *Differential diagnosis of diseases of the oral mucosa,* Chicago, 1988, Quintessence.

Sonis ST, Fazio RC, Fang L: *Principles and practice of oral medicine,* ed 5, Philadelphia, 1995, WB Saunders.

Topazian RG, Goldberg MH: *Oral and maxillofacial infections,* ed 2, Philadelphia, 1994, WB Saunders.

Wood NK, Goaz PW: *Differential diagnosis of oral and maxillofacial lesions,* ed 5, St Louis, 1997, Mosby.

Photography

Bengel W: The ideal dental photographic system, *Quintessence Int* 24:251, 1993.

Freehe CL: Photography in dentistry: equipment and technique, *Dent Clin North Am* 27:3, 1983.

Oral biopsy

Dajani AS et al: Prevention of bacterial endocarditis: recommendations by the American Heart Association, clinical cardiology, *JAMA* 264:2919, 1990.

Eisen D: The oral mucosal punch biopsy: a report of 140 cases, *Arch Dermatol* 128:815, 1992.

Ficarra G, McClintock B, Hansen LS: Artifacts created during oral biopsy procedures, *J Craniomaxillofac Surg* 15:34, 1987.

Harahap M: How to biopsy oral lesions, *J Dermatol Surg Oncol* 15:1077, 1989.

Lynch DP, Morris LF: The oral mucosal punch biopsy: indications and technique, *J Am Dent Assoc* 121:145, 1990.

Malamed SF: *Handbook of local anesthesia,* ed 4, St Louis, 1997, Mosby.

Moenning JE, Tomich CE: A technique for fixation of oral mucosal lesions, *J Oral Maxillofac Surg* 50:1345, 1992.

Robinson JK et al: *Atlas of cutaneous surgery,* Philadelphia, 1996, WB Saunders.

Roth RJ: An instrument and technique to facilitate biopsies of lesions of the structures of the mouth and within the oral cavity, *J Dermatol Surg Oncol* 7:862, 1981.

Immunofluorescence tests

Dahl MV: *Clinical immunodermatology,* ed 2, St Louis, 1988, Mosby.

Firth NA et al: Assessment of the value of immunofluorescence microscopy in the diagnosis of oral mucosal lichen planus, *J Oral Pathol Med* 19:295, 1990.

Firth NA et al: Direct immunofluorescence of oral mucosal biopsies: a comparison of fresh-frozen tissue and formalin-fixed, paraffin-embedded tissue, *J Oral Pathol Med* 21:358, 1992.

Helander SD, Rogers RS III: The sensitivity and specificity of direct immunofluorescence testing in disorders of mucous membranes, *J Am Acad Dermatol* 30:65, 1994.

Kilpi AM et al: Direct immunofluorescence in the diagnosis of oral mucosal diseases, *Int J Oral Maxillofac Surg* 17:6, 1988.

Siegel MA: Intraoral biopsy technique for direct immunofluorescence studies, *Oral Surg Oral Med Oral Pathol* 72:681, 1991.

Siegel MA, Anhalt GJ: Direct immunofluorescence of detached gingival epithelium for diagnosis of cicatricial pemphigoid: report of five cases, *Oral Surg Oral Med Oral Pathol* 75:296, 1993.

Verma KK, Khaitan BK, Singh MK: Antibody deposits in Tzanck smears in pemphigus vulgaris, *J Cutan Pathol* 20:317, 1993.

Viral diagnostic tests

Bagg J et al: Rapid diagnosis of oral herpes simplex or zoster virus infections by immunofluorescence: comparison with Tzanck cell preparations and viral culture, *Br Dent J* 167:235, 1989.

Brodell RT, Helms SE, Devine M: Office dermatologic testing: the Tzanck preparation, *Am Fam Physician* 44:857, 1991.

Cohen PR: Tests for detecting herpes simplex virus and varicella-zoster virus infections, *Dermatol Clin* 12:51, 1994.

Cubie HA et al: Application of molecular techniques in the rapid diagnosis of EBV-associated oral hairy leukoplakia, *J Oral Pathol Med* 20:271, 1991.

Dhariwal SK, Cubie HA, Southam JC: Detection of human papillomavirus in oral lesions using commercially developed typing kits, *Oral Microbiol Immunol* 10:60, 1995.

Epstein JB et al: The role of an immunoperoxidase technique in the diagnosis of oral herpes simplex virus infection in patients with leukemia, *Diagn Cytopathol* 3:205, 1987.

Flaitz CM, Hammond HL: The immunoperoxidase method for the rapid diagnosis of intraoral herpes simplex virus infection in patients receiving bone marrow transplants, *Spec Care Dentist* 8:82, 1988.

Kimura H et al: Detection and direct typing of herpes simplex virus by polymerase chain reaction, *Med Microbiol Immunol Berl* 179:177, 1990.

MacPhail LA et al: Direct immunofluorescence vs. culture for detecting HSV i oral ulcers: a comparison, *J Am Dent Assoc* 126:74, 1995.

Migliorati CA, Jones AC, Baughman PA: Use of exfoliative cytology in the diagnosis of oral hairy leukoplakia, *Oral Surg Oral Med Oral Pathol* 76:704, 1993.

Miller CS, Zeuss MS, White DK: In situ detection of HPV DNA in oral mucosal lesions: a comparison of two hybridization kits, *J Oral Pathol Med* 20:403, 1991.

Mintz GA, Rose SL: Diagnosis of oral herpes simplex virus infections: practical aspects of viral culture, *Oral Surg Oral Med Oral Pathol* 58:486, 1984.

Fungal diagnostic tests

Allen CM: Diagnosing and managing oral candidiasis, *J Am Dent Assoc* 123:77, 1992.

Axell T et al: Evaluation of a simplified diagnostic aid (Oricult-N) for detection of oral candidoses, *Scand J Dent Res* 93:52, 1985.

Bergman JJ et al: Clinical comparison of microscopic and culture techniques in the diagnosis of Candida vaginitis, *J Fam Pract* 18:549, 1984.

Jeganathan S, Chan YC: Immunodiagnosis in oral candidiasis: a review, *Oral Surg Oral Med Oral Pathol* 74:451, 1992.

Lewis MAO, Samaranayake LP, Lamey PJ: Diagnosis and treatment of oral candidosis, *J Oral Maxillofac Surg* 49:996, 1991.

Lynch DP, Gibson DK: The use of calcofluor white in the histopathologic diagnosis of oral candidiasis, *Oral Surg Oral Med Oral Pathol* 63:698, 1987.

Olsen I, Stenderup A: Clinical-mycologic diagnosis of oral yeast infections, *Acta Odontol Scand* 48:11, 1990.

Reed BD, Pierson CL: Evaluation of a latex agglutination test for the identification of Candida species in vaginal discharge, *J Am Board Fam Pract* 5:375, 1992.

Skoglund A, Sunzel B, Lerner UH: Comparison of three test methods used for the diagnosis of candidiasis, *Scand J Dent Res* 102:295, 1994.

CHAPTER 3

Reactive Processes and Injuries

HAIRY TONGUE

Hairy tongue is a common reactive process that results from various precipitating factors including the use of broad-spectrum antibiotics for a systemic infection, radiation therapy for head and neck malignancies, and poor oral hygiene. This tongue abnormality is also observed with much greater frequency in drug addicts, alcohol and tobacco users, and patients infected with human immunodeficiency virus (HIV).

Clinically, a matted layer forms on the dorsal surface of the tongue as a result of hypertrophy and elongation of the filiform papillae and lack of normal desquamation. Normal filiform papillae are approximately 1 mm long compared with the papillae in hairy tongue, which reach lengths of 12 to 18 mm. The papillae appear as lengthened hairs that may be yellow, white, brown, or, most commonly, black, depending on their staining from foods, tobacco, medications, and pigment-producing bacteria (Fig. 3-1). Overgrowth of *Candida albicans* is common and contributes to the severity of the condition.

Hairy tongue is rarely symptomatic, although patients may be concerned or disturbed with the unsightly appearance of the lesions. Infrequently, hairy tongue may result in gagging, halitosis, and taste alterations. Desquamation of the papillae can be encouraged by meticulous oral hygiene and brushing the tongue regularly. Topical application of retinoids and antifungal medications hastens the resolution of the condition. Keratolytic agents, reported to be of benefit, are usually not necessary and may be irritating. The simple excision of the papillae with scissors should be undertaken when topical therapy fails.

TRAUMATIC ULCERS

Traumatic ulcers comprise one of the most common oral abnormalities encountered. The etiology is most often due to an injury sustained from either the teeth or an external irritant. During mastication, the lateral borders of the tongue, buccal mucosa, and lips endure the greatest degree of trauma, accounting for the high frequency of traumatic ulcerations on these sites (Fig. 3-2). Common iatrogenic ulcerations acquired during dental treatment may result from the removal of a dry cotton roll from the vestibule, tearing the mucosa. Additionally, necrosis of the hard palate, characterized by a well-defined ulcer, may result from the overly rapid injection of local anesthetic, producing ischemia (Fig. 3-3). Dental appliances, especially in children, commonly produce oral ulcerations as do newly placed dentures that rub against the mucosa. Habitual causes of ulcerations, such as the unconscious biting of the buccal mucosa or lips, are much easier to diagnose than factitial ulcerations (Fig. 3-4), which require a complete evaluation to exclude other causes. Cheek biting is also accompanied by irregularly shaped white plaques with desquamation. The size of a traumatic ulcer may vary from a few millimeters to several centimeters, depending on the insult. The lesions are usually painful and superficial, displaying a yellow center with a red margin. Healing results rapidly in the majority of instances. A traumatic ulceration, however, may become chronic if the underlying cause is not cor-

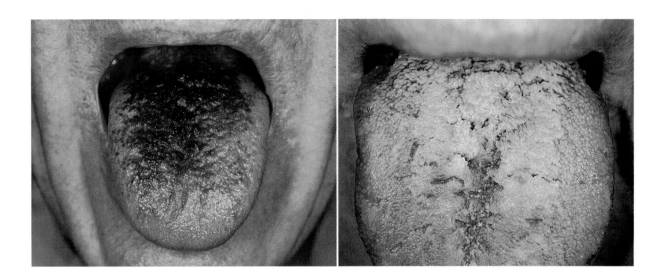

FIG. 3-1   Black and white hairy tongues resulting from elongation and lack of desquamation of the filiform papillae.

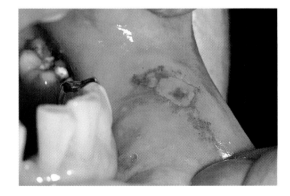

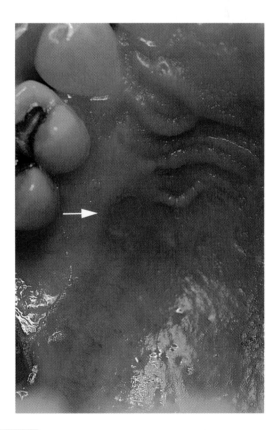

FIG. 3-2   After a local anesthetic is administered, the lip and buccal mucosa are commonly traumatized accidentally during mastication.

FIG. 3-3   Well-demarcated ulcer of the palate occasionally results from the rapid injection of local anesthetic, causing local ischemia.

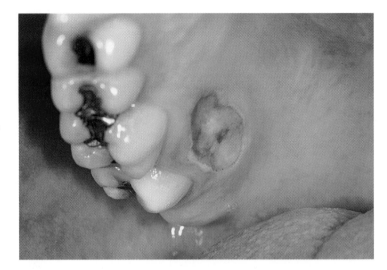

FIG. 3-4   Factitial ulcer from placement of foreign objects such as a pencil eraser in the oral cavity.

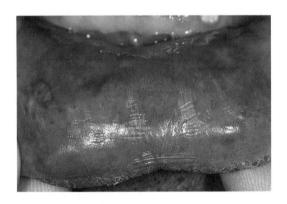

FIG. 3-5   Chronic habitual biting of lower lip resulting in frictional hyperkeratosis.

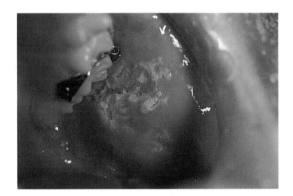

FIG. 3-6   Frictional hyperkeratosis caused by chronic irritation from an orthodontic bracket rubbing against the buccal mucosa.

rected. For example, chronic ulcerations may result from sharp-edged or fractured teeth. Excessive rubbing of the tongue, as occurs in patients with Parkinson's disease or patients whose dental restorations infringe on the tongue space, will result in chronic traumatic ulceration of the tongue. These ulcers become surrounded by a white margin, are often deep and indurated, and may resemble a malignancy. Ulcerations that persist after the cause has been identified and eliminated should always be subjected to biopsy.

FRICTIONAL HYPERKERATOSIS

As with chronic irritation of the skin, the oral mucosal surfaces reveal characteristic morphologic changes when subjected to chronic trauma. Chronic cheek or lip biting, poorly fitting dentures, sharp teeth cusps, broken dental restorations, and tongue movement habits can all result in white patches or plaques (Figs. 3-5 and 3-6). In fact, trauma is the most common etiologic factor in the development of asymptomatic white lesions in the oral cavity. The lesions can vary significantly in size, shape, and thickness depending on the degree of trauma and occur most frequently on the tongue, labial mucosa, alveolar ridge, and buccal mucosa. Single or multiple areas may be involved. The diagnosis of frictional hyperkeratosis should be made only when there is an obvious and direct rela-

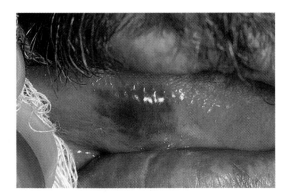

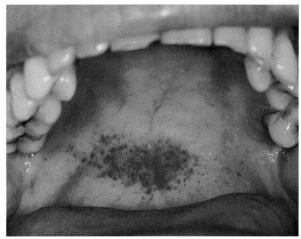

FIG. 3-7   Acute hematoma on the tongue resulting from a direct mechanical blow to the mouth.

FIG. 3-8   Fellatio commonly results in petechiae at the junction of the hard and soft palates.

tionship between trauma and a white plaque. Irregularly shaped verrucous or proliferative lesions or those displaying speckled erythema should be viewed with suspicion and subjected to biopsy. Unlike leukoplakia (see Chapter 5), which is defined as a precancerous white lesion occurring without an apparent cause, traumatic white lesions result in benign hyperkeratosis of the epithelium without evidence of dysplasia. Treatment should be directed at eliminating the underlying cause, and if the lesions do not resolve, a biopsy is mandatory to exclude other causes including carcinoma.

PETECHIAE, ECCHYMOSES, AND HEMATOMAS

A large number of systemic disorders that result in hematologic abnormalities may manifest in the oral cavity as petechiae and ecchymoses (see Chapter 12). These submucosal hemorrhages do not blanch on pressure and occur in varying sizes and shapes. Unexplained causes of such oral lesions, especially when discovered on the palate, should be thoroughly evaluated with laboratory testing. Traumatic causes, however, are responsible for the majority of oral petechiae and ecchymoses. The buccal mucosa, tongue, and lips are often sites of accidental bites or mechanical traumatic events that result in painless hematomas, petechiae, or blood blisters (Fig. 3-7). In these instances a history of trauma can almost always be elicited from the patient. The lesions resolve spontaneously within several days.

Specific causes of trauma result in characteristic patterns of petechiae. For example, petechiae and ecchymosis at the junction of the hard and soft palate may frequently be noted after fellatio (Fig. 3-8). Vigorous coughing and vomiting result in similar findings. Viral infections, especially mononucleosis, bacterial infections, and vasculitis, may all be accompanied by palatal petechiae. The history generally reveals the cause in these cases.

Superficial hematomas arise most often on the tongue as rubbery, blue masses and commonly follow traumatic incidents. The lesions may also develop inferior to the extraction site following a tooth extraction. As the hematoma clots, it becomes firm and dark but eventually resolves spontaneously. Hematomas may become infected or may require aspiration if they are expanding.

DRUG REACTIONS

A significant number of commonly prescribed drugs cause direct and indirect adverse reactions that are manifested in the oral cavity. Chemotherapy, for example, may alter the oral environment, making patients susceptible to opportunistic oral infections, or it may have direct cytotoxic effects resulting in ulcerations. The direct stomatotoxic effects of chemotherapy are discussed in Chapter 9. Many medications may induce oral pigmentation; the importance of differentiating drug-induced oral pigmentation from systemic causes is evaluated in Chapter 10. Clearly, the most frequent drug-related side effect reported in the oral cavity is xerostomia (see Chapter 14), most often as a result of anticholinergic, antidepressant, antihypertensive, antipsychotic, antihistaminic, and sympathomimetic agents. Dry mouth may lead to mucosal erythema and ulcerations, secondary bacterial and fungal infections, and an increased rate of caries. The diagnosis of any oral drug reaction produces a high index of suspicion, necessitating thorough history taking and physical examination.

Stomatitis Medicamentosa

Stomatitis medicamentosa is a general term that refers to an inflammatory oral eruption caused by a systemically administered drug. This adverse hypersensitivity reaction may result from an extensive number of medications, most commonly antibiotics, antiinflammatory agents, anticonvulsants, antihypertensives, and antidepressants. Initially, patients may complain of burning and pain followed by the development of widespread oral ulcerations and stomatitis. In general, the oral features are

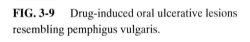

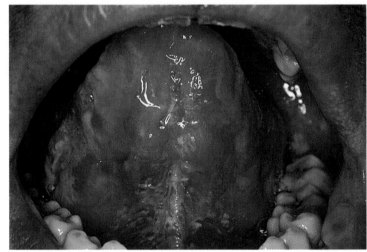

FIG. 3-9   Drug-induced oral ulcerative lesions resembling pemphigus vulgaris.

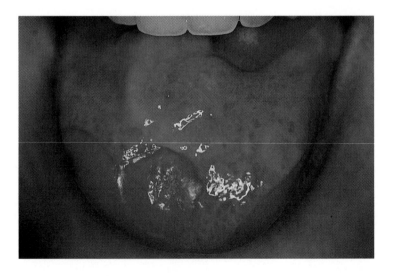

FIG. 3-10   Erythema multiforme reaction secondary to the administration of antibiotics.

specific and may be accompanied by a skin eruption and systemic symptoms. Alternatively, characteristic oral features clinically and histologically resembling autoimmune diseases such as hydralazine- or procainamide-induced lupus erythematosus, penicillamine- or captopril-induced lichen planus, and pemphigus vulgaris- or sulfonamide-induced erythema multiforme may ensue (Figs. 3-9 and 3-10). Oral involvement may often be the first sign of these disorders and infrequently the only manifestation. Although many of these reported drug-induced autoimmune oral eruptions have been poorly documented, a thorough drug history should be obtained in all patients with unexplained oral stomatitis or those exhibiting clinical features of the autoimmune diseases. The withdrawal of the offending drug results in complete resolution of the oral eruption.

Drug-Induced Gingival Hyperplasia

Phenytoin, cyclosporine, and a variety of calcium channel blockers commonly result in clinically and histologically identical enlargement of the gingivae (Figs. 3-11 to 3-13). Although the mechanism of gingival hyperplasia is elusive, all of these agents deplete intracellular calcium, thereby theoretically diminishing the synthesis of collagenase and decreasing the rate of gingival connective tissue turnover.

The incidence of gingival overgrowth in patients treated with phenytoin approximates 50% and is influenced by the dose and duration of treatment in the majority of cases. The severity of the hyperplasia also directly correlates with the serum levels and dose of phenytoin as well as length of treatment. The enlargement usually appears several months after the initiation of phenytoin and peaks in severity after approximately 1 year of treatment. The interdental papillae are affected first, and the hyperplasia progresses gradually and painlessly, sometimes extending to full coverage of the teeth by the gingivae. The labial gingivae of the upper and lower anterior teeth are most commonly affected, and the enlargement is strikingly absent at edentulous sites. The changes may be localized or generalized. The gingival tissues are firm, nodular, and lobulated and may frequently be associated with inflammation. Several months may elapse before improvement is noted after discontinuation of the drug. Substitution with other anticonvulsant medications may also result in gingival enlargement but far less frequently and with much less severity.

All of the calcium channel blockers can result in gingival hyperplasia, although nifedipine accounts for the majority of reported cases. The exact incidence of this adverse reaction is unknown, but the total number of cases is significant and the enlargement is commonly observed. Unlike

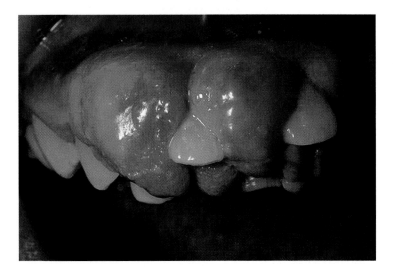

FIG. 3-11   Phenytoin-induced gingival hyperplasia can cover the entire tooth surfaces and is exacerbated by poor oral hygiene.

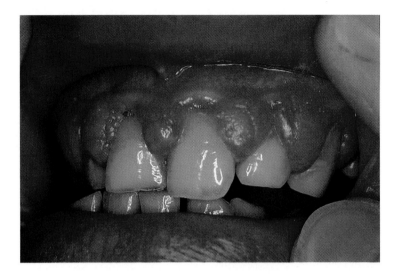

FIG. 3-12   All of the calcium channel blockers can result in gingival hyperplasia, but nifedipine accounts for the majority of reported cases.

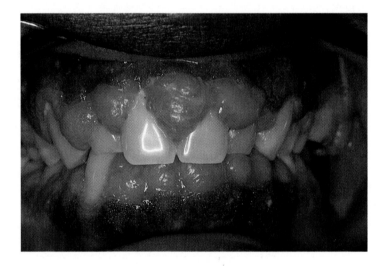

FIG. 3-13   Cyclosporine-induced gingival hyperplasia is a well-recognized adverse reaction.

phenytoin-induced hyperplasia, there is no dose-dependent effect of calcium channel blockers on the severity or incidence of the gingival enlargement. The gingival changes resemble those induced by phenytoin and usually appear within the first 9 months of therapy.

The incidence of gingival hyperplasia in patients receiving cyclosporine ranges from 8% to 70%. The wide disparity may be because of the diverse group of autoimmune diseases treated with this drug and the variations in host susceptibility. A dose-dependent response occurs when serum cyclosporine levels exceed 170 to 200 mg/ml, although not in all patients. The gingival alterations are observed more frequently in children than in adults.

The histologic appearance of drug-induced hyperplasia is the same regardless of the offending drug. Characteristics include elongation and reticulation of the rete ridges, proliferation of fibro-

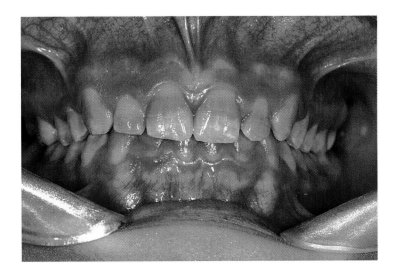

FIG. 3-14   Tetracycline staining of teeth manifests as shades of gray and yellow, which worsens with aging.

blasts and increased formation of collagen fibers, as well as noncollagenous proteins such as glycosaminoglycans.

The greatest risk factor for the development of drug-induced gingival hyperplasia is poor oral hygiene. The prevention or reduction of drug-induced gingival enlargement by the thorough removal of dental plaque, calculus, and inflammation and the concomitant maintenance of an optimal oral hygiene program has been well established, especially in patients taking phenytoin or nifedipine. Surgical correction may be needed to improve function and aesthetics when the gingivae enlarge despite these measures.

Tetracycline-Induced Tooth Discoloration

Tetracycline has a high affinity for deposition in bones and teeth. Discoloration of the developing teeth may result if tetracycline is administered during the mother's pregnancy or before the child is 8 years old. The portion of the teeth stained and the number of teeth discolored are dependent on the length of treatment, dosage, and precise stage of tooth development at the time of drug administration. The affected teeth may initially display shades of yellow, brown, or gray, which darken with aging and sun exposure (Fig. 3-14). The administration of doxycycline and minocycline during mineralization of the deciduous or permanent teeth also produces tooth discoloration. Minocycline, however, can cause a distinct blue band of discoloration when chronically administered to adolescents or adults for the treatment of acne. The blue pigment is most evident in the middle portion of the crowns in contrast to tetracycline stain, which is most pronounced at the gingival third. Minocycline staining of erupted permanent teeth occurs rarely and usually in patients taking more than 100 mg/day. All drug-induced pigmentation of the teeth is permanent and can be masked by cosmetic dental procedures.

ANGIOEDEMA

Angioedema is characterized by episodic bouts of well-circumscribed, nonpitting subepithelial edema and occurs as both hereditary and nonhereditary forms. Hereditary angioedema is an autosomal dominant condition and is characterized by functional levels of C1 inhibitor activity in the blood that are approximately 30% of normal values, resulting in low levels of complement compo-

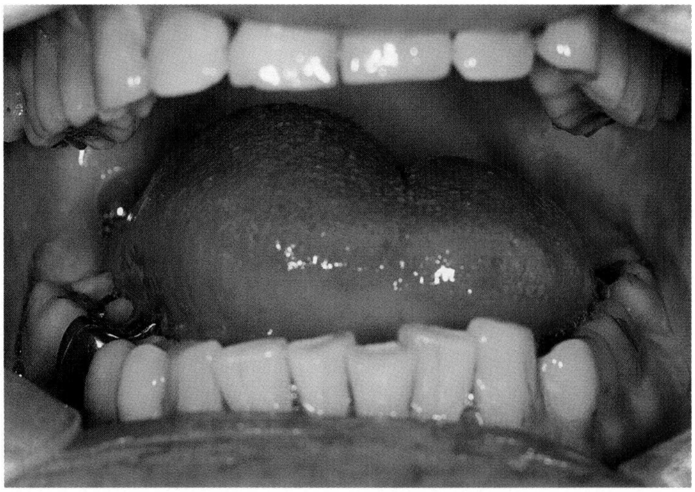

FIG. 3-15   Intraoral angioedema characterized by asymmetric swelling of the tongue.

nents C4 and C2. The first episode usually occurs in childhood, and the frequency and severity of attacks increase significantly during adolescence. Repeated and irregularly occurring attacks last 1 or more days and involve the gastrointestinal tract, extremities, and oropharynx. Although the extremity swelling is painless, abdominal attacks are accompanied by severe pain resulting from edema of the bowel. All patients with hereditary angioedema are at increased risk for attacks of laryngeal edema during and after procedures involving the oral cavity. Oral manipulation including extractions, biopsy, and the use of local anesthetics can result in serious, life-threatening complications. Any form of minor trauma may result in an attack, and approximately one third of attacks are precipitated by emotional stress.

The nonhereditary form of angioedema is the result of an IgE-mediated hypersensitivity reaction without complement activation, most frequently to foods, medications, and inhalants. As in the hereditary form, the sudden onset and rapid progression of an attack may result in upper airway obstruction, but its occurrence is uncommon. In contrast to hereditary angioedema, urticarial skin lesions arise frequently, whereas abdominal and extremity involvement do not occur. Quincke's disease refers to a localized, nonhereditary form of angioedema of the uvula.

In all forms of angioedema, the oral cavity is commonly involved. The uvula is nonerythematous, swollen, and distended. One or both lips may be grossly enlarged and often crack if the swelling does not resolve within a day. Tongue, buccal mucosal, and gingival swelling may develop but are generally asymptomatic (Fig. 3-15).

Infusion of a vapor-heated, C1-inhibitor concentrate is the safest and perhaps most effective means of preventing attacks of hereditary angioedema and treating acute attacks. Continuous administration of the androgenic hormone danazol may result in fewer episodes. Nonhereditary angioedema is most commonly treated with corticosteroids and antihistamines, although a diverse group of agents may also be beneficial. Epinephrine is required only in attacks causing upper airway obstruction. Recurrences may be eliminated by identifying and avoiding precipitating factors.

CONTACT AND IRRITANT STOMATITIS

Contact stomatitis involving the oral mucosa is well recognized but frequently difficult to diagnose. The oral changes that result from a primary irritant stomatitis may be hard to distinguish from contact stomatitis. Furthermore, the characteristic clinical features of an allergy evident on the skin may

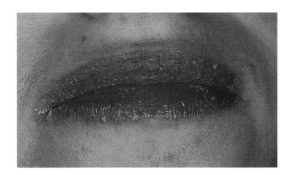

FIG. 3-16   Scaly, erythematous, and painful lips characteristic of contact stomatitis to lipstick.

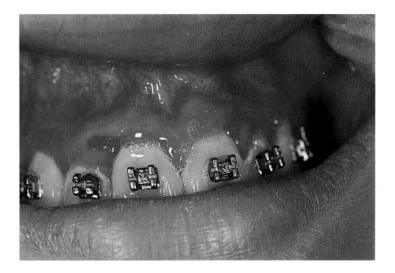

FIG. 3-17   Areas of erythema and erosion caused by orthodontic metal contacting the mucosal surfaces.

be minimal in the mouth. A diverse array of contactants may be responsible for an oral hypersensitivity reaction, necessitating a detailed history and correlation with the oral examination. Frequent known allergens include mouthwashes and dentifrices, which contain an assortment of antimicrobial agents, essential oils, flavoring and coloring agents, preservatives, and astringents and are used for cosmetic and therapeutic purposes (Fig. 3-16). One of the most consistently reported allergies in the mouth is to cinnamon compounds, which, like all allergens, produce an acute stomatitis characterized by swelling, vesiculation, ulceration, erythema, and pain. Allergic reactions to acrylic compounds, resins, and metals in dentures, partial dentures, orthodontic appliances, and dental restorations are easily recognized because the mucosal changes are limited to the areas in direct contact with the allergenic material (Fig. 3-17). This phenomenon has been more prevalent in recent years as nonprecious metals have substituted for gold in dental crowns, resulting in a significant increase in nickel hypersensitivity reactions in the mouth. The allergy manifests as gingival inflammation at the site of contact between the crown and mucosa. Allergies to foods and chewing gums, topical anesthetics, and numerous exogenous agents placed in the mouth may result in a burning sensation. With chronic exposure, lesions tend to be keratotic, desquamative, and lichenoid. Rarely, systemic symptoms and a cutaneous eruption may develop secondary to an oral allergic reaction. The diagnosis of contact stomatitis can be supported by a positive skin test without the need to test the oral mucosa. Each ingredient in the preparation should be tested, whether it is active or inert.

Allergic reactions may also produce clinical features that mimic a variety of oral diseases. For example, dental restorations may, on occasion, produce allergic reactions that result in oral morphologic changes identical to lichen planus (see Chapter 9). This is supported by studies that reveal significantly higher hypersensitivity reactions to mercury in patients with oral lichen planus than control patients and the resolution of lesions in these patients when mercury is removed. Additionally, patients with positive patch tests to gold experience improvement in their oral lichenoid eruption when their gold restorations are replaced. These reactions, however, are uncommon, and before any dental restoration is removed, careful evaluation and patch-testing should be performed. Plasma cell gingivitis is another unique allergic manifestation characterized by sharply demarcated, fiery red, edematous marginal and attached gingivae. Various agents have been implicated, most commonly in chewing gums. Resolution of the gingival changes occurs when the etiologic agent is identified. The chronic administration of an oral contactant, such as cinnamon in toothpaste or mouthwash, can result in oral lesions resembling lupus erythematosus, necessitating a high index of suspicion. Histopathologic changes suggestive of a chronic contact stomatitis include hyperkeratosis, chronic lichenoid mucositis with plasmacytic infiltration, and chronic perivascular inflammation. Recognition of the clinical and histopathologic changes prompting a withdrawal of the suspected compound will result in disappearance of the lesions.

Irritant stomatitis may commonly develop from the inadvertent contact of various dental chemicals with the oral mucosa. For example, phenol, eugenol, bleaching agents, or sodium hypochlorite may cause superficial erosions at their site of contact with the oral mucosa (Fig. 3-18). To achieve pain relief from an aching tooth, patients frequently apply aspirin preparations directly on painful teeth and on the adjacent mucosa in the labial or buccal vestibule (Fig. 3-19). This results in the formation of a painful, white, necrotic surface, which desquamates and erodes. Other chemicals applied

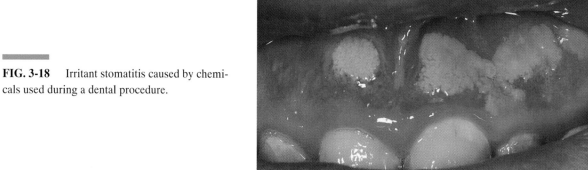

FIG. 3-18   Irritant stomatitis caused by chemicals used during a dental procedure.

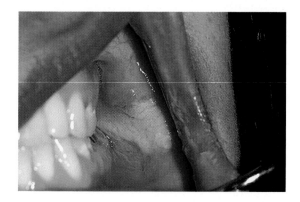

FIG. 3-19   Aspirin burn resulting from placement of aspirin directly on buccal mucosa.

in the oral cavity may produce similar clinical features. All irritant reactions spontaneously resolve, but the administration of topical corticosteroids hastens resolution.

DENTURE INJURIES

Denture Stomatitis

Denture stomatitis or denture sore mouth results from the continuous 24-hour-a-day wearing of complete or partial dentures. The condition usually affects the maxillary alveolar ridge and palate and is clinically characterized by a sharply outlined, deeply reddened, edematous area coinciding with the mucosa directly contacting the denture (Figs. 3-20). Hyperemic pinpoint foci or white patches may be observed within the affected site. The condition is relatively painless, although some patients experience burning. The exact etiology is unknown but is not usually an allergy to the denture material. Denture wearers of blood group O are more susceptible to denture stomatitis, suggesting a genetic predisposition. The role of candidiasis as an etiologic agent is supported by the positive cultures obtained in nearly all cases from affected areas and from the offending dentures. Recently, cases resistant to antifungal therapy have been reported, and in such cases, other microorganisms have been isolated. Thus infection, trauma, and probably a defect in the host defense mechanism are all significant in the pathogenesis of denture stomatitis. Treatment should be directed at eliminating candidiasis with topical and possibly systemic agents, depending on the severity, and simultaneously improving oral hygiene.

Papillary Hyperplasia of the Palate

Papillary hyperplasia of the palate is a common and chronic condition that is observed almost exclusively in denture wearers. Predisposing factors include ill-fitting dentures, poor oral hygiene, and continuously wearing dentures, even while sleeping. Recently, cases of *Candida*-associated palatal hyperplasia occurring in dentate patients infected with HIV and in healthy subjects with poor oral hygiene have been reported. Clinically, 1- to 2-mm red and edematous papules coalesce into plaques and cover the hard palate (Fig. 3-21). The lesions resemble warts and are firm on palpation. Chronic irritation from the dentures may result in significant inflammation, although in the majority of cases the lesions are pink and painless. Microscopically, the papillary projections consist of inflammatory

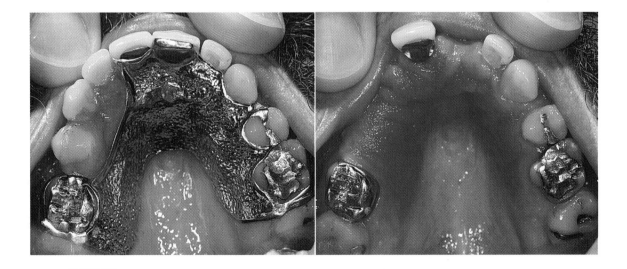

FIG. 3-20   Denture stomatitis. Sharply outlined area of erythema on denture-bearing surface of alveolar mucosa and palate.

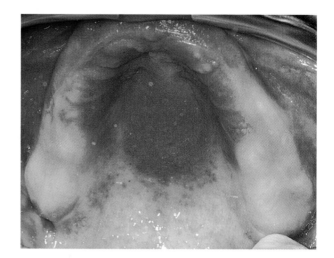

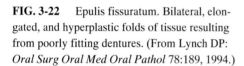

FIG. 3-21 Papillary hyperplasia characterized by coalescing red, minute papules on the palate in a denture wearer.

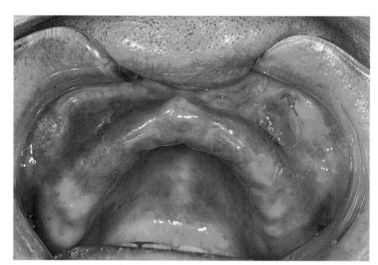

FIG. 3-22 Epulis fissuratum. Bilateral, elongated, and hyperplastic folds of tissue resulting from poorly fitting dentures. (From Lynch DP: *Oral Surg Oral Med Oral Pathol* 78:189, 1994.)

hyperplastic connective tissue with overlying pseudoepitheliomatous hyperplasia. When proper oral hygiene is maintained and the dentures are regularly removed, the condition may resolve. Surgical removal of the papillations is required for persistent lesions.

Epulis Fissuratum

Epulis fissuratum is a common reactive process whereby redundant tissue develops from prolonged irritation from the edge of a poorly fitting denture. Chronic trauma and movement of the denture induce a hyperplastic fold of connective tissue to proliferate at the base of the alveolar ridge where the denture rests. The lesions are elongated, mobile, pink ridges and are usually 1 to 3 cm long (Fig. 3-22). Epulis fissuratum has a propensity to occur labially and anteriorly rather than lingually and posteriorly. Multiple, redundant folds of tissue may be observed at one or more sites depending on the degree of irritation. If untreated, these painless lesions may become firm and eventually ulcerate. Microscopically, a mixed inflammatory infiltrate surrounds coarse collagen bundles overlying a normal epithelium. The folds of tissue should be surgically excised while the denture is being replaced or adjusted to fit properly.

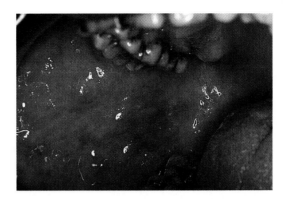

FIG. 3-23   Smoker's melanosis characterized by hyperpigmentation of the buccal mucosa and tobacco staining of the teeth.

THERMAL INJURIES

Smoker's Melanosis

Aside from physiologic pigmentation that is observed in dark-skinned individuals, tobacco use is the most common cause of oral melanin pigmentation. The prevalence of oral pigmentation is significantly higher in smokers who smoke more than 10 cigarettes a day than in nonsmokers, and melanin pigmentation increases proportionately with tobacco consumption.

Smoker's melanosis predominantly affects the anterior mandibular gingiva and interdental papillae, although pigmentation may also develop on the palate and buccal mucosa (Fig. 3-23). Diffuse areas of pigmentation or multiple and uniformly dark macules coalesce on the anterior gingiva and on other oral sites. The condition has been reported to occur more commonly in women and after the third decade of life. It is estimated that approximately one fourth of smokers display some hyperpigmentation on the lower gingiva. The pigmentation resembles physiologic pigmentation both clinically and histologically. Melanin deposition within the basal cell layer and lamina propria can be demonstrated on biopsy and differentiates this cause of pigmentation from neoplastic processes such as malignant melanoma. The cessation of smoking generally results in disappearance of the pigmentation.

Nicotine Stomatitis

Also known as smoker's palate, nicotine stomatitis is a reactive process that occurs almost exclusively in long-term pipe smokers. The condition is also observed in reverse smokers (lit end placed in the mouth), suggesting that thermal effects are responsible for the observed changes. Nicotine stomatitis has a characteristic appearance and is generally confined to the hard palate. Initially, the palate becomes erythematous before the recognizable changes occur. With continued thermal insult, the mucosa of the palate is transformed into a diffuse, white, and thickened surface. The palate is nodular and composed of numerous 1- to 2-mm papules, many with a small, central, red punctum, representing an inflamed minor salivary gland orifice (Fig. 3-24). The papules on the palate are separated from one another by fissures, creating a wrinkled and rough appearance. The entire process is asymptomatic and is usually discovered during a dental examination. Biopsy from patients who are reverse smokers reveals significant dyskeratosis and epithelial atypism that is acanthotic, hyperkeratotic, and parakeratotic. The risk for transformation into squamous cell carcinomas should not be ignored in these patients. However, nicotine stomatitis in pipe smokers is a benign reactive process that has no malignant potential. Cessation of smoking usually results in complete resolution within several months.

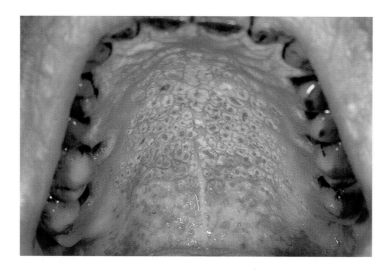

FIG. 3-24   Nicotine stomatitis. Numerous small palatal papules with red puncta separated by fissures are the result of pipe smoking.

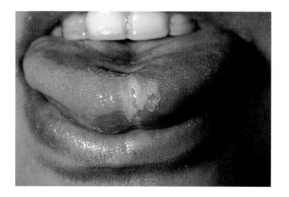

FIG. 3-25   An acute burn of the tongue resulting from contact with a hot food item.

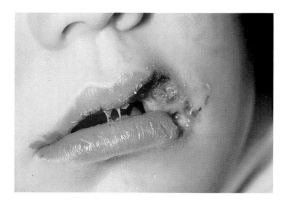

FIG. 3-26   Electrical burns most frequently involve the lip commissure and often result in severe destruction.

Burns

Burns in the oral cavity are commonly encountered after the ingestion of hot food or drink. The palate and tongue are most frequently affected, especially the mucosa overlying a palatal torus. Pain, erythema, and sloughing mucosa are manifestations of mild burns (Fig. 3-25); however, vesicles and ulcerations may develop in severe cases. The rich vascular nature of the oral cavity results in rapid healing, usually within 1 week.

Unfortunately, electrical burns of the oral cavity are one of the most frequent types of burns seen in children. The accident usually occurs in children under 2 years of age and is the result of chewing on an electrical cord, with eventual contact of live bare wire. The burn can cause severe necrosis and destruction of the upper and lower lips, especially at the oral commissures (Fig. 3-26). The injured area is painless and blood-free and develops a black eschar. When the burn extends intraorally, the tongue and gingiva are most severely affected, as are the developing tooth germs. Systemic complications including shock and cardiac arrhythmias are rare. Permanent disfigurement may be minimized by prosthodontic treatment using an oral splint within 10 to 14 days after the initial injury and with reconstructive surgical procedures.

SUGGESTED READINGS

Hairy tongue

Langtry JA et al: Topical tretinoin: a new treatment for black hairy tongue, *Clin Exp Dermatol* 17:163, 1992.

Salonen L, Axell T, Hellden L: Occurrence of oral mucosal lesions, the influence of tobacco habits and an estimate of treatment time in an adult Swedish population, *J Oral Pathol Med* 19:170, 1990.

Sarti GM et al: Black hairy tongue, *Am Fam Physician* 41:1751, 1990.

Traumatic ulcers

Cohen SG, Sirois DA, Sollecito TP: The differentiation of intraoral ulcers, *Hosp Pract* 26:101, 1991.

Damm DD, White DK, Brinker CM: Variations of palatal erythema secondary to fellatio, *Oral Surg* 52:417, 1981.

Hartenian KM, Stenger TG: Postanesthetic palatal ulceration, *Oral Surg* 42:447, 1976.

Kvam E, Bondevik O, Gjerdet NR: Traumatic ulcers and pain in adults during orthodontic treatment, *Community Dent Oral Epidemiol* 17: 154, 1989.

Woods MA et al: Oral ulcerations, *Quintessence Int* 21:141, 1990.

Stomatitis medicamentosa

Gallagher GT: Oral mucous membrane reactions to drugs and chemicals, *Curr Opinion Dent* 1:777, 1991.

Smith RG, Burtner AP: Oral side-effects of the most frequently prescribed drugs, *Special Care Dent* 14:96, 1994.

Zelickson BD, Rogers RS: Oral drug reactions, *Dermatol Clin* 5:695, 1987.

Drug-induced gingival hyperplasia

Dongari A, McDonnell HT, Langlais RP: Drug-induced gingival overgrowth, *Oral Surg Oral Med Oral Pathol* 76:543, 1993.

Harel-Raviv M et al: Nifedipine-induced gingival hyperplasia, *Oral Surg Oral Med Oral Pathol Oral Radiol Endod* 79:715, 1995.

Seymour RA, Smith DG: The effect of a plaque control program on the incidence and severity of cyclosporin-induced gingival changes, *J Clin Periodontol* 18:107, 1991.

Tetracycline-induced tooth discoloration

Siller GM, Tod MA, Savage NW: Minocycline-induced oral pigmentation, *J Am Acad Dermatol* 30:350, 1994.

Wallman IS, Hilton HB: Teeth pigmented by tetracycline, *Lancet* 1:827, 1962.

Angioedema

Atkinson JC, Frank MM: Oral manifestations and dental management of patients with hereditary angioedema, *J Oral Pathol Med* 20:139, 1991.

Mattingly G, Rodu B, Alling R: Quincke's disease: nonhereditary angioneurotic edema of the uvula, *Oral Surg Oral Med Oral Pathol* 75:292, 1993.

Waytes AT, Rosen FS, Frank MM: Treatment of hereditary angioedema with a vapor-heated C1 inhibitor concentrate, *N Engl J Med* 334:1630, 1996.

Contact and irritant stomatitis

Bruce GJ, Hall WB: Nickel hypersensitivity-related periodontitis, *Compendium* 16:178, 1995.

Fisher AA: Contact stomatitis, *Dermatol Clin* 5:709, 1987.

Hedin CA, Karpe B, Larson A: Plasma-cell gingivitis in children and adults: a clinical and histological description, *Swed Dent J* 18:117, 1994.

Miller RL, Gould AR, Bernstein ML: Cinnamon-induced stomatitis venenata: clinical and characteristic histopathologic features, *Oral Surg Oral Med Oral Pathol* 73:708, 1992.

Ostman PO, Anneroth G, Skoglund A: Oral lichen planus in contact with amalgam fillings: a clinical, histologic, and immunohistochemical study, *Scand J Dent Res* 102:172, 1994.

Stanley HR: Effects of dental restorative materials: local and systemic responses reviewed, *J Am Dent Assoc* 124:76, 1993.

Van Loon LA, Bos JD, Davidson CL: Clinical evaluation of fifty-six patients referred with symptoms tentatively related to allergic contact stomatitis, *Oral Surg Oral Med Oral Pathol* 74:572, 1992.

Denture injuries

Bhaskar SN, Beasley JD, Cutright DE: Inflammatory papillary hyperplasia of the oral mucosa: report of 341 cases, *J Am Dent Assoc* 81:949, 1970.

Buchner A, Helft M: Pathologic conditions of the oral mucosa associated with ill-fitting dentures: III. Epulis fissuratum and flabby ridge, *Isr J Dent Med* 28:7, 1979.

Budtz-Jørgensen E: Oral mucosal lesions associated with the wearing of removable dentures, *J Oral Pathol* 10:65, 1981.

Cutright DE: The histopathologic findings in 583 cases of epulis fissuratum, *Oral Surg* 37:410, 1974.

Iacopino AM, Wathen WF: Oral candidal infection and denture stomatitis: a comprehensive review, *J Am Dent Assoc* 123:46, 1992.

Jeganathan S, Lin CC: Denture stomatitis—a review of the aetiology, diagnosis and management, *Aust Dent J* 37:107, 1992.

Nikawa H et al: Denture stomatitis and ABO blood types, *J Prosthet Dent* 66:391, 1991.

Reichart PA et al: Candida-associated palatal papillary hyperplasia in HIV infection, *J Oral Pathol Med* 23:403, 1994.

Thermal injuries

Hedin CA, Axell T: Oral melanin pigmentation in 467 Thai and Malaysian people with special emphasis on smoker's melanosis, *J Oral Pathol Med* 20:8, 1991.

Hedin CA, Pindborg JJ, Axell T: Disappearance of smoker's melanosis after reducing smoking, *J Oral Pathol Med* 12:228, 1993.

Linebaugh ML, Koka S: Oral electrical burns: etiology, histopathology, and prosthodontic treatment, *J Prosthodont* 2:136, 1993.

Ramulu C et al: Nicotine stomatitis and its relation to carcinoma of the hard palate in reverse smokers of chuttas, *J Dent Res* 52:711, 1973.

Reddy CR, Rajakumari K, Ramulu C: Regression of stomatitis nicotina in persons with a long-standing habit of reverse smoking. Morphologic evidence of the role of ducts, *Oral Surg Oral Med Oral Pathol* 38:570, 1974.

CHAPTER 4

Developmental Disorders

Cysts of the oral cavity and perioral soft tissues can develop in several ways. All cysts, by definition, are epithelial lined cavities; however, the etiology of oral cysts can be divided into three major categories. Fissural cysts are thought to arise from epithelium that is enclaved during the process of embryonic mesenchymal fusion. Developmental cysts arise from proliferating epithelium within connective tissue in utero, infancy, childhood, or adulthood. The third category contains the odontogenic cysts, which arise in conjunction with developing and erupting teeth.

Although most "developmental" cysts become evident before adulthood, they all share a common tendency to increase in size gradually, presumably as a result of increased intraluminal hydrostatic pressure with localized bone resorption.

The majority of cysts do not manifest in the oral cavity but are detected radiographically or extraorally during a head and neck examination. The following description of cysts is provided for completeness, with emphasis on oral manifestations.

FISSURAL CYSTS

Palatal Cysts of the Newborn (Epstein's Pearls, Bohn's Nodules)

Palatal cysts of the newborn is the consensus term used to describe small developmental cysts noted on the palates of newborn infants. Epstein's pearls were originally described as small cystic lesions arising along the median palatal raphe and were thus fissural in nature. Bohn's nodules are found primarily near the junction of the hard and soft palates and are thought to be derived from minor salivary glands. Because *Epstein's pearls* and *Bohn's nodules* are two terms that have been used interchangeably in the literature and the entities are frequently difficult to distinguish clinically, the term *palatal cysts of the newborn* is more acceptable.

Palatal cysts of the newborn are common, present in over two thirds of all neonates examined. The lesions are small, cream-colored papules that are most often found at the junction of the hard and soft palates near the midline (Fig. 4-1). Similar lesions have been reported more anteriorly in the midline of the hard palate, as well as more posteriorly, adjacent to the midline.

Palatal cysts of the newborn are keratinizing, as evidenced by their clinical color. No treatment is required because they either degenerate shortly after birth or fuse with the overlying mucosal surface, rupture, and disgorge their contents.

Nasolabial Cysts

The nasolabial cyst is an uncommon lesion that occurs laterally in the upper lip. Although it was originally thought that this cyst was purely fissural, arising from entrapped epithelium at the fusion of the maxillary median nasal and lateral nasal processes, it has also been proposed to develop from aberrant nasal lacrimal duct epithelium.

Clinically, the nasolabial cyst appears as a swelling of the lateral upper lip, often with mild displacement of the ala of the nose. Intraorally, there is often obliteration of the maxillary mucolabial

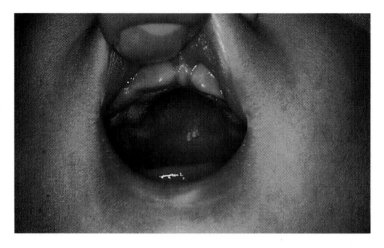

FIG. 4-1 Multiple palatal cysts of the newborn are characterized by cream-colored papules that develop most frequently on the palate.

fold. Nasolabial cysts are usually asymptomatic; however, they have been reported to rupture spontaneously, with subsequent oral or nasal drainage. In addition, these lesions may become secondarily infected and symptomatic.

Nasolabial cysts have been most commonly reported in adults with a high female predominance (3:1). A small percentage may occur bilaterally. Unlike most of the other fissural cysts, bone resorption is uncommon, although cases of pressure resorption of the underlying maxilla have been reported.

Nasolabial cysts are usually treated with surgical excision, and recurrence is rare.

Globulomaxillary Cysts

Traditionally, it was taught that the globulomaxillary cyst arose from epithelium trapped during the fusion of the globular portion of the medial nasal process and the maxillary process. This etiologic theory has fallen into disrepute because there is no true fusion between median nasal and maxillary processes. Instead, it appears that globulomaxillary cysts are actually of odontogenic origin, representing either a periapical or lateral periodontal cyst.

Characteristically, the globulomaxillary cyst presents as an inverted, pear-shaped radiolucency between the roots of the maxillary lateral incisor and cuspid teeth. Root displacement may occur, resulting in clinical malalignment of the teeth. In most cases, however, the lesion is detected radiographically, with no clinical indication of its presence.

Microscopically, most globulomaxillary cysts are lined with stratified squamous epithelium supporting their putative origin as periapical cysts. Occasionally, these lesions share histopathologic features of either odontogenic keratocysts or lateral periodontal cysts. Lesions that contain respiratory epithelium may, in fact, be truly fissural in nature; however, this may also be caused by the close proximity of the lesions to the maxillary sinus. It should also be noted that respiratory epithelium can occasionally be found in odontogenic cysts in other anatomic locations.

Globulomaxillary cysts are treated by surgical removal. The vitality of the adjacent maxillary lateral incisor and cuspid teeth must always be evaluated and endodontic therapy administered as needed. The recurrence rate of globulomaxillary cysts is low; lesions that share histopathologic features of odontogenic keratocysts should be monitored more closely because their recurrence rate is higher.

Nasopalatine Duct Cysts

The nasopalatine duct cyst occurs in approximately 1% of the population, making it the most common nonodontogenic cyst of the oral cavity. The lesion is thought to arise from cystic degeneration of remnants of the nasopalatine duct. Other proposed, yet unlikely etiologies for the nasopalatine duct cyst are the cystic degeneration of residual epithelium of the organ of Jacobson, cystic degeneration of traumatized or infected minor salivary gland ducts, and mucus retention phenomena of minor salivary glands.

Nasopalatine duct cysts are slightly more common in males and most frequently found in middle adulthood. In fact, their description during infancy and childhood is uncommon.

Most nasopalatine duct cysts are asymptomatic, intrabony, and found on routine radiographic examination. Clinically apparent lesions manifest as smooth, dome-shaped swellings in the area of the incisive foramen. The compressibility of the cyst is variable, depending on what percentage of the lesion is intrabony. Occasionally, the lesion will become infected or drain into the oral cavity. In rare cases there is a significant expansion of the cyst with marked pressure necrosis of the anterior palate.

Typically, nasopalatine duct cysts appear radiographically as well-circumscribed, inverted pear-shaped radiolucencies between the roots of the maxillary incisor teeth. Root resorption rarely occurs. The lesion also frequently exhibits a heart-shaped radiographic appearance as a result of indentation of its superior aspect by the nasal spine. It should be noted that the incisive foramen is a normal anatomic finding in this area. Occasionally, it is difficult to determine whether a radiolucency is a large incisive foramen or a small nasopalatine duct cyst. By convention, in the absence of other clinical signs and symptoms, radiolucencies less than 6 mm in diameter represent the incisive foramen.

The lining of nasopalatine duct cysts ranges from stratified squamous to respiratory epithelia. The percentage of respiratory epithelium present is proportional to the anatomic location of the cyst in the nasopalatine duct. For example, more superior lesions contain a higher percentage of respiratory epithelium.

Nasopalatine duct cysts are treated by surgical enucleation with an extremely low rate of recurrence.

Median Palatal Cysts

The median palatal cyst is a controversial lesion that was proposed to arise from epithelium trapped during the fusion of the lateral maxillary palatal shelves. Most investigators believe, however, that the lesion represents a posteriorly positioned nasopalatine duct cyst rather than a unique entity.

Unlike nasopalatine duct cysts, median palatal cysts are normally seen in younger adults, occasionally attaining a diameter of several centimeters. The histopathologic features of median palatal cysts are identical to those found in nasopalatine duct cysts. They are also treated by surgical excision with minimal risk of recurrence.

Median Mandibular Cysts

As with the globulomaxillary cyst, the median mandibular cyst may, in fact, not be developmental in origin. It has been theorized that the lesion represents cystic degeneration of epithelium trapped during the embryonic fusion of the mandible. Embryologically, however, the mandible develops as a single, bilobed proliferation of mesenchyme. Therefore no fusion of epithelium-lined processes occurs. Accordingly, median mandibular cysts are most likely of odontogenic origin.

As its name implies, the median mandibular cyst is found in the anterior mandible. The lesions are normally asymptomatic and noted as an incidental finding during a routine radiographic examination. Occasionally, cortical expansion results. Even more rare is the presence of cortical erosion.

The histopathologic features of the median mandibular cyst are identical to those of globulomaxillary cysts, further strengthening the theory of odontogenic origin of these lesions that is similar to periapical cysts, lateral periodontal cysts, and odontogenic keratocysts. These lesions also rarely contain respiratory epithelium, but, as has been noted, respiratory epithelium can also be found in other nonfissural oral cysts.

Surgical removal is the treatment of choice for median mandibular cysts. Reported recurrence rates are extremely low. It is essential to test adjacent teeth for vitality in the event that conjoint endodontic therapy is necessary.

DEVELOPMENTAL CYSTS

Epidermoid Cysts

Epidermoid cysts are common dermatologic lesions that arise from the follicular infundibulum. These cysts frequently arise after inflammation of the hair follicle as a secondary complication of the healing process. They are occasionally referred to as *sebaceous cysts;* however, this term should be avoided because of derivation of the epidermoid cyst from the hair follicle, rather than the associated sebaceous glands.

Epidermoid cysts are more common in males than females, usually arising on the skin of the head and neck as well as the back. They are primarily seen in adults, but they are also found in children, in association with Gardner's syndrome, for example. The lesions present as dome-shaped nodules in the subcutaneous tissues with variable fluctuance and inflammation. Histologically, the lesions are keratinizing, which results in their cream-colored clinical appearance. Analogous lesions may occur in the mouth after traumatic implantation of oral mucosal epithelium.

Epidermoid cysts are best treated by conservative surgical excision. Recurrence is uncommon.

Dermoid Cysts

The dermoid cyst, or benign cystic teratoma, is an uncommon lesion characterized by the presence of tissues derived from ectoderm, mesoderm, and endoderm. The amount of tissue differentiation varies greatly, ranging from microscopically distinguishable tissues to anatomically recognizable structures (e.g., teeth). Classic teratomas of the ovary typically contain not only teeth, but also adnexal skin appendages, muscle, bone, and gastrointestinal mucosa.

Oral dermoid, or teratoid, cysts are uncommon. They normally occur in the midline of the floor of the mouth. Those above the geniohyoid muscle frequently displace the tongue superiorly, occasionally resulting in significant functional impairment. Lesions that occur below the geniohyoid muscle are apparent clinically as a submental swelling.

Oral dermoid cysts vary in size from several millimeters to involving the entire floor of the mouth. They are most commonly diagnosed in young adults as slow-growing, painless, firm masses. Occasionally, they have been reported to drain intraorally and may become secondarily infected. The cyst lining consists of keratinizing epithelium with skin appendages prominent in the cyst wall.

Dermoid cysts are treated by surgical removal. Recurrence is uncommon.

Thyroglossal Duct Cysts

Thyroglossal duct cysts arise from residual thyroglossal duct epithelium that remains after the embryologic development of the thyroid and its descent from the base of the tongue to the anterior neck. The actual impetus for cystic degeneration of this residual epithelium may be caused by either inflammation secondary to head and neck infections or retention of secretory products within the thyroglossal duct.

Typically, thyroglossal duct cysts develop in the midline of the neck, anywhere along the path of the thyroglossal duct, from the base of the tongue to the suprasternal notch. The majority of lesions develop inferior to the hyoid bone. Most thyroglossal duct cysts become apparent by adolescence or early adulthood and are equally prevalent in males and females. Clinically, the lesions usually present as small, asymptomatic, fluctuant masses of the submental region or anterior neck. Intraorally, they are found on the dorsum of the tongue near the foramen caecum. Frequently, thyroglossal duct cysts develop fistulous tracts, both intraorally and extraorally. Microscopically, the

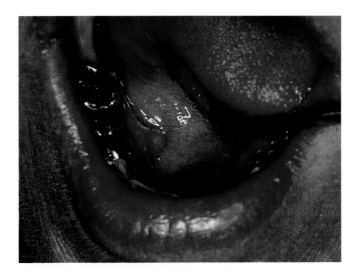

FIG. 4-2   A common location for the occurrence of a lymphoepithelial cyst.

cyst is lined by either stratified squamous or columnar epithelium, although other types of epithelium have been reported. The presence of thyroid tissue in the cyst wall is a variable finding.

Thyroglossal duct cysts have a tendency to recur if they are not treated with aggressive surgery; however, appropriately treated lesions have a recurrence rate of less than 10%.

Lymphoepithelial Cysts

Lymphoepithelial cysts can develop both intraorally and extraorally. The cervical lymphoepithelial cyst or branchial cleft cyst develops in the lateral neck and is either caused by residua of the branchial clefts or cystic changes in parotid gland epithelium, which becomes trapped during embryogenesis in superior cervical lymph nodes.

Branchial cleft cysts are most frequently diagnosed in the third and fourth decades of life. They manifest as soft, fluctuant masses in the superior lateral neck, which is adjacent to the anterior border of the sternocleidomastoid muscle. Occasionally, the lesions can become secondarily infected and symptomatic.

The oral lymphoepithelial cyst is thought to arise from epithelium entrapped within Waldeyer's ring. In contrast to the branchial cleft cyst, oral lymphoepithelial cysts are usually small and lined by keratinizing mucosa, resulting in a cream-colored clinical appearance. They are most frequently found in the floor of the mouth (Fig. 4-2) but have also been reported on the posterior lateral tongue, tonsillar pillars, and soft palate.

Both branchial cleft cysts and oral lymphoepithelial cysts are treated surgically and have a low incidence of recurrence.

Heterotopic Gastrointestinal Cysts

Heterotopic gastrointestinal cysts are rare developmental lesions that are considered to be choristomas rather than teratomas because of the normal histologic appearance of the gastrointestinal mucosa. The cysts are comprised of heterotopic islands of gastrointestinal mucosa representing misplaced embryonal tissue. Heterotopic gastrointestinal cysts have been found in the esophagus, small bowel, pancreas, gallbladder, and in Meckel's diverticulum. Oral lesions are characterized by small nodules, usually just several millimeters, occurring most frequently on the tongue, floor of the mouth,

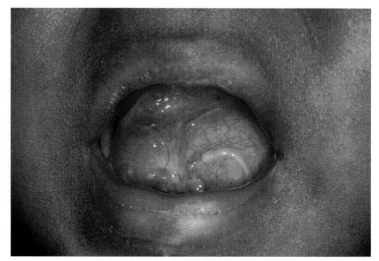

FIG. 4-3   Heterotopic gastrointestinal cysts are rare and develop most frequently on the tongue in infancy or childhood.

Table 4-1   Inflammatory Odontogenic Cysts

CYST	FEATURES
Radicular cyst	Well-defined radiolucency that varies in size. Cysts arise from epithelium of a periapical granuloma, an inflammatory lesion of the periapical tissues.
Residual radicular cyst	Cyst arises from epithelium that persists after extraction of an infected tooth with previous apical pathosis. Radiographically, a radiolucency is evident at the site of the extracted tooth.
Paradental cyst	Occurs in relation to partly or fully erupted teeth and is almost exclusively confined to the mandible. The radiographic characteristics are variable.

and lip (Fig. 4-3). The majority of cysts develop in males and are detected during infancy or childhood. Histologically, the cysts are lined partly by gastric mucosa and, less commonly, by intestinal epithelium. The cysts generally do not recur after excision.

ODONTOGENIC CYSTS

Odontogenic cysts are unique in that they arise as a by-product of odontogenesis. Many of the odontogenic cysts described are intrabony and, therefore, are not apparent during a clinical examination. The characteristics of inflammatory odontogenic cysts are outlined in Table 4-1.

Dentigerous Cysts

The dentigerous or follicular cyst is the most common developmental odontogenic cyst, comprising approximately 20% of all jaw cysts. The lesions arise because of the separation of the developing tooth follicle from the crown of an unerupted tooth. Its precise pathogenesis is unclear. Dentigerous cysts can arise in conjunction with the development of any tooth, although mandibular third molars are most commonly affected, followed by maxillary canines. Most dentigerous cysts are diagnosed in adolescents and young adults. In the absence of clinical expansion of the jaws, they are most fre-

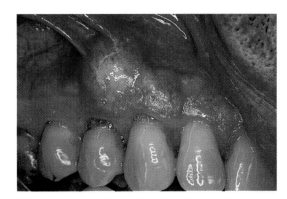

FIG. 4-4   Odontogenic keratocysts typically manifest radiographically, although occasionally they may be evident in the oral soft tissues.

quently noted as part of a routine radiographic examination. Dentigerous cysts are slightly more common in males and in blacks. Occasionally, dentigerous cysts can become secondarily infected and subsequently symptomatic.

Dentigerous cysts in association with maxillary third molars are normally treated by enucleation of the cyst and extraction of the tooth. In situations in which extraction of the tooth is unadvisable, as with a cuspid tooth, the cyst wall can be removed and the tooth allowed to erupt. Large, expansile cysts may be treated by marsupialization with a subsequent second-stage excision of residual cyst lining.

The prognosis for most dentigerous cysts is excellent, and the recurrence rate is extremely low, provided that all of the cyst lining is removed.

Eruption Cysts

The eruption cyst is analogous to the dentigerous cyst, differing only in that it occurs in soft tissue rather than bone. Eruption cysts are almost always diagnosed in children. They present clinically as soft, fluctuant, frequently translucent swellings of the gingival mucosa overlying the crown of an unerupted tooth. The lesions are most commonly found in association with erupting mandibular molars. Occasionally, the lumina of the cyst contains a small amount of traumatic hemorrhage, which gives the lesion a dark brown or purplish hue. If the lesions do not spontaneously rupture, they are treated by unroofing the cyst. In essentially all cases the eruption of the underlying tooth continues without complication.

Odontogenic Keratocysts

The odontogenic keratocyst is a developmental odontogenic cyst that is unique in its ability to keratinize and in its high recurrence rate. The lesions comprise approximately 10% of all developmental odontogenic cysts. Approximately three fourths of odontogenic keratocysts involve the posterior body and ascending ramus of the mandible. They are most commonly diagnosed in the second through fourth decades of life with a marked male predilection. Small odontogenic keratocysts are only evident radiographically; however, larger lesions are frequently associated with pain, expansion of the mandible, and, occasionally, drainage. The lesions may manifest orally as a dome-shaped cystic mass (Fig. 4-4). Multiple odontogenic keratocysts are associated with cutaneous basal cell carcinomas in the nevoid basal cell carcinoma or Gorlin-Goltz syndrome. Most odontogenic keratocysts are lined with perikeratinizing epithelium with frequent daughter cysts or islands of odontogenic epithelium in the cyst wall. It is believed that the presence of these daughter cysts and odontogenic epithelial islands contribute to the high rate of recurrence in the absence of aggressive surgical removal.

Approximately one third of odontogenic keratocysts recur, necessitating aggressive surgical removal rather than simple enucleation. An orthokeratinized variant of odontogenic keratocysts is unique in that the lesions do not tend to recur, even after simple enucleation. In addition, they have not been reported in association with the nevoid basal cell carcinoma syndrome. It has been suggested that the orthokeratinized variant be classified separately from odontogenic keratocysts and designated as an orthokeratinized odontogenic cyst.

Nevoid Basal Cell Carcinoma Syndrome

The nevoid basal cell carcinoma syndrome, or Gorlin-Goltz syndrome, is an autosomal dominant disorder characterized by multiple cutaneous basal cell carcinomas, odontogenic keratocysts of the jaws, rib and vertebral anomalies, and intracranial calcifications. Numerous other anomalies comprising alternate manifestations of the syndrome have also been reported.

Affected individuals frequently have a characteristic facial appearance consisting of frontal bossing, ocular hypertelorism, and mandibular prognathism. Cutaneous basal cell carcinomas usually appear in young adulthood but have also been reported in children. They are frequently present on skin not exposed to the sun. In addition, the majority of patients have both palmar and plantar pits that represent altered maturation of basal epithelial cells. Basal cell carcinomas may develop within these pits. Most affected individuals also exhibit skeletal anomalies including bifid ribs and kyphoscoliosis. Cranial radiographs frequently reveal a unique lamellar calcification of the falx cerebri.

One of the hallmarks of the nevoid basal cell carcinoma syndrome is the presence of odontogenic keratocysts in the jaws, occurring in over three fourths of affected individuals. Unlike non-syndrome-related odontogenic keratocysts, these lesions are often multiple and arise at a much younger age, often in adolescence.

Although mortality associated with the nevoid basal cell carcinoma syndrome is very low, a significant amount of morbidity is associated with both the skin lesions and jaw cysts. Because of the inheritance pattern of the syndrome, genetic counseling of patients' parents is appropriate.

Gingival Cysts of the Newborn

Gingival or alveolar cysts of the newborn are small (less than 2 to 3 mm), superficial, cream-colored, keratinizing cysts that are occasionally noted on the alveolar mucosa of infants. The lesions are more prominent in the maxillary alveolar mucosa. They arise from epithelial rests of Serres, which are residua of the developing dental lamina. The lesions frequently disappear spontaneously, either by spontaneous rupture or fusion with the overlying mucosa. No treatment is indicated.

Gingival Cysts of the Adult

Gingival cysts of the adult are uncommon lesions, similar to the gingival cysts of the newborn, and represent a soft tissue counterpart of the lateral periodontal cyst. Like lateral periodontal cysts, gingival cysts of the adult are most commonly found in the mandibular canine-premolar area, usually in older adults (Fig. 4-5). The facial surface of the gingiva is much more commonly involved than the lingual surface. Maxillary gingival cysts are much less frequent, comprising fewer than one third of reported cases. When present, they are most frequently located in the anterior portion of the maxilla.

Gingival cysts of the adult appear clinically as asymptomatic, dome-shaped swellings with normal overlying mucosa. The lesions are usually less than 0.5 cm in diameter and often have a bluish, translucent appearance. Occasionally, the lesions cause resorption of the underlying bone, resulting in saucerization. Gingival cysts of the adult are best treated with surgical excision and have an excellent prognosis with minimal risk of recurrence.

Lateral Periodontal Cysts

Lateral periodontal cysts are uncommon, intrabony analogs to gingival cysts of the adult. They are thought to arise from cystic degeneration of epithelial rests of Malassez, which remain in alveolar bone after maturation of the dental lamina. The lesion is normally found in adults on routine radiographic examination. Similar to their soft-tissue counterparts, lateral periodontal cysts arise most frequently in the mandibular canine-premolar area, with maxillary lesions most frequently noted in the anterior region. There is a slight male predilection for lateral periodontal cysts. A variant of the lat-

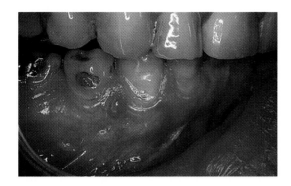

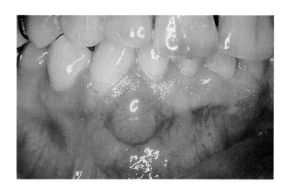

FIG. 4-5 The gingival cyst of the adult most frequently develops on the lower anterior gingiva and is a small, translucent mass.

FIG. 4-6 The lateral periodontal cyst rarely presents intraorally as an expansile mass. Most lesions manifest radiographically.

eral periodontal cyst, the botryoid odontogenic cyst, has also been described. It differs from the lateral periodontal cyst in that it is multilocular, and its clinical appearance resembles a grapelike cluster of fused, individual, lateral periodontal cysts. Rarely, both lateral periodontal cysts and botryoid odontogenic cysts present clinically as firm, expansile lesions apparent on the facial gingiva (Fig. 4-6). Surgical enucleation of the lateral periodontal cyst is curative, with a low incidence of recurrence.

It should be noted that lesions that are clinically and radiographically consistent with both gingival cysts of the adult and lateral periodontal cysts may have a histopathologic diagnosis of odontogenic keratocysts. For this reason, all such lesions should be submitted for histopathologic examination.

Calcifying Odontogenic Cysts

The calcifying odontogenic cyst, or Gorlin cyst, is an uncommon odontogenic cyst with a great diversity of histopathologic features and clinical presentations. Many investigators consider the lesion a neoplasm, as does the World Health Organization. Nevertheless, because of its variability, it is being presented in association with the other odontogenic cysts.

The calcifying odontogenic cyst is primarily an intraosseous lesion; however, approximately 20% of these cysts occur peripherally. They have been described in a wide age range of patients, from infancy to advanced age. The majority of lesions, however, are diagnosed in young adults. Calcifying odontogenic cysts are distributed equally between the maxilla and mandible, although the majority of lesions are found anteriorly rather than posteriorly. When the lesions occur in soft tissue, they have no distinctive clinical features and may be confused with a variety of benign gingival cysts and neoplasms (Fig. 4-7). Intraosseous lesions can be unilocular or multilocular with well-circumscribed borders and central calcifications. They are frequently associated with the crown of an unerupted tooth, usually the canine tooth.

Although calcifying odontogenic cysts are normally small, they have occasionally been reported to undergo significant enlargement with subsequent root resorption, root divergence of adjacent teeth, and malocclusion.

Calcifying odontogenic cysts are characterized histologically by the presence of ghost cells within the epithelial component of the lesion. It is unclear whether the cells represent necrotic epithelial cells or a manifestation of aberrant keratinization. Frequently, the ghost cells are calcified. Occasionally, dysplastic dentin is present in the adjacent connective tissue and is thought to represent odontogenic epithelial induction of pluripotent odontogenic mesenchymal tissue. Approximately 20% of calcifying odontogenic cysts are associated with odontomas.

Calcifying odontogenic cysts are treated by surgical enucleation. The prognosis is excellent with minimal chance of recurrence.

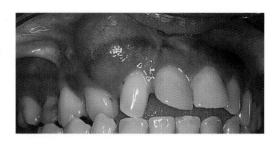

FIG. 4-7 A large and expanding calcified odontogenic cyst causing displacement of the lateral incisor.

Glandular Odontogenic Cysts

The glandular odontogenic cyst is a rare variant of a developmental odontogenic cyst. It normally presents as a unilocular radiolucency of the anterior mandible, which may cause bony expansion. This cyst is differentiated from other developmental odontogenic cysts by the presence of mucus cells and, occasionally, cilia. Microscopically, these lesions bear some resemblance to low-grade mucoepidermoid carcinomas. Although the number of reported cases of glandular odontogenic cysts is low, simple curettage appears to be curative.

VASCULAR-LYMPHATIC LESIONS

Until recently, the nomenclature and classification of vascular birthmarks have been confusing. A new classification of these lesions recognizes two distinct groups taking into account histopathology, pathogenesis, and natural history. Old terms including *cavernous, strawberry,* and *capillary hemangiomas* were descriptive and have been abandoned. The new classification of vascular birthmarks recognizes either hemangiomas or vascular malformations based on their presentation, natural history, and histologic features. A large and diverse group of acquired vascular proliferations in adulthood has been described. This group includes the hemangioma and angioma, as well as various hamartomatous, hyperplastic, and neoplastic tumors. These have not been precisely defined or classified.

Hemangiomas

Hemangiomas in infancy are benign vascular neoplasms comprised of capillaries and venules. Acquired lesions in adults may represent hamartomas. Hemangiomas are the most common tumor of infancy and childhood and are diagnosed in approximately 2% of newborns. Most lesions are first noted during early infancy, but by age 2, 10% of all children exhibit a hemangioma. The most common anatomic location for hemangiomas is the head and neck, which accounts for approximately 50% of all reported cases.

Hemangiomas proliferate during the first year of life. Dermal lesions are bright red, raised, firm, and well demarcated, whereas subcutaneous lesions appear blue and are soft on palpation. Precursor lesions of hemangiomas appear as pale patches that are often easily overlooked. Proliferation of hemangiomas occurs for approximately 1 to 2 years before reaching a plateau phase and finally involuting gradually. By age 10, complete resolution occurs in approximately 90% of hemangiomas.

Hemangiomas represent one of the most common lesions of the oral cavity. They may be single or multiple and occur most frequently on the tongue, buccal mucosa, and lips. Superficial lesions are dark blue or red and easily recognized (Fig. 4-8), whereas deep-seated hemangiomas are usually pink, dome shaped, and nondescript until aspirated (Fig. 4-9). Therapeutic intervention of oral hemangiomas is frequently unnecessary unless they result in serious complications. Ulceration, expansion, obstruction, or interference with feeding or breathing necessitates treatment with systemic corticosteroids, usually at doses of 2 to 4 mg/kg/day, and intralesional corticosteroids. Interferon-α may be used in treating life-threatening hemangiomas. The need for intervention also depends on the size and location of the lesion, as well as the aesthetic concerns of the patient. Chemical sclerosis,

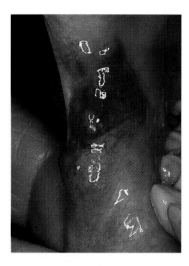

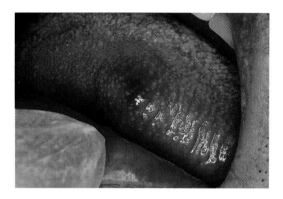

FIG. 4-8   Superficial hemangiomas are dark purple and easily recognized, resembling cutaneous lesions.

FIG. 4-9   Deep hemangiomas are lighter in color than superficial lesions and may not be recognized until aspirated.

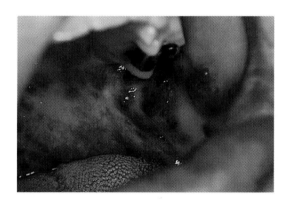

FIG. 4-10   Extensive vascular malformation of the oral cavity structures.

embolization, and laser therapy have all been used in the treatment of oral hemangiomas. Oral vascular lesions may be seen in a number of systemic conditions as described in Chapter 11.

Vascular Malformations

Vascular malformations are always present at birth, never proliferate, and never involute. They may be comprised of abnormal capillaries, veins, arteries, lymphatics, or a combination of these. Capillary malformations, also known as port-wine stains, are the most frequently occurring cutaneous malformation and may involve the underlying structures including the oral cavity (encephalotrigeminal angiomatosis) (see Chapter 11). Venous malformations and arteriovenous malformations of the oral cavity often go undetected until adulthood (Fig. 4-10). Whereas venous malformations are low-flow vascular lesions that may require treatment as a result of compression of adjacent structures, arteriovenous malformations are high-flow vascular lesions that may result in ischemia, pain, hemorrhage, and cardiac complications. The latter lesions may be detected by the presence of a pulsating thrill and warmth overlying the lesion, findings that may help differentiate arteriovenous malformations from hemangiomas.

Low-flow oral vascular malformations have been successfully treated with a combination of sclerotherapy and ablative surgery, as well as laser therapy.

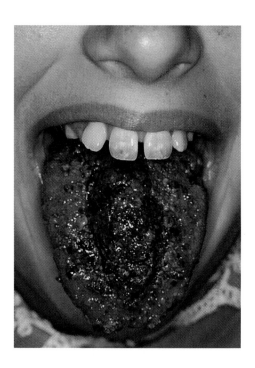

FIG. 4-11 Lymphangiomas in the oral cavity most frequently involve the tongue and consist of multinodules that may be translucent and hemorrhagic.

Lymphangioma

Lymphangiomas, like other vascular malformations, are developmental anomalies that occur during embryogenesis. Like hemangiomas, these lesions present with diverse clinical and histologic features ranging from small capillary-size vessels to large cystic lesions with significant involvement of adjacent anatomic structures.

The vast majority of lymphangiomas occur in the head and neck. Over half of all lymphangiomas are diagnosed at birth, with essentially all lesions being noted clinically by 2 years of age. Extraoral lymphangiomas are more common in the posterior neck. They present clinically as compressible soft tissue masses that have the capacity to undergo significant enlargement, extending superiorly into the oral cavity and inferiorly to involve the mediastinum. These cystic lymphangiomas, often referred to as cystic hygromas, can result in marked functional impairment and disfigurement.

Intraoral lymphangiomas are most frequently found in the anterior tongue and present clinically with macroglossia. Lymphangiomas can also occur in other oral sites including the floor of the mouth and buccal mucosa. Tongue lesions are usually superficial and frequently involve the papillae, although extensive lymphangiomas affecting the entire dorsal surface may also be seen. Clinically, lingual lesions have a multinodular surface texture. The individual nodules are often translucent; however, intralesional hemorrhage is frequently present, resulting in a variegated color pattern (Fig. 4-11). On palpation the lesions are somewhat firm with ill-defined borders.

The treatment of lymphangiomas depends on their size and location. Small lesions can be easily removed; however, the indistinct borders of lymphangiomas make recurrences common, especially with more infiltrative cavernous lesions. Unlike hemangiomas, lymphangiomas do not respond well to sclerosing agents, nor do they spontaneously regress.

MISCELLANEOUS DEVELOPMENTAL DISORDERS
Geographic Tongue

Geographic tongue or benign migratory glossitis is a common inflammatory disorder of the tongue affecting all age groups. The condition occurs in 1% to 2% of the population and is more common in females. Although the etiology is unknown, genetic factors may be significant, as evidenced by a

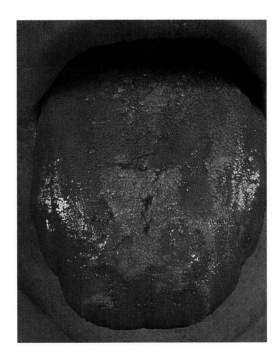

FIG. 4-12   Geographic tongue. Multiple areas of denuded, erythematous patches surrounded by a well-defined, white, raised border occur most frequently on the dorsal and lateral tongue.

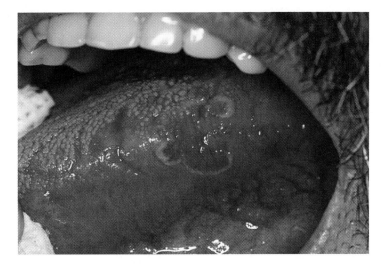

FIG. 4-13   A solitary lesion of benign migratory glossitis on the lateral tongue demonstrating loss of filiform papillae and a white hyperkeratotic border.

strong familial tendency and an increased frequency of the disease in individuals with HLA-DR5 and DRW6 genotypes. In addition, geographic tongue has been reported to occur more frequently in patients with other hereditary cutaneous disorders including psoriasis, Reiter's syndrome, and pityriasis rubra pilaris, supporting a genetic predisposition. An association with fissured tongue is well documented, but the link with atopy and allergies may be fortuitous.

Clinically, single or multiple irregularly shaped, erythematous patches that are often outlined with a well-defined, white, raised border occur most commonly on the lateral and dorsal surfaces of the tongue (Figs. 4-12 and 4-13). The red lesions are the same color as the remainder of the tongue but are apparent because the affected areas are devoid of filiform papillae. Within the red, atrophic,

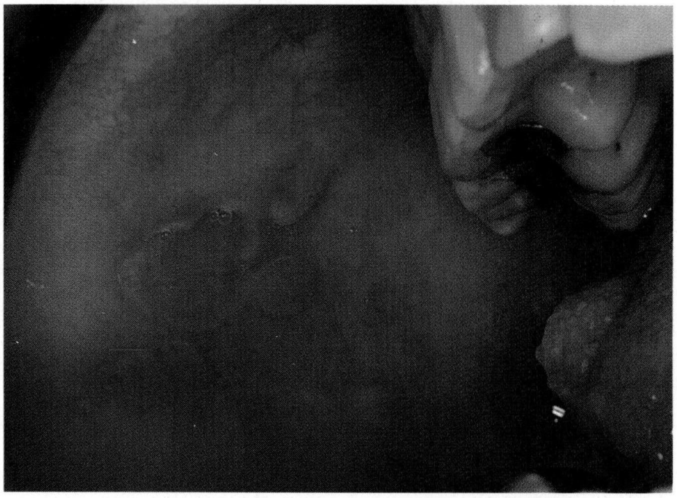

FIG. 4-14 Ectopic geographic tongue refers to lesions with morphologic features identical to geographic tongue occurring on mucosal surfaces other than the tongue.

and denuded mucosal patches, the fungiform papillae persist and appear elevated and red. The lesions of geographic tongue are circinate and vary in size from several millimeters to several centimeters and cover the entire dorsal surface. The desquamation of filiform papillae persists for hours or days before resolving spontaneously and returning to a normal appearance. The lesions are replaced by new patches of varying sizes and configurations that develop at other sites on the tongue. Infrequently, patients may be noted to display characteristic lesions of geographic tongue on surfaces other than the tongue (Fig. 4-14), most commonly on the lips, palate, and buccal mucosa. In these instances of ectopic geographic tongue, the tongue is usually simultaneously affected.

Histologically, the glossitis demonstrates a loss of filiform papillae with marginal hyperkeratosis and an intense inflammatory infiltrate. Microabscess formation near the epithelial surface is commonly noted and is identical to the histologic changes in psoriasis, supporting studies that document a close association between these entities.

In the majority of cases the lesions are asymptomatic and require no therapy. Occasionally, patients complain of burning and pain of varying severity, which can be greatly relieved by the frequent application of potent topical corticosteroids. Geographic tongue may persist for months or, more characteristically, for years before undergoing spontaneous resolution.

Fissured Tongue

Also known as scrotal or plicated tongue, fissured tongue is a common finding occurring in 5% to 10% of the population. The incidence of fissured tongue increases with age and is therefore thought to be a reactive process. Although the etiology is unknown, electrolyte imbalances in saliva and mild hematologic abnormalities have been noted in patients with fissured tongue. The condition is commonly observed in association with geographic tongue, supporting a genetic etiology. Fissured tongue occurs more commonly in patients with Down's syndrome and constitutes one aspect of the triad in the Melkersson-Rosenthal syndrome (see Chapter 12).

Clinically, multiple grooves and fissures are present on the dorsal surface of the tongue. Usually, a central groove is present in the midline with smaller grooves radiating from it and distributed symmetrically and independently (Fig. 4-15). However, an assortment of patterns may be noted with fissures of various lengths, depth, and number. The clinical appearance of fissured tongue worsens

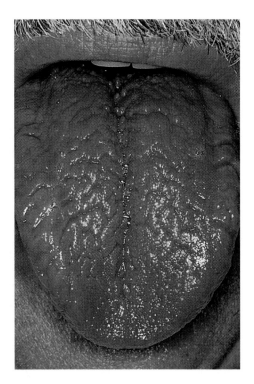

FIG. 4-15   A central groove with smaller radiating grooves is the most common presentation of fissured tongue; this anomaly frequently coexists with geographic tongue.

Table 4-2   Selected Syndromes with Lip Pits

SYNDROME	LIP PITS	ASSOCIATED FINDINGS
Popliteal pterygium syndrome	Midline	Cleft palate, popliteal web, toenail dysplasia, syndactyly, genital anomalies, and oral webs
Van der Woude syndrome	Midline	Cleft lip and palate, skeletal and heart defects, hypodontia, Hirschsprung's disease
Oral-facial-digital syndrome	Midline	Clefting of tongue, jaw, and lips; digital malformations including clinodactyly, brachydactyly, and polydactyly; ocular hypertelorism, and micrognathia (see Chapter 11)
Marres and Cremers syndrome	Commisural	Congenital conductive or mixed deafness, preauricular sinus, external ear anomaly
Miscellaneous associations	Midline or commisural	Clubfoot, preauricular fistulas, ankyloglossia, ichthyosis, nail deformities

with age, but, fortunately, the condition is painless. Patients should be encouraged to clean their tongues regularly to avoid the retention of food debris in the fissures.

Lip Pits

Lip pits are developmental anomalies that occur either as an isolated defect or in association with other developmental disturbances (Table 4-2). Usually, bilateral and symmetric depressions develop on the vermilion border of the lower lip (Fig. 4-16). These depressions represent fistulas that trans-

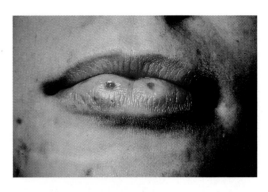

FIG. 4-16   Bilateral pits on the vermilion border of the lip represent fistulas that connect with the underlying minor salivary glands.

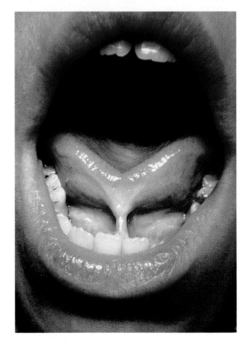

FIG. 4-17   This type of tongue tie anomaly represents a form of partial ankyloglossia and may be easily corrected by surgically releasing the frenum.

verse the underlying muscles and communicate with minor salivary glands through their excretory ducts. Viscous saliva can be expressed from the sinuses with pressure. Approximately three fourths of patients with central lip pits have an associated cleft lip, cleft palate, or both. This syndrome is often inherited as an autosomal dominant trait with variable penetrance.

A much more common location for lip pits to develop is at the commisures of the lips, either unilaterally or bilaterally. Fluid may be expressed from these fistulas as well. The condition is sometimes hereditary and associated with preauricular pits.

Lip pits may be surgically excised if repeated infections become problematic or for cosmetic reasons.

Ankyloglossia

Complete ankyloglossia, characterized by the fusion of the tongue to the floor of the mouth, is rare and may be seen with increased frequency in certain disorders including the Pierre-Robin syndrome or trisomy 13 syndrome. The more common tongue tie anomaly represents a partial ankyloglossia. This malformation may develop as a consequence of a short lingual frenum or a frenum that is anchored toward the tip of the tongue (Fig. 4-17). The incidence of ankyloglossia is increased in newborns by the mother's use of cocaine during pregnancy. Speech difficulties, the maintenance of proper

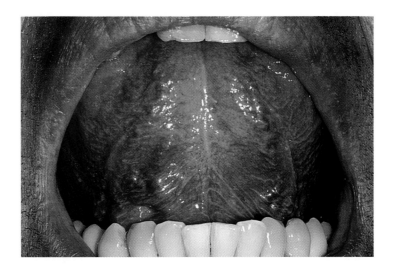

FIG. 4-18   Oral varices are most common sublingually and appear in adulthood.

oral hygiene, and even breast feeding may be compromised as a result of restricted tongue movements. Many patients have no difficulties and may be unaware of their defect. The lingual frenum may be surgically released, allowing the tongue full range of motion.

Oral Varices

Oral varices are common vascular developmental anomalies most frequently noted in older adults. The precise pathogenesis of oral varices is unclear. It was once though that oral varices were associated with hypertension or cardiovascular disease, but this is not the case. A relationship with varicose veins of the leg is probably fortuitous.

Oral varicosities are most frequently noted in the sublingual tissues. They present clinically as asymptomatic, compressible, violaceous elevations of the ventral-lateral tongue (Fig. 4-18). Occasionally, the lesions thrombose and become firm to palpation. Occasionally, oral varices are noted in other areas of the mouth, most frequently on the lips and buccal mucosa.

The histopathologic features of oral varices reveal only dilated and tortuous veins. Occasionally, the lesions may undergo thrombosis with recanalization or dystrophic calcification with the development of a phlebolith. Such calcifications are rarely, if ever, noted radiographically.

In the absence of symptoms or concern from the patient, lingual varices require no treatment. Lesions involving the vermilion borders of the lips may be removed for aesthetic reasons by conservative surgical excision.

SUGGESTED READINGS

General

Kreidler JF, Raubenheimer EJ, van Heerden WF: A retrospective analysis of 367 cystic lesions of the jaw: the Ulm experience, *J Craniomaxillofac Surg* 21:339, 1993.

Main DM: Epithelial jaw cysts: 10 years of the WHO classification, *J Oral Pathol Med* 14:1, 1985.

Shear M: Developmental odontogenic cysts: an update, *J Oral Pathol Med* 23:1, 1994.

Fissural cysts

Palatal cysts of the newborn (Epstein's pearls, Bohn's nodules)

Flinck A et al: Oral findings in a group of newborn Swedish children, *Int J Paediatr Dent* 4:67, 1994.

Ikemura K et al: Cysts of the oral mucosa in newborns: a clinical observation, *Sangyo Ika Daigaku Zasshi* 5:163, 1983.

Jorgenson RJ et al: Intraoral findings and anomalies in neonates, *Pediatrics* 69:577, 1982.

Nasolabial cysts

Allard RHB: Nasolabial cyst: review of the literature and report of 7 cases, *Int J Oral Surg* 11:351, 1982.

Kuriloff DB: The nasolabial cyst—nasal hamartoma, *Otolaryngol Head Neck Surg* 96:268, 1987.

Globulomaxillary cysts

Christ TF: The globulomaxillary cyst: an embryologic misconception, *Oral Surg Oral Med Oral Pathol* 30:315, 1970.

D'Silva NJ, Anderson L: Globulomaxillary cyst revisited [see comments], *Oral Surg Oral Med Oral Pathol* 76:182, 1993.

Wysocki GP, Goldblatt LI: The so called "globulomaxillary cyst" is extinct, *Oral Surg Oral Med Oral Pathol* 76:185, 1993.

Nasopalatine duct cysts

Chapple IL, Ord RA: Patent nasopalatine ducts: four case presentations and review of the literature, *Oral Surg Oral Med Oral Pathol* 69:554, 1990.

Swanson KS, Kaugars GE, Gunsolley JG: Nasopalatine duct cyst: an analysis of 334 cases, *J Oral Maxillofac Surg* 49:268, 1991.

Median palatal cysts

Courage GF, North AF, Hansen LS: Median palatal cysts, *Oral Surg Oral Med Oral Pathol* 37:745, 1974.

Donnelly JC, Koudelka BM, Hartwell GR: Median palatal cyst, *J Endod* 12:546, 1986.

Zachariades N, Papanicolaou S: The median palatal cyst: does it exist? Report of three cases with oromedical implications, *J Oral Med* 39:173, 1984.

Median mandibular cysts

Gardner DG: An evaluation of reported cases of median mandibular cysts, *Oral Surg Oral Med Oral Pathol* 65:208, 1988.

White DK, Lucas RM, Miller AS: Median mandibular cyst: review of the literature and report of two cases, *J Oral Surg* 33:372, 1975.

Developmental cysts

Epidermoid cysts

Cortezzi W, de Albuquerque EB: Secondarily infected epidermoid cyst in the floor of the mouth causing a life threatening situation: report of a case, *Oral Maxillofac Surg* 52:762, 1994.

Dohvoma CN: Epidermoid cyst: an unusual cause of obstructive sialadenitis, *Br J Oral Maxillofac Surg* 30:125, 1992.

Rajayogeswaran V, Eveson JW: Epidermoid cyst of the buccal mucosa, *Oral Surg Oral Med Oral Pathol* 67:181, 1989.

Dermoid cysts

King RC, Smith BR, Burk JL: Dermoid cyst in the floor of the mouth. Review of the literature and case reports, *Oral Surg Oral Med Oral Pathol* 78:567, 1994.

Lalwani AK, Engel TL: Teratoma of the tongue: a case report and review of the literature, *Int J Pediatr Otorhinolaryngol* 24:261, 1992.

Lyssett J, Sparnon AL, Byard RW: Embryogenesis of enterocystomas—enteric duplication cysts of the jaws, *Oral Surg Oral Med Oral Pathol* 75:626, 1993.

Triantafillidou E, Karakasis D, Laskin J: Swelling of the floor of the mouth. *J Oral Maxillofac Surg* 47:733, 1989.

Thyroglossal duct cysts

Allard RHB: The thyroglossal duct cyst, *Head Neck Surg* 5:134, 1982.

Dolata J: Thyroglossal duct cyst in the mouth floor: an unusual location, *Otolaryngol Head Neck Surg* 110:580, 1994.

Girard M, DeLuca SA: Thyroglossal duct cyst, *Am Fam Physician* 42:665, 1990.

Katz AD, Hochigian M: Thyroglossal duct cysts: a thirty-year experience with emphasis on occurrence in older patients, *Am J Surg* 155:741, 1988.

Samuel M, Freeman NV, Sajwany MJ: Lingual thyroglossal duct cyst presenting in infancy, *J Pediatr Surg* 28:891, 1993.

Sturgis EM, Miller RH: Thyroglossal duct cysts, *J La State Med Soc* 145:459, 1993.

Vincent SD, Synhorst JB II: Adenocarcinoma arising in a thyroglossal duct cyst: report of a case and literature review, *J Oral Maxillofac Surg* 47:633, 1989.

Lymphoepithelial cysts

Bhaskar SN: Lymphoepithelial cysts of the oral cavity: report of twenty-four cases, *Oral Surg Oral Med Oral Pathol* 21:120, 1996.

Buchner A, Hansen LS: Lymphoepithelial cysts of the oral cavity, *Oral Surg Oral Med Oral Pathol* 50:441, 1980.

Camilleri AC, Lloyd RE: Lymphoepithelial cyst of the parotid gland, *Br J Oral Maxillofac Surg* 28:329, 1990.

Kumara GR, Gillgrass TJ, Bridgman JB: A lymphoepithelial cyst (branchial cyst) in the floor of the mouth, *N Z Dent J* 91:14, 1995.

Sakoda S, Kodama Y, Shiba R: Lymphoepithelial cyst of oral cavity: report of a case and review of the literature, *Int J Oral Surg* 12:127, 1983.

Heterotopic gastrointestinal cysts

Balakrishnan A, Bailey CM: Lymphangioma of the tongue: a review of pathogenesis, treatment and the use of surface laser photocoagulation, *J Laryngol Otol* 105:924, 1991.

Oygur T et al: Oral congenital dermoid cyst in the floor of the mouth of a newborn: the significance of gastrointestinal-type epithelium, *Oral Surg Oral Med Oral Pathol* 174:627, 1992.

Odontogenic cysts

Dentigerous cysts

McMillan MD, Smillie AC: Ameloblastomas associated with dentigerous cysts, *Oral Surg Oral Med Oral Pathol* 51:489, 1981.

Shear M: Cysts of the jaws: recent advances, *J Oral Pathol Med* 14:43, 1985.

Eruption cysts

Clark CA: A survey of eruption cysts of the newborn, *Oral Surg Oral Med Oral Pathol* 15:917, 1962.

Das S, Das AK: A review of pediatric oral biopsies from a surgical pathology service in a dental school, *Pediatr Dent* 15:208, 1993.

Seward MH: Eruption cyst: an analysis of its clinical features, *J Oral Surg* 31:31, 1973.

Odontogenic keratocysts

Anand VK, Arrowood JP Jr, Krolls SO: Odontogenic keratocysts: a study of 50 patients, *Laryngoscope* 105:14, 1995.

Brannon RB: The odontogenic keratocyst—a clinicopathologic study of 312 cases. Part I. Clinical features, *Oral Surg Oral Med Oral Pathol* 42:54, 1976.

Brannon RB: The odontogenic keratocyst—a clinicopathologic study of 312 cases. Part II. Histologic features, *Oral Surg Oral Med Oral Pathol* 43:233, 1976.

Chehade A et al: Peripheral odontogenic keratocyst, *Oral Surg Oral Med Oral Pathol* 77:494, 1994.

Crowley TE, Kaugars GE, Gunsolley JC: Odontogenic keratocysts: a clinical and histologic comparison of the parakeratin and orthokeratin variants, *J Oral Maxillofac Surg* 50:22, 1992.

Meara JG et al: Odontogenic keratocysts in the pediatric population, *Arch Otolaryngol Head Neck Surg* 122:725, 1996.

Zachariades N, Papanicolaou S, Triantafyllou D: Odontogenic keratocysts: review of the literature and report of sixteen cases, *J Oral Maxillofac Surg* 43:177, 1985.

Nevoid basal cell carcinoma syndrome

Cohen MM Jr: Perspectives on craniofacial asymmetry. III. Common and/or well-known causes of asymmetry, *Int J Oral Maxillofac Surg* 24:127, 1995.

Gorlin RJ, Goltz R: Multiple nevoid basal cell epithelioma, jaw cysts and bifid rib syndrome, *N Engl J Med* 262:908, 1960.

Gorlin RJ: Nevoid basal cell carcinoma syndrome, *Medicine* 66:98, 1987.

Kuster W, Happle R: Neurocutaneous disorders in children, *Curr Opin Pediatr* 5:436, 1993.

Orlow SJ, Watsky KL, Bolognia JL: Skin and bones. I, *J Am Acad Dermatol* 25:205, 1991.

Shanley S et al: Nevoid basal cell carcinoma syndrome: review of 118 affected individuals, *Am J Med Genet* 50:282, 1994.

Gingival cysts of the newborn

Cataldo E, Berkman M: Cysts of the oral mucosa in newborns, *Am J Dis Child* 116:44, 1968.

Gingival cysts of the adult

Buchner A, Hansen LS: The histomorphologic spectrum of the gingival cyst in the adult, *Oral Surg Oral Med Oral Pathol* 48:532, 1979.

Moskow BS, Bloom A: Embryogenesis of the gingival cyst, *J Clin Periodontol* 10:119, 1983.

Nxumalo TN, Shear M: Gingival cyst in adults, *J Oral Pathol Med* 21:309, 1992.

Shade NL, Carpenter WM, Delzer DD: Gingival cyst of the adult: case report of a bilateral presentation, *Periodontology* 58:796, 1987.

Lateral periodontal cysts

Altini M, Shear M: The lateral periodontal cyst: an update, *J Oral Pathol Med* 21:245, 1992.

Angelopoulou E, Angelopoulos AP: Lateral periodontal cyst: review of the literature and report of a case, *J Periodontol* 61:126, 1990.

Carter LC, Carney YL, Perez-Pudlewski D: Lateral periodontal cyst: multifactorial analysis of a previously unreported series, *Oral Surg Oral Med Oral Pathol Oral Radiol Endod* 81:210, 1996.

Cohen DA et al: The lateral periodontal cyst: a report of 37 cases, *J Periodontol* 55:230, 1984.

Fantasia JE: Lateral periodontal cyst: analysis of forty-six cases, *Oral Surg Oral Med Oral Pathol* 48:237, 1975.

Greer RO Jr, Johnson M: Botryoid odontogenic cyst: clinicopathologic analysis of ten cases with three recurrences, *J Oral Maxillofac Surg* 46:574, 1988.

Gurol M, Burkes EJ Jr, Jacoway J: Botryoid odontogenic cyst: analysis of 33 cases, *J Periodontol* 66:1069, 1995.

Lynch DP, Madden CR: The botryoid odontogenic cyst: report of a case and review of the literature, *J Periodontol* 56:163, 1985.

Wysocki GP et al: Histogenesis of the lateral periodontal cyst and the gingival cyst of the adult, *Oral Surg Oral Med Oral Pathol* 50:327, 1980.

Calcifying odontogenic cysts

Buchner A: The central (intraosseous) calcifying odontogenic cyst: an analysis of 215 cases, *J Oral Maxillofac Surg* 49:330, 1991.

Buchner A et al: Peripheral (extraosseous) calcifying odontogenic cyst: a review of forty five cases, *Oral Surg Oral Med Oral Pathol* 72:65, 1991.

el Beialy RR, el Mofty S, Refai H: Calcifying odontogenic cyst: case report and review of literature, *J Oral Maxillofac Surg* 48:637, 1990.

Hong SP, Ellis GL, Hartman KS: Calcifying odontogenic cyst: a review of ninety two cases with reevaluation of their nature as cysts or neoplasms, the nature of ghost cells, and subclassification, *Oral Surg Oral Med Oral Pathol* 72:56, 1991.

Kaugars CC, Kaugars GE, DeBiasi GF: Extraosseous calcifying odontogenic cyst: report of case and review of literature, *J Am Dent Assoc* 119:715, 1989.

Glandular odontogenic cysts

Gardner DG et al: The glandular odontogenic cyst: an apparent entity, *J Oral Pathol Med* 17:359, 1988.

Hussain K, Edmondson HD, Browne RM: Glandular odontogenic cysts: diagnosis and treatment, *Oral Surg Oral Med Oral Pathol Oral Radiol Endod* 79:593, 1995.

Patron M, Colmenero C, Larrauri J: Glandular odontogenic cyst: clinicopathologic analysis of three cases, *Oral Surg Oral Med Oral Pathol* 72:1, 1991.

Toida M et al: Glandular odontogenic cyst: a case report and literature review, *J Oral Maxillofac Surg* 52:1312, 1994.

Vascular-lymphatic lesions

Bartlett JA, Riding KH, Salkeld LJ: Management of hemangiomas of the head and neck in children, *J Otolaryngol* 17:111, 1988.

Kaban LB, Mulliken JB: Vascular anomalies of the maxillofacial region, *J Oral Maxillofac Surg* 44:203, 1986.

Kane WJ et al: Significant hemangiomas and vascular malformations of the head and neck: clinical management and treatment outcomes, *Ann Plast Surg* 35:133, 1995.

Mantravadi J, Roth LM, Kafrawy AH: Vascular neoplasms of the parotid gland: parotid vascular tumors, *Oral Surg Oral Med Oral Pathol* 75:70, 1993.

Mulliken JB, Glowacki J: Hemangiomas and vascular malformations in infants and children: a classification based on endothelial characteristics, *Plast Reconstr Surg* 69:894, 1982.

Nigro J et al: Angiogenesis, vascular malformations and proliferations. In Arndt KA et al, editors: *Cutaneous medicine and surgery: an integrated program in dermatology,* Philadelphia, 1996, WB Saunders.

Sadan N, Wolach B: Treatment of hemangiomas of infants with high dose of prednisone, *J Pediatr* 128:141, 1996.

Silverman RA: Hemangiomas and vascular malformations, *Pediatr Clin North Am* 38:811, 1991.

Stal S, Hamilton S, Spira M: Hemangiomas, lymphangiomas, and vascular malformations of the head and neck, *Otolaryngol Clin North Am* 19:769, 1986.

Wagner M, Suen JY: Management of congenital vascular lesions of the head and neck, *Oncology* 9:989, 1995.

Waner M, Suen JY, Dinehart S: Treatment of hemangiomas of the head and neck, *Laryngoscope* 102:1123, 1992.

Lymphangioma

Balakrishnan A, Bailey CM: Lymphangioma of the tongue: a review of pathogenesis, treatment and the use of surface laser photocoagulation, *J Laryngol Otolaryngol* 105:924, 1991.

Kennedy TL: Cystic hygroma lymphangioma: a rare and still unclear entity, *Laryngoscope* 99:1, 1989.

Levin LS, Jorgenson RJ, Jarvey BA: Lymphangiomas of the alveolar ridges in neonates, *Pediatrics* 58:881, 1976.

Lobitz B, Lang T: Lymphangioma of the tongue, *Pediatr Emerg Care* 11:183, 1995.

Ogita S et al: OK-432 therapy for unresectable lymphangiomas in children, *J Pediatr Surg* 26:263, 1991.

Osborne TE et al: Surgical correction of mandibular deformities secondary to large cervical cystic hygromas, *J Oral Maxillofac Surg* 45:1015, 1987.

Ricciardelli EJ, Richardson MA: Cervicofacial cystic hygroma: patterns of recurrence and management of the difficult case, *Arch Otolaryngol Head Neck Surg* 117:546, 1991.

Wilson S, Gould AR, Wolff C: Multiple lymphangiomas of the alveolar ridge in a neonate: case study, *Pediatr Dent* 8:231, 1986.

Miscellaneous developmental disorders

Geographic tongue

Banoczy J, Szabo L, Csiba A: Migratory glossitis: a clinical-histologic review in seventy cases, *Oral Surg Oral Med Oral Pathol* 39:113, 1975.

Fenerli A et al: Histocompatibility and geographic tongue, *Oral Surg Oral Med Oral Pathol* 76:476, 1993.

Hume WJ: Geographic stomatitis: a critical review, *J Dent* 3:25, 1975.

Sigal MJ, Mock D: Symptomatic benign migratory glossitis: report of two cases and literature review, *Pediatr Dent* 14:392, 1986.

Fissured tongue

Jia YH, Guan RY, Li LX: Relationship between fissured tongue with flow and components of saliva, *Chung-Kuo Chung Hsi I Chieh Ho Tsa Chih* 14:31, 1994.

Kullaa-Mikkonen A, Penttila I, Kotilainen R: Haematological and immunological features with fissured tongue syndrome, *Br J Oral Maxillofac Surg* 25:481, 1987.

Powell FC: Glossodynia and other disorders of the tongue, *Dermatol Clin* 5:687, 1987.

Lip pits

Cervenka J, Gorlin RJ, Anderson VE: The syndrome of pits of the lower lip and cleft lip and/or palate, *Am J Hum Genet* 19:416, 1967.

Herold HZ, Shmueli G, Baruchin AM: Popliteal pterygium syndrome, *Clin Orthop* 209:194, 1986.

Marres HA, Cremers CW: Congenital conductive or mixed deafness, preauricular sinus, external ear anomaly, and commissural lip pits: an autosomal dominant inherited syndrome, *Ann Otol Rhinol Laryngol* 100:928, 1991.

Schinezel A, Kläusler M: The Van der Woude syndrome (dominantly inherited lip pits and clefts), *J Med Genet* 23:291, 1986.

Taylor WB, Mich AA, Lane DK: Congenital fistulas of the lower lips: associations with cleft lip-palate and anomalies of extremities, *Arch Dermatol* 94:421, 1966.

Ankyloglossia

Harris EF, Friend GW, Tolley EA: Enhanced prevalence of ankyloglossia with maternal cocaine use, *Cleft Palate Craniofac J* 29:72, 1992.

Notestine GE: The importance of the identification of ankyloglossia (short lingual frenulum) as a cause of breastfeeding problems, *J Hum Lact* 6:113, 1990.

Warden PJ: Ankyloglossia: a review of the literature, *Gen Dent* 39:252, 1991.

Wright JE: Tongue-tie, *J Paediatr Child Health* 31:276, 1995.

Oral varices

Ettinger RL, Manderson RD: A clinical study of sublingual varices, *Oral Surg Oral Med Oral Pathol* 38:540, 1974.

Kleinman HZ: Lingual varicosities, *Oral Surg Oral Med Oral Pathol* 23:546, 1967.

Southam IC, Ettinger RL: A histologic study of sublingual varices, *Oral Surg Oral Med Oral Pathol* 38:879, 1974.

Weathers DR, Fine RM: Thrombosed varix of oral cavity, *Arch Dermatol* 104:427, 1971.

CHAPTER 5

Benign, Premalignant, and Malignant Lesions

The oral mucosal surfaces are subjected to daily irritation through normal masticatory functions and hygiene measures. Furthermore, patients who neglect their oral health allow plaque and calculus, which serve as additional irritants, to accumulate on their teeth. Various oral habits such as lip and cheek biting are common in both children and adults and are a source of daily oral trauma. It is not surprising that the majority of masses encountered in the oral cavity actually represent reactive processes to these various forms of trauma rather than true neoplastic lesions. A careful history and physical examination may often reveal the underlying source of the injury. Table 5-1 features uncommon benign and malignant lesions that may arise in the oral cavity.

BENIGN LESIONS
Pyogenic Granuloma

Pyogenic granulomas are not infectious in origin and do not exhibit granulomatous inflammation histologically. Rather, these common lesions represent reactive processes to trauma, most often from the accumulation of calcified dental plaque (calculus) on teeth surfaces or trauma sustained during mastication or oral hygiene procedures. Hormonal stimulation of pyogenic granulomas is supported by their increased frequency in gravid women. These "pregnancy tumors," which are clinically and histologically identical to pyogenic granulomas, usually develop at the end of the first trimester and continue to increase in size throughout pregnancy. Intraoral pyogenic granulomas are also associated with systemic causes, as evidenced by their emergence after allogenic bone marrow transplantation. The development of an array of satellite pyogenic granulomas around the site of attempted ablation of a single lesion supports a traumatic etiology. A diverse group of vascular lesions that develops in the mouth and on the skin sharing similar microscopic features of the pyogenic granuloma has been classified under the term *lobular capillary hemangioma*. This concept links the intraoral pyogenic granuloma and pregnancy tumors with pyogenic granuloma-like tumors occurring in the mouth and on the skin.

Clinically, oral pyogenic granulomas are exophytic, intensely red, and, occasionally, ulcerated masses (Fig. 5-1). The lesions are often pedunculated, bleeding easily and at times profusely with provocation. Like pyogenic granulomas of the skin, they evolve rapidly, attaining a size of 0.5 to 2 cm. Although they can arise at any age, they develop most frequently in young adults and in females more than males. The maxillary anterior marginal gingiva is a favored site, with 75% of cases occurring in this location. Patients with gingival lesions often do not have a history of preceding trauma because the lesions are generally a result of dental calculus, whereas extragingival pyogenic granulomas are frequently preceded by an oral traumatic event.

Histologically, early lesions of oral pyogenic granulomas display granulation tissue in a polypoid configuration; mature lesions feature lobular clusters of capillaries separated by intersecting bands of fibrosis. Ulceration of the overlying surface with formation of a fibrinous membrane is a frequent finding.

Table 5-1   Uncommon Benign and Malignant Lesions of the Oral Cavity

LESION	CLINICAL FEATURES
Angiomyoma	Benign hamartoma consisting of smooth muscle and blood vessels. The lesions may arise on any mucosal surface and often appear vascular.
Chondrosarcoma	Malignant tumor of cartilaginous tissue may appear as a large and rapidly expanding, erythematous, ulcerated mass. The lesions arise primarily on the alveolar ridges.
Congenital epulis of the newborn	A reactive process developing almost exclusively on the alveolar ridges as a solitary, painless, pedunculated nodule.
Fibrosarcoma	Malignant mesenchymal tumor may present as a firm exophytic mass, often ulcerated, most frequently on the gingiva, tongue, and lips.
Hemangiopericytoma	Benign and malignant forms originate from blood vessel pericytes. The lesions are usually reddish, firm nodules that may rapidly enlarge.
Leiomyoma	Benign, smooth-muscle tumor characterized by a slow-growing, mucosal-colored nodule arising typically on the tongue, buccal mucosa, and lip.
Myxoma	Benign, mesenchymal tumor characterized by a soft nodule that appears most frequently on the buccal mucosa, floor of the mouth, and palate.
Osseous choristoma	Benign tumor of histologically normal osseous tissue occurring most frequently on the posterior dorsal surface of the tongue.
Rhabdomyosarcoma	Malignant skeletal muscle tumor may involve the oral structures, usually by direct tumor invasion. The lesions, which are usually indurated and rapidly expansive, typically involve the buccal mucosa and palate.
Warty dyskeratoma	An uncommon tumor of the skin and oral cavity that is histologically identical to Darier's disease. Nodules that are occasionally ulcerated arise most frequently on the hard palate and alveolar ridge.

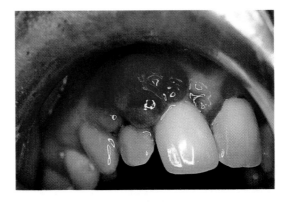

FIG. 5-1   Pyogenic granulomas of the oral cavity typically occur on the anterior maxillary gingiva and are characterized by intensely red, exophytic masses.

FIG. 5-2 Peripheral giant cell granulomas arise almost exclusively on the gingiva, mandibular more than maxillary, and are often bluish-purple.

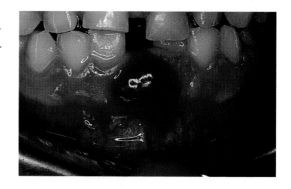

Pyogenic granulomas should be completely excised to the depth of the periosteum, and the adjacent teeth should be professionally cleaned to prevent recurrences of gingival lesions. Pregnancy tumors often spontaneously resolve after parturition, and surgery should be performed only for persistent lesions. As with skin lesions, recurrences of oral pyogenic granulomas are not uncommon.

Peripheral Giant Cell Granuloma

The peripheral giant cell granuloma, like the oral pyogenic granuloma, is common and arises as a result of trauma. Oral irritating factors that precipitate the development of the peripheral giant cell granuloma include tooth extractions, poorly fitting dental prostheses, faulty dental restorations, and, most important, the accumulation of dental plaque and calculus. Almost all cases develop on the gingiva or alveolar mucosa; approximately 10% occur in edentulous areas. The lesions are slightly more common in the mandible than in the maxilla and develop twice as often in the posterior segment as in the anterior segment, concentrated in the area around the premolar and molar teeth. The peripheral giant cell granuloma affects people of all age groups but has a peak incidence in the fourth and fifth decades of life and occurs much more frequently in women than in men.

Clinically, the lesions are deep red or sometimes bluish-purple, pedunculated or sessile masses usually 0.5 to 2 cm in diameter (Fig. 5-2). The consistency of peripheral giant cell granulomas may be soft, but more commonly they are firm and display a smooth surface. Occasionally, they ulcerate or bleed profusely. The lesions are often clinically indistinguishable from pyogenic granulomas.

Histologically, characteristic features include a nonencapsulated, highly cellular mass with abundant giant cells, inflammation, interstitial hemorrhage, and hemosiderin deposits. Mature bone or osteoid can be found in 50% of samples. Immunohistochemical and ultrastructural studies reveal that peripheral giant cell granulomas are comprised mainly of cells of the mononuclear phagocyte system and that Langerhans cells are present in two thirds of lesions.

Treatment is by surgical excision; however, the recurrence rate is greater than 10%, primarily because of failure to eliminate underlying irritating factors.

Keratoacanthoma

The keratoacanthoma is a self-limiting proliferative process that mimics squamous cell carcinomas both clinically and microscopically. Keratoacanthomas arise more frequently in men and rarely develop before the sixth decade of life. Increased numbers of keratoacanthomas may occur in immunosuppressed patients, and a number of well-documented variants with generally distributed eruptive keratoacanthomas have been described. More than 90% of keratoacanthomas originate on sun-exposed skin, with nearly 10% occurring periorally or on the vermilion border of the lips. Lesions occur on both the upper and lower lips with equal frequency.

Clinically, cutaneous keratoacanthomas appear as distinctive, indurated, painless, dome-shaped nodules displaying a characteristic central, keratin-filled crater. The keratin plug is crusted, irregular,

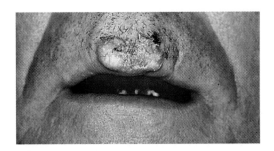

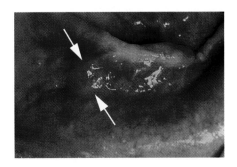

FIG. 5-3   Keratoacanthomas commonly arise on the lips and clinically resemble squamous cell carcinomas in their appearance and rapid growth pattern.

FIG. 5-4   Traumatic neuromas occur as small, mucosal-colored nodules commonly on the alveolar ridge in edentulous patients after a tooth extraction.

and frequently darkened or discolored. Keratoacanthomas grow at a rapid rate, attaining an average size of 1.0 to 2.5 cm. If untreated, keratoacanthomas typically undergo spontaneous involution over 4 to 8 weeks.

Intraoral keratoacanthomas have been described occurring as either an isolated lesion or in association with the eruptive forms. Like their cutaneous counterpart, oral lesions grow rapidly and resemble oral squamous cell carcinomas (Fig. 5-3). By contrast, oral lesions are painful.

Some investigators believe that keratoacanthomas represent extremely well-differentiated squamous cell carcinomas. Recently, significant differences between these entities have been demonstrated using a new monoclonal antibody, MIB-1, and studying the loss of heterozygosity at a number of loci. Human papillomavirus has been suggested as an etiologic agent; however, actinic damage is more likely to be of significance in the pathogenesis of these lesions. This is supported by the fact that the vast majority occur on sun-exposed skin.

Keratoacanthomas occurring on the lips or intraorally require biopsy to differentiate them from squamous cell carcinomas. Delaying biopsy and waiting for spontaneous involution are not warranted when keratoacanthomas occur at these sites because metastasis from carcinomas of the lips and mucous membranes occurs frequently. Excision should include clinically normal adjacent tissue to allow for adequate histopathologic evaluation. A significant amount of dyskeratosis is frequently noted deep within the lesion accompanied by a pronounced chronic inflammatory infiltrate. The histologic features can closely resemble well-differentiated squamous cell carcinomas. In cross section, keratoacanthomas are cup-shaped, with an infiltrating epithelial base.

Excisional surgery is currently the treatment of choice for oral and lip keratoacanthomas, resulting in a recurrence rate of less than 5%. When the diagnosis has been established, intralesional therapy of keratoacanthomas with methotrexate or 5-fluorouracil can be used and produces excellent results.

Amputation Neuroma

Also known as a traumatic neuroma, amputation neuroma represents a reactive proliferation of neural tissue after trauma. The lesions arise after a nerve is transected, most commonly after a traumatic injury to the mouth or after a tooth extraction. These traumatic events account for the high incidence of amputation neuromas developing around the mental foramen and on the alveolar ridge in edentulous patients. Traumatic neuromas are also commonly observed on the lip or tongue following a deep laceration. Clinically, the lesion is characterized as a slow-growing nodule, usually just several millimeters in size (Fig. 5-4). The surface is smooth and covered by normal mucosa. Although a useful feature in diagnosing the lesion is the presence of pain on palpation, the majority of lesions are asymptomatic. Traumatic neuromas located around the mental foramen appear to cause the greatest degree of discomfort, especially when irritated by dentures. The pain may be localized to the neuroma or referred to the anatomic structures innervated by the damaged nerve. Histologically, traumatic neuromas are comprised of irregularly arranged nerve fascicles containing neurofibrils and Schwann cells surrounded by a well-developed perineurium.

Surgical excision is the treatment of choice for traumatic neuromas. Although the recurrence rate is low, residual pain occasionally persists despite adequate removal.

Verruciform Xanthoma

Verruciform xanthoma is an uncommon lesion of unknown etiology that occurs predominantly on the oral mucosa and less frequently on the skin and anogenital area. Many believe that the verruciform xanthoma represents a reactive process of oral epithelium to trauma rather than a true neoplasm. This is supported by its association with nevi, dysplastic epithelium, blistering diseases of the oral mucosa, and graft-versus-host disease, as well as its occurrence after bone marrow transplantation.

Verruciform xanthomas are most commonly seen in adults and occur equally in men and women. They develop most frequently on the gingiva, alveolar mucosa, and hard palate, although they can arise on any mucosal site. Clinically, verruciform xanthomas typically appear as asymptomatic, soft, sessile plaques. The lesions are well circumscribed with a warty or verruciform surface texture (Fig. 5-5). Verruciform xanthomas are usually whiter than the surrounding mucosa, although their color may range from red to varying shades of orange or yellow. The lesions rarely enlarge beyond 2.0 cm, and multiple lesions occur infrequently.

Verruciform xanthomas may frequently be confused with human papillomavirus–associated lesions (e.g., wart or condyloma acuminatum) and squamous cell carcinoma. A biopsy, revealing papillomatosis, acanthosis, and hyperparakeratosis accompanied by the presence of foamy lipid-laden cells filling the connective tissue, is required for diagnosis. The origin of these foam cells is unknown, although they most likely represent macrophages. Unlike other forms of xanthomas that may be associated with lipid abnormalities and diabetes, verruciform xanthomas are not associated with any systemic abnormalities.

Malignant transformation does not occur, and recurrences of excised lesions are rare.

Fibrous Histiocytoma

The fibrous histiocytomas represent a unique conglomeration of lesions comprised of histiocytes and fibroblasts. Because the tumors display variable clinical presentations and assume many forms, considerable confusion surrounds their classification. Fibrous histiocytomas occurring on the skin have also been called *dermatofibromas, fibroxanthomas,* and *sclerosing hemangiomas,* although it is unclear whether fibrous histiocytomas in the mouth are the same entities. Current evidence suggests that the cell of origin of all these lesions may be the tissue histiocyte, which, over time, assumes fibroblastic characteristics.

The majority of fibrous histiocytomas occur on the lower extremities. Oral lesions are relatively uncommon and develop most frequently on the buccal mucosa followed by the tongue, gingiva, and lip. The oral lesions are usually solitary, painless, firm nodules without distinctive clinical features that range in size from 1 to 2 cm (Fig. 5-6). The surface, usually smooth and nonulcerated, is covered by pink epithelium. Whereas cutaneous lesions arise most frequently in young adults, oral lesions develop more commonly in the fifth to sixth decades of life.

Histologic examination reveals plump fibroblasts arranged as intersecting fascicles with foamy histiocytes. Immunologic stains may be needed to differentiate the fibrous histiocytoma from other fibrous tumors.

Conservative surgical excision is curative for fibrous histiocytomas. Recurrences are uncommon with the exception of deep-seated lesions, which are often incompletely excised.

Lipoma

The lipoma is a benign neoplasm of fat. It is the most common mesenchymal neoplasm, developing in the subcutaneous tissues of upper trunk and proximal extremities. Oral mucosal lipomas are con-

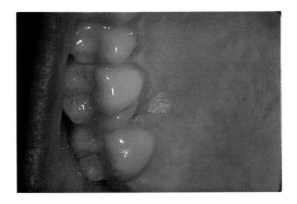

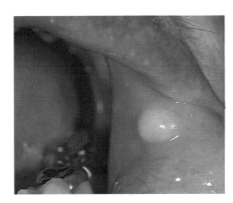

FIG. 5-5   Verruciform xanthomas are usually whiter than the surrounding mucosa and are well circumscribed with a warty or verruciform surface texture.

FIG. 5-6   Oral fibrous histiocytomas are usually diagnosed from biopsy because they display no distinctive clinical features.

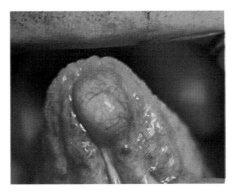

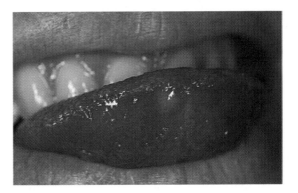

FIG. 5-7   Yellow submucosal nodules may be easily recognized as superficial oral lipomas.

FIG. 5-8   Granular cell tumors develop typically on the tongue and appear as firm, pink, asymptomatic nodules.

sidered to be uncommon, although their incidence is probably higher than that reported. Although lipomas appear to be more prevalent in obese individuals, changes in body weight do not alter the clinical appearance of the lesions.

Oral lipomas usually present as asymptomatic, slow-growing, smooth-surfaced sessile or pedunculated nodules and are 1 to 2 cm in size (Fig. 5-7). Typically, superficial oral lipomas are either yellow or white, whereas deep-seated lesions are covered by normal-appearing mucosa. More than 50% of oral lipomas occur on the buccal and vestibular mucosa, although the tongue, floor of mouth, and lips are also favored sites. The majority of oral lipomas develop in middle-aged adults and are uncommon in children. Histologic features resemble normal adipose tissue, with fat lobules appearing larger than normal. Variations of oral lipomas including fibrolipomas, myxolipomas, and angiolipomas may be encountered, depending on the proportion of other cellular elements present.

Lipomas that are surgically excised generally do not recur.

Granular Cell Tumor

The granular cell tumor is a relatively uncommon neoplasm occurring predominantly on the skin and oral mucosa. Although the majority develop on the head and neck, approximately 30% are confined to the tongue. Lesions may infrequently arise on the buccal mucosa and other oral sites. Intraoral granular cell tumors most frequently occur in middle-aged adults and twice as often in women than men.

Clinically, the oral granular cell tumor presents as a solitary, firm, sessile, asymptomatic nodule

(Fig. 5-8). Tumors range in size from 0.5 to 3 cm and are rarely ulcerated. More commonly, their surface is smooth and of normal color, although occasionally, lesions may appear yellow. Multiple lesions may also occur.

Originally, the granular cell tumor lesion was thought to arise from skeletal muscle and was termed *granular cell myoblastoma.* More recent evidence, confirming the presence of S-100 protein and Leu-7 antigen supports its origin from Schwann cells. Microscopically, the lesions are characterized by large, eosinophilic granular cells arranged in clusters and fascicles blending into adjacent skeletal muscle. The granules stain positive with periodic acid-Schiff but are diastase resistant. Approximately half of all cases of granular cell tumors exhibit pseudoepitheliomatous hyperplasia of the overlying epithelium. This feature may result in a mistaken diagnosis of squamous cell carcinoma, especially if the biopsy specimen is superficial and does not reveal the underlying pathologic changes. Recurrences are uncommon after the lesions are surgically excised.

Neurilemoma (Schwannoma)

The neurilemoma is a benign neoplasm originating from periaxonal or endoneural Schwann cells. It is a relatively uncommon tumor with up to one half of all cases occurring in the head and neck region.

Clinically, the oral neurilemoma is an asymptomatic, slow-growing mass that develops most frequently in the third to fifth decades of life. Neurilemomas are variable in size. ranging from a few millimeters to several centimeters. Their surface is usually covered by normal epithelium, and they are firm to palpation (Fig. 5-9). Although neurilemomas can occur anywhere in the mouth, they are most frequently discovered on the tongue. Lesions may also arise centrally within bone.

Microscopically, neurilemomas are encapsulated and comprised of distinctive Antoni A (hypercellular areas) and Antoni B cells (hypocellular areas). Verocay bodies, characterized by the arrangement of palisaded nuclei in double rows, are also characteristically present.

The tumor is benign and malignant transformation does not occur. The lesions may be surgically excised with a low recurrence rate.

Neurofibroma

The neurofibroma is a benign proliferation of neuromesenchymal tissue composed of Schwann cells, perineural cells, fibroblasts, and mast cells. It can arise as either a solitary tumor or in association with neurofibromatosis. Solitary neurofibromas of the skin and oral cavity develop most frequently in the third and fourth decades. Whereas their occurrence in skin is common, oral cavity lesions are infrequent and appear as asymptomatic, slow-growing, soft nodules (Fig. 5-10). Oral neurofibromas

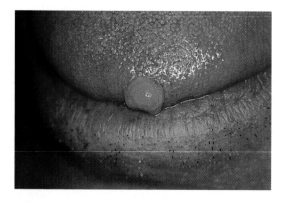

FIG. 5-9   Neurilemomas occur almost exclusively on the tongue and clinically resemble granular cell tumors.

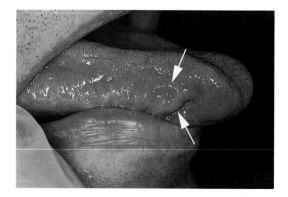

FIG. 5-10   Oral neurofibromas, appearing as soft masses, retain the same color as the normal mucosa and arise most commonly on the tongue.

retain the same color as the normal mucosa. They can achieve a size of 2 to 3 cm. Despite their large size, which predisposes them to trauma, they generally remain nonulcerated. Common sites for development include the tongue, buccal mucosa, and palate. Diffuse involvement of the tongue may result in macroglossia and is often accompanied by enlargement of the fungiform papillae. The incidence of oral involvement in patients with neurofibromatosis approximates 30%, with multiple oral lesions frequently present. Intrabony neurofibromas, predominantly in the mandible, may also occur. Malignant transformation of oral neurofibromas has been reported but is rare.

Histologically, the lesions are unencapsulated and composed of haphazardly arranged spindle cells. Fibroblasts and mast cells are also present.

Oral neurofibromas may be surgically excised and rarely recur. Recognition of these oral tumors may help establish the diagnosis of neurofibromatosis, especially in forme fruste cases when other stigmata are not apparent.

Fibrous Hyperplasia and Other Fibrous Tumors (Fibroma, Giant Cell Fibroma, Peripheral Ossifying Fibroma)

Once confused with the oral fibroma, which is an exceedingly rare true neoplasm, fibrous hyperplasia represents a reactive process to trauma and is the most common tumor in the oral cavity. It occurs in all age groups but has a peak incidence in the fourth to sixth decades of life, with a higher incidence in women. The lesions are firm, exophytic, nodular, or pedunculated and are covered by normal pink mucosa (Fig. 5-11). Hyperkeratosis secondary to chronic trauma may make the lesions white. Fibrous hyperplasia develops most frequently in areas subjected to trauma such as the inner aspect of the lips, the buccal mucosa, and the tongue. Lesions are painless and usually range in size from several millimeters to a centimeter. Histologically, the mass consists of hyperplastic fibrous connective tissue with minimal inflammation. Immunohistochemical studies reveal that the differentiated and ordered pattern of extracellular matrix proteins is characteristic of normal oral mucosa, supporting a reactive process.

The giant cell fibroma and the peripheral ossifying fibroma represent variants of fibrous hyperplasia. It has been postulated that peripheral ossifying fibromas represent pyogenic granulomas that have matured, fibrosed, and undergone focal calcification. In contrast to fibrous hyperplasia, the giant cell fibroma and the peripheral ossifying fibroma occur most frequently in young adults and twice as often in women as men and develop predominantly on the gingiva. Clinically, the giant cell fibroma is identical to fibrous hyperplasia but larger and broadly attached to the underlying mucosal surface. The peripheral ossifying fibroma may resemble either a large fibrous hyperplasia or a pyo-

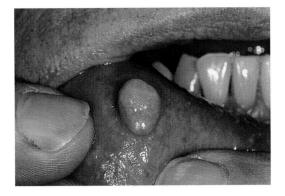

FIG. 5-11   Fibrous hyperplasias, the most common tumors of the oral cavity, represent a reaction to trauma, accounting for their high prevalence on the labial and buccal mucosa and tongue.

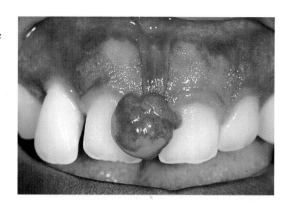

FIG. 5-12   Peripheral ossifying fibromas often clinically resemble pyogenic granulomas and develop typically on the gingiva.

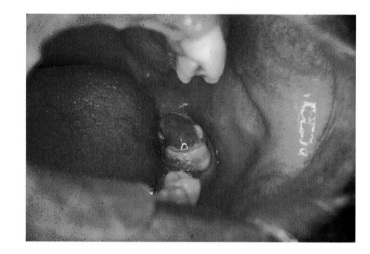

FIG. 5-13   Pulp polyps are a reactive process to dental decay and are characterized by an intensely red mass protruding from the pulp chamber, often filling the entire cavity of the tooth.

genic granuloma because it often arises from the interdental papillae (Fig. 5-12). Surface ulceration is also frequently present. Histologically, the giant cell fibroma contains stellate and multinucleated cells, which have been shown to be of fibroblastic origin, whereas the peripheral ossifying fibroma features epithelial nests and deposits of cementum, bone, and dystrophic calcification throughout the fibrous tissue. These histologic features may occasionally be found in fibrous hyperplasia, supporting the association of these entities.

The lesions may be surgically excised, but if the underlying traumatic cause is not eliminated, they occasionally recur.

Pulp Polyp

The dental pulp, comprised of blood vessels, nerves, lymphatics, and connective tissue, is protected by the calcified dental structures. When dental caries destroys this protective layer exposing the pulp chamber, a reactive process known as chronic hyperplastic pulpitis may develop. This lesion, also known as a *pulp polyp,* is comprised of excessive granulation tissue and occurs almost exclusively in children and adolescents. An intensely red mass protrudes from the pulp chamber and often fills the entire cavity of the tooth (Fig. 5-13). The rich vascular supply of the primary and permanent first molar teeth accounts for these as favored sites for the development of an inflammatory hyperplastic response.

Pulp polyps may remain unchanged for long periods if the carious lesion is not restored. The tooth may be treated by endodontic therapy with pulp extirpation or by extraction.

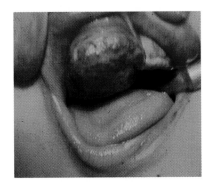

FIG. 5-14   Melanotic neuroectodermal tumors of infancy typically occur on the anterior maxillary ridge and achieve a significant size that may result in underlying bone destruction.

Melanotic Neuroectodermal Tumor of Infancy

The melanotic neuroectodermal tumor of infancy is a primitive neuroectodermal tumor with polyphenotypic expression of neural and epithelial markers, melanin production, occasional glial, and rhabdomyoblastic differentiation. It arises in infancy, usually before 6 months of age and affects males and females equally. Greater than half of all cases develop on the anterior maxillary alveolar ridge, but the tumor may also appear on the mandible, epididymis, dura, brain, and uterus. Clinically, oral lesions grow rapidly, achieving an average size of 2 to 3 cm (Fig. 5-14). The surface is smooth and covered with either normal or pigmented mucosa. As the lesions progress, they destroy the underlying bone, resulting in displacement of the teeth.

Histologically, the lesions are distinctive and comprised of tubular or alveolar formations of large melanin-containing cells possessing scant or fibrillar cytoplasm. Characteristic laboratory abnormalities include high levels of vanillymandelic acid and serum α-fetoprotein.

The melanotic neuroectodermal tumor of infancy is a benign growth that can be locally invasive and destructive, simulating malignancy. Rare cases of metastases and death have been reported, and recurrences are not uncommon after excision. The behavior of the tumor cannot be predicted from morphologic findings or flow cytometry studies.

PREMALIGNANT LESIONS
Leukoplakia

Oral mucosal leukoplakia is undoubtedly the most misused term in clinical oral diagnosis. It is defined by the World Health Organization as "a white patch or plaque that cannot be characterized clinically or pathologically as any other disease." As such, *leukoplakia* is exclusively a clinically descriptive term that does not connote the benign, premalignant, or malignant characteristics of the lesion either clinically or microscopically. Solitary white lesions or diseases displaying white plaques or patches whose diagnosis as distinct entities is based on clinical and histologic features, such as lichen planus, frictional hyperkeratosis, nicotinic stomatitis, and white sponge nevus, should not be designated as leukoplakia. When the same lesions cannot be clinically identified, they may be referred to as leukoplakia pending definitive histopathologic diagnosis.

Leukoplakia, the most common chronic lesion of oral mucous membranes, is noted in approximately 5% of adults, with the great majority of cases occurring in men. The lesions usually arise after age 40, and the incidence of oral leukoplakia increases with age, affecting approximately 8% of men over 70 years of age.

Although leukoplakia is considered a premalignant lesion, it does not imply that epithelial dysplasia is always histologically present. In fact, less than one fourth of all leukoplakia has a microscopically dysplastic component. Long-term clinical studies suggest a risk of malignant transformation ranging from 5% to nearly 50%, depending on the clinical type of leukoplakia and the presence of risk factors for malignant transformation.

The specific cause of leukoplakia remains unclear, although several etiologic factors are strongly correlated with its development. Unquestionably, cigarette, cigar, and pipe smoking are most closely associated with the formation of oral leukoplakia. More than 80% of individuals with oral leukoplakia consume tobacco in some form. In addition, the severity of oral leukoplakia is directly proportional to the duration and quantity of tobacco use. When leukoplakia results from tobacco use, a significant percentage of lesions, especially early ones, will completely regress or partially disappear after cessation of the habit. Nicotine stomatitis (see Chapter 3), resulting from thermal irritation produced by pipe smoking, represents a nonleukoplakic keratosis that, unlike leukoplakia, is completely reversible and not precancerous regardless of the magnitude and duration of habit.

Alcohol is another known risk factor for the development of oral leukoplakia. Alcohol and tobacco exhibit profound synergism in the malignant transformation of leukoplakia into squamous cell carcinoma. White plaques on the buccal mucosa that result from the use of mouth rinses with high alcohol content do not represent leukoplakia and are not considered premalignant.

Ultraviolet radiation is a well-accepted etiologic factor in the development of leukoplakia on the vermilion border of the lower lip. This type of leukoplakia is associated with changes that are observed in actinic cheilitis.

Several microorganisms have been associated with the development of oral leukoplakia. Historically, chronic *Treponema pallidum* infections in tertiary syphilis were frequently associated with leukoplakia, primarily of the dorsal tongue. Fortunately, such lesions are rare because of the early diagnosis and treatment of syphilis. *Candida* infections may also be responsible for the development of leukoplakia. Chronic hyperplastic candidiasis, also referred to as candidal leukoplakia, results in verrucous white plaques often associated with inflammation. The lesions arise most frequently on the buccal mucosa, although any site may be affected. It is unclear whether dysplastic changes observed microscopically are directly related to the yeast infection or whether *Candida* secondarily infects previously altered epithelium. Human papillomaviruses, especially HPV type 16 and HPV type 18, have also been discovered in some plaques of oral leukoplakia. Interestingly, these specific subtypes have been associated with the development of cervical carcinoma, as well as oral carcinoma. The role of human papillomavirus in the development of oral malignancy is unclear, as these organisms can also be detected in normal epithelial cells.

Approximately three fourths of all oral leukoplakias are found on the vermilion border of the lips, buccal mucosa, and gingiva. Oral leukoplakia can assume one of several clinical forms that frequently change over time. The lesions may range in size from a few millimeters to several centimeters, and the surface may be smooth or verrucous. Thin leukoplakia, as its name implies, is clinically characterized by a slightly elevated, white, hyperkeratotic plaque that is usually translucent with sharply demarcated borders (Fig. 5-15). Histologically, the majority of lesions reveal no dysplasia

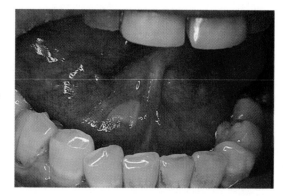

FIG. 5-15   Thin leukoplakia is characterized by a slightly elevated, white, hyperkeratotic plaque.

on biopsy. In tobacco smokers who discontinue their habit, thin leukoplakias almost always resolve. In those that do not, over half enlarge, thicken, and assume a corrugated or leathery appearance (Fig. 5-16). The majority of these thick lesions remain unchanged, with some progressing to a more severe form and yet others regressing if the etiologic factor is eliminated. The granular or nodular forms of leukoplakia, characterized by the presence of proliferative, nodular, or verrucous white plaques (Fig. 5-17), represent more advanced, severe lesions that have a higher rate of malignant transformation. A particularly ominous variation of leukoplakia is the presence of erythematous or erosive lesions within the white plaque, termed *speckled leukoplakia* or *erythroleukoplakia* (Fig. 5-18). Of all of the different types of oral leukoplakia, this type has the highest propensity for malignant degeneration.

A rare variant, proliferative verrucous leukoplakia, is characterized by the presence of irregularly shaped hyperkeratotic areas of leukoplakia, which slowly progress to involve multiple mucosal surfaces. Unlike other forms of oral leukoplakia, the majority of patients with proliferative verrucous

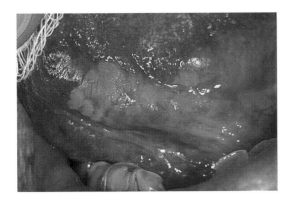

FIG. 5-16   As leukoplakia enlarges, it often assumes a thickened, corrugated, and leathery appearance.

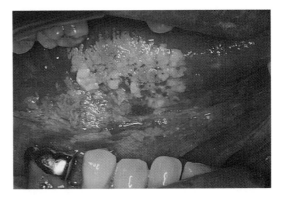

FIG. 5-17   The nodular forms of leukoplakia, characterized by the presence of proliferative, nodular, or verrucous white plaques, represent more advanced, severe lesions, which have a higher rate of malignant transformation.

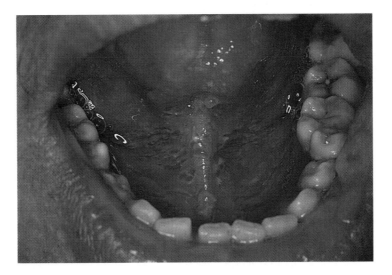

FIG. 5-18   Erythroleukoplakia, consisting of a red and white plaque arising, in the floor of the mouth.

leukoplakia are women. Proliferative verrucous leukoplakia has a propensity to develop into a transitional stage of verrucous carcinoma; however, the vast majority eventually become frank squamous cell carcinomas. Additionally, proliferative verrucous leukoplakia does not regress, even when all contributing factors have been eliminated. The proliferative verrucous leukoplakia spectrum includes the various forms of leukoplakia that have been defined based on their histologic alterations including verrucous hyperplasia, verrucous leukoplakia, and florid oral papillomatosis.

The microscopic features of oral mucosal leukoplakia comprise a wide spectrum of findings that are distinct for each clinical variant. With the exception of speckled leukoplakia, all forms exhibit hyperkeratosis to some degree. Approximately 10% to 20% of all leukoplakias exhibit epithelial dysplasia, carcinoma in situ, or frank carcinoma on initial biopsy. Dysplastic changes are frequently present when candidal leukoplakia is biopsied. Erythroleukoplakia or speckled leukoplakia reveals significant anaplasia, representing sites in which immature epithelial cells can no longer produce keratin.

It cannot be overemphasized that all oral mucosal leukoplakias require biopsy. Repeated biopsies may be required for large lesions or cases of multiple lesions. In the evaluation of patients with leukoplakia, it is also important to stress the significance of location of the lesion. More than 90% of oral leukoplakias that exhibit microscopic evidence of dysplasia or carcinoma occur on the tongue, vermilion border of the lip, and floor of the mouth. Leukoplakias on these sites should be viewed with great suspicion. Clinical studies of patients with oral leukoplakia indicate that 3% to 5% eventually result in squamous cell carcinoma. Malignant transformation usually occurs within several years after the diagnosis of leukoplakia, although the time frame ranges from several months to several decades. Long-standing lesions have a greater risk of malignancy than those of recent origin. The likelihood of malignant degeneration is most closely correlated with the type of leukoplakia. Thin leukoplakias have a low malignant potential, whereas thick leukoplakias undergo malignant degeneration with greater frequency. As many as one in seven cases of verrucous leukoplakias eventually become malignant, and approximately 25% to 50% of all erythroleukoplakias transform into squamous cell carcinomas. As expected, the incidence of malignant degeneration correlates with the severity of dysplasia noted in the initial biopsy. Thus approximately 10% of leukoplakias with moderate dysplasia eventually undergo malignant degeneration, whereas 25% of plaques displaying severe dysplasia become malignant.

The treatment of choice for oral mucosa leukoplakia is excision. In addition to surgical excision, leukoplakia may be treated by electrocautery, cryosurgery, or laser surgery. Leukoplakia may recur after eradication, necessitating careful follow-up. In individuals with ongoing risk factors, semiannual surveillance is necessary.

In the absence of histologically demonstrated dysplasia, leukoplakia may be carefully followed in conjunction with the elimination of any potential etiologic factors, especially tobacco. Chemoprevention with topical and systemic retinoids, as well as with dietary and nutritional supplements containing antioxidants, may prove useful in these cases and eventually become a viable alternative to surgery. Studies involving newer agents with fewer adverse reactions are currently being evaluated. Additionally, a number of genetic and biologic alterations in patients exhibiting premalignant leukoplakias have been identified and may serve as markers for cancer risk assessment and effectiveness of cancer-chemopreventive agents. These include increased levels of proteolytic activities, microsatellite alterations at chromosome 9p21 and 3p14, increased expression of cytokeratins CK8 and CK19, and gene deletions in premalignant oral lesions.

Erythroplakia (Erythroplasia of Queyrat)

By definition, erythroplakia is a red patch that cannot be clinically or pathologically diagnosed as any other condition and is not inflammatory in origin. Oral mucosal lesions are analogous to premalignant erythematous lesions on the penis.

Oral mucosal erythroplakia is much less common than leukoplakia and develops at a later age, usually in the sixth to eighth decades of life. Like leukoplakia, the lesions are observed more commonly in men and in those who consume tobacco and alcohol.

The floor of the mouth is the most common site for erythroplakia, followed by the lateral and ventral tongue and soft palate. The lesions may be single or multiple and range in color from light pink to fiery red. The surface of the lesions may be either smooth, papular, or velvety. The lesions may be well circumscribed or they may blend with the surrounding tissue, making them difficult to detect. Speckled erythroplakia is analogous to speckled leukoplakia and describes a plaque of erythroplakia mixed with specks of leukoplakia (Fig. 5-18). A variety of other oral conditions may mimic erythroplakia including mucositis, erythematous candidiasis, and acute trauma. Because more than three fourths of erythroplakia histologically exhibit severe dysplasia, carcinoma in situ, or frank carcinoma, a biopsy is essential to differentiate treatable inflammatory causes from the more serious lesion—erythroplakia. These lesions should be regarded as the earliest manifestation of oral carcinoma.

When examined microscopically, the epithelial cells are anaplastic and lose their capability to produce keratin. The underlying vasculature imparts the characteristic red color, which is intensified by chronic inflammation that is frequently present.

Wherever possible, persistent red areas should be subjected to biopsy and, when identified histologically as dysplastic, should be completely excised. Although destructive modalities commonly used for the treatment of leukoplakia may be appropriate, the specimen should be preserved for histopathologic examination and detection of microscopically invasive carcinoma. Recurrences are possible and require careful, long-term follow-up.

Smokeless Tobacco Lesions (Snuff Dipper's Hyperkeratosis, Tobacco Pouch Lesion)

The use of smokeless tobacco is practiced worldwide and is especially prevalent in Southeast Asia and the Indian subcontinent. The use of this extremely addictive substance has tripled in the last 20 years, and it is estimated that more than 5% of the population currently engages in chewing tobacco or dipping snuff. The incidence may be even higher, approximating 20% in selected southeastern states. The majority of individuals who use smokeless tobacco begin their habit in late childhood or early adolescence and rarely in adulthood.

A variety of oral alterations result from the indulgence in smokeless tobacco. Frequently, there is localized gingival recession in the areas where the tobacco or snuff is placed, often associated with destruction of the underlying alveolar bone. The incidence of dental caries in teeth that come in contact with the tobacco products is increased, presumably because of the sugar that is added to these substances. Extrinsic brown or black staining of the teeth, as well as physical abrasion of the enamel, may also commonly occur.

A distinctive hyperkeratosis develops on the mucosal surfaces that contact the tobacco products. This tobacco pouch keratosis is found in approximately 10% to 20% of chewing tobacco users and in roughly two thirds of snuff dippers. In western Europe and North America, tobacco pouch keratosis is observed mostly in young adults and geriatric men. Usually, the lesion is restricted to the mucosal surfaces of the inner lip or cheek that come in direct contact with the smokeless tobacco. Clinically, the mucosa appears grayish-white, with an indistinct border, and is frequently surrounded by erythema (Fig. 5-19). The surface of the mucosa has a velvety texture, often with a cobblestone appearance. The lesions are asymptomatic and patients are often unaware of their presence. Long-standing lesions in heavy smokeless tobacco users may become thickened and verrucous, although in the majority of cases the lesions never progress beyond the velvety stage. The extent and severity of the lesions vary greatly and are influenced by many factors. Significantly large lesions result from increased number of years of tobacco use, large amounts of tobacco consumed on a daily basis, long duration of daily use, placement of tobacco at a single site, and the use of certain brands of smokeless tobacco.

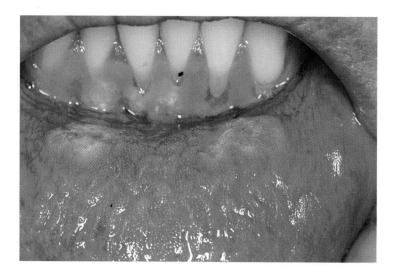

FIG. 5-19   Snuff dipper's hyperkeratosis. Localized gingival recession and characteristic hyperkeratotic and velvety appearance of labial mucosa are restricted to the area in contact with snuff.

In several Asian countries, most notably India, tobacco pouch keratosis develops much more commonly because of the high prevalence of smokeless tobacco use and the concomitant use of other carcinogenic agents including betel leaves, slaked lime, and areca nuts. The use of this mixture of tobacco products has been associated with the development of oral submucous fibrosis.

The microscopic appearance of tobacco pouch keratosis is nonspecific and characterized by acanthosis, orthokeratosis, and marked parakeratosis. The parakeratin layer is comprised of distinctively large, pale, partly vacuolated cells containing keratohyalin granules. Although the epithelium is hyperplastic, dysplasia is uncommon.

Although historically the use of smokeless tobacco has been associated with the development of verrucous carcinoma, the true carcinogenic potential of smokeless tobacco is low and estimated to be less than a 5% lifetime risk. It is suggested that only lesions that are markedly thickened or that exhibit other features suggestive of malignant transformation, including induration, ulceration, or rapid change, should be biopsied. When the diagnosis is uncertain, it is advisable to obtain histopathologic confirmation of this presumably benign lesion.

Fortunately, the vast majority of tobacco pouch keratoses resolve in 2 to 3 weeks after cessation of tobacco use. In those individuals who are unable to discontinue their habit, the smokeless tobacco should be placed in alternating areas of the mouth, although this may result in gingival and periodontal complications affecting multiple areas. All lesions that persist after discontinuation of tobacco use should be subjected to biopsy.

Oral Submucous Fibrosis

Oral submucous fibrosis is a precancerous collagen disorder that occurs almost exclusively in India and Southeast Asia. The condition is chronic and characterized by inflammation and a progressive fibrosis of the lamina propria and deeper connective tissues. Clinically, oral submucous fibrosis is characterized initially by the presence of multiple oral vesicles and erosions, most frequently on the palate and tongue. The disease may extend to the pharynx and esophagus and commonly results in severe tongue burning. The clinical hallmark of the condition is the formation of numerous fibrous bands that eventually severely restrict movement of the tongue and other oral structures. Patients have difficulty in opening the mouth (trismus), masticating, and swallowing. The tongue and other oral

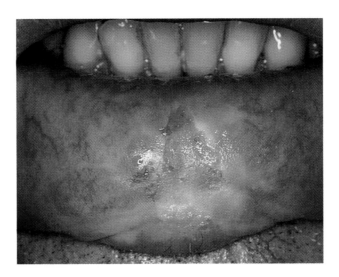

FIG. 5-20   Atrophy, erythema, and keratotic changes are characteristic of actinic cheilitis.

mucosal surfaces become atrophic and painful, and taste impairment may be demonstrated by electrogustometry. Mucosal melanosis and xerostomia are advanced features of the disease.

The precise cause of submucous fibrosis is unknown, although the culturally characteristic use of betel quid (consisting of powdered tobacco, slaked lime, areca nuts, and betel leaves) in the oral cavity has been strongly implicated in the development of the disease.

Microscopically, oral submucous fibrosis is characterized by marked scarification of the connective tissue associated with a dense, chronic inflammatory infiltrate. The epithelium is typically hyperkeratotic, although atrophy with loss of rete ridges is also frequently noted. Of greatest significance is the high incidence of epithelial dysplasia and carcinoma detected in patients with oral submucous fibrosis. Up to 15% of all cases display evidence of dysplasia, with 5% to 10% revealing invasive carcinoma.

Unlike tobacco pouch keratosis, oral submucous fibrosis does not resolve after cessation of contact with the carcinogenic agents. Early cases may be treated with intralesional and topical corticosteroids, whereas surgical excision of the fibrotic bands is required to alleviate trismus in the advanced stages. Periodic and long-term follow-up are essential in the early detection of oral carcinoma.

Actinic Cheilitis

Actinic cheilitis is a precancerous lesion that develops on the vermilion border of the lower lip. The lesion is analogous to the actinic keratosis that occurs on the skin, and both lesions represent manifestations of chronic ultraviolet radiation exposure. Like its cutaneous counterpart, actinic cheilitis seldom occurs in young individuals and is much more common in men than in women.

Clinically, actinic cheilitis manifests as atrophy of the vermilion border, with alterations in the color and texture of the lip. Acute lesions display erythema, edema, and fine scaling, although chronic lesions exhibit areas of leukoplakia, atrophy, and roughened, keratotic changes (Fig. 5-20). The mucocutaneous junction is often obliterated. Lesions demonstrating erosions or induration are suggestive of severe dysplasia or malignancy and require biopsy. Because the vermilion border of the lip does not display the same anatomic landmarks as skin, the differentiation of a hyperplastic actinic cheilitis from an early squamous cell carcinoma becomes more difficult.

Microscopically, actinic cheilitis exhibits the presence of atypical keratinocytes along the basal cell layer and disordered cornification and maturation. The amount of atypia present varies, and prominent hyperplasia extending around the superficial capillaries should be considered an early feature of squamous cell carcinoma. Variable degrees of chronic inflammation and solar elastosis are present in the superficial lamina propria and underlying connective tissue, respectively.

Actinic cheilitis is generally an irreversible condition, reflecting actinic damage that occurred over a period of 20 to 30 years before development of the lesion. The use of topical sunscreens should be encouraged to prevent additional damage. Suspicious areas should be subjected to biopsy because the risk of metastases from squamous cell carcinomas arising on the lips is significantly greater than those developing on facial skin. Squamous cell carcinoma has been reported to occur in actinic cheilitis in up to 10% of cases. Cryosurgery is an effective treatment for localized lesions. Diffuse involvement of the lower lip can be treated by laser, vermilionectomy, or topical chemotherapy using 5-flu-orouracil.

MALIGNANT NEOPLASMS
Squamous Cell Carcinoma

Epidemiology. Squamous cell carcinomas account for more than 90% of all oral malignancies. It is the sixth most common cancer in men and the twelfth in women. Nearly 30,000 new cases of oral cancer, constituting 3% to 5% of all malignancies, are diagnosed yearly in the United States, and approximately 8000 deaths per year are attributed to this malignancy. The rate is significantly higher in some regions of the world including India, Hong Kong, France, and Puerto Rico.

As with most malignancies, the risk of oral cancer increases with age; it occurs mainly in persons over 40 years of age. Excluding pharyngeal and vermilion border malignancies, the annual rate of oral cancer in the United States is 7.7 per 100,000 individuals. The incidence of oral cancer has been increasing dramatically in African-American males and decreasing in all other groups of Americans. Oral cancer develops three times more commonly in men than in women.

Squamous cell carcinoma of the vermilion border of the lower lip, unlike intraoral carcinoma, is closely associated with chronic sun exposure. Although only 4 per 100,000 people develop lower lip carcinomas, this rate increases over sevenfold for men in their eighth decade of life. The incidence of squamous cell carcinoma of the vermilion border of the lower lip is distinctly uncommon in women and nonwhite men.

Etiology. The etiology of oral squamous cell carcinoma is diverse and related to multiple factors that contribute to its development. Extrinsic factors include combustible tobacco, ethanol, and ultraviolet radiation (for vermilion border lesions). Intrinsic factors include systemic conditions such as generalized debilitation, nutritional deficiencies, syphilis, and iron-deficiency anemia. A genetic predisposition does not appear to be significant in the development of squamous cell carcinoma of the oral cavity.

During the last 50 years there has been a dramatic decrease in tobacco smoking. Currently, less than one fourth of adults in the United States smoke cigarettes, although those who continue to do so appear to be much heavier smokers than their predecessors. For this reason, the effects of tobacco in the development of oral cancers may be greater than previously reported.

A significant body of epidemiologic data has demonstrated an association between cigarette smoking and oral cancer. Over three fourths of patients with oral cancer are smokers, a figure three times greater than that in the general population. The risk of developing oral cancer from cigarette smoking is proportional to the frequency and duration of the habit. Patients with known oral cancer who continue to smoke have an approximately five times greater risk for developing a second primary cancer compared with those who quit smoking.

Aside from cigarettes, other forms of combustible tobacco, including cigars and pipes, predispose to the development of oral cancer. Reverse smoking (the lit end of a cigar or a cigarette held inside the mouth) is performed in certain Indian and Hispanic populations. This habit, particularly common in women, poses a great risk for the development of oral cancer. Approximately one half of all oral cancers that result from reverse smoking are found on the hard palate, an atypical site for squamous cell carcinomas to develop in the United States.

Smokeless tobacco users have a fourfold increased risk of developing squamous cell carcinoma. In certain populations, women are the predominant users of this tobacco product and, not surprisingly, the incidence of oral cancer is proportionately higher in this group. The majority of oral cancers in smokeless tobacco users are found at the site where the tobacco is habitually held in the mouth.

The use of alcohol by itself has not been shown to be carcinogenic, although it appears to be a significant potentiator of other known carcinogens, especially tobacco. Specifically, there is a fifteenfold increased risk for those who consume both alcohol and tobacco. Studies have also revealed that individuals who consume large quantities of alcohol are frequently heavy smokers. The effects of alcohol in the development of oral cancer are both dose- and time-dependent.

The relationship of ultraviolet radiation and actinic cheilitis has been well established and discussed previously. Therapeutic radiation to the head and neck has also been documented to increase the number of oral cancers, although the risk is small when compared with the effects of alcohol and tobacco. Nevertheless, patients with a history of radiation therapy involving the head and neck should have their oral cavity regularly examined. Diagnostic dental radiographs are not implicated as causative in the development of oral squamous cell carcinoma.

Plummer-Vinson syndrome (see Chapter 12) is a unique condition associated with defective cell-mediated immunity, esophageal scarring and webbing, and iron deficiency anemia. Affected individuals are at a higher risk for squamous cell carcinoma of the mouth and upper aerodigestive tract.

Syphilis of the oral cavity has been associated with a fourfold increase in the risk of squamous cell carcinoma of the tongue. Unlike tobacco-associated tongue cancers, lesions developing in association with tertiary syphilis occur on the dorsal surface of the tongue.

Some of the medications used to treat syphilis in the nineteenth and early twentieth centuries, including arsenic and heavy metals, were themselves carcinogenic and may have been responsible for the observed changes. Fortunately, early diagnosis and treatment of syphilis have all but eliminated this complication.

Chronic hyperplastic candidiasis or candidal leukoplakia is considered to be a premalignant lesion. Experimental hyperkeratotic lesions can be reproduced on the dorsal tongues of rats inoculated with *Candida albicans,* organisms known to produce carcinogenic nitrosamines. Furthermore, squamous cell carcinomas have been reported to develop in humans with candidal leukoplakia without other risk factors. The evidence implicating *Candida* in the initiation of oral squamous cell carcinoma is circumstantial and necessitates additional substantiation.

A number of oncogenic viruses may be associated with the development of oral cancer, but a significant correlation exists mainly with the human papillomavirus. This virus has also been implicated as an etiologic agent in carcinomas of other portions of the aerodigestive tract, uterus, cervix, vulva, and penis. HPV type 16 has been demonstrated to have the capability of maintaining the proliferative state of epithelial cells, contributing to the production of malignant phenotypes. Furthermore, the virus may bind to and inactivate tumor suppressor genes while stimulating oncogenes and proto-oncogenes. There is no experimental evidence to suggest that herpes simplex virus plays any role in the development of oral squamous cell carcinoma.

It has been well established that immunosuppressed individuals are at higher risk for developing various malignancies, including oral squamous cell carcinomas. Patients undergoing immunosuppressive chemotherapy or conditioning for bone marrow transplantation or those infected with the human immunodeficiency virus (HIV) are at increased risk for oral squamous cell carcinoma.

Nutritional deficiencies have been implicated as an important predisposing factor in the development of oral cancers. In several epidemiologic studies, low intakes of vitamin E, carotenoids, or both have been associated with a higher oral cancer risk. Alcohol and tobacco use and malnutrition promote impaired salivary gland function and oral mucosal immunity, reduce helper CD4 cells, and depress natural killer cell activity. These result in impaired tumor surveillance.

Research is currently being focused on the role of oncogenes in the development of oral can-

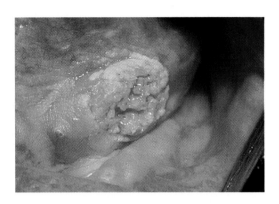

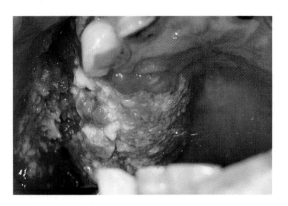

FIG. 5-21 Squamous cell carcinoma developing within a plaque of leukoplakia.

FIG. 5-22 Hyperkeratotic red and white masses on the maxillary gingiva and palate are typical of an oral squamous cell carcinoma.

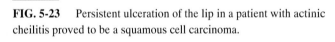

FIG. 5-23 Persistent ulceration of the lip in a patient with actinic cheilitis proved to be a squamous cell carcinoma.

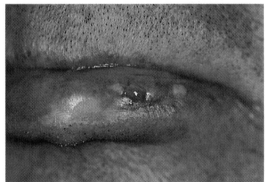

cers. Additionally, inactivation or alterations of tumor-suppressor genes have been associated with an increased incidence and progression of oral squamous cell carcinomas. The p53 gene is a tumor-suppressor gene found in mutated form in various cancers, and it is well established that a high incidence of p53 mutations exist in oral cavity squamous cell carcinomas. A higher incidence of these mutations has also been noted in tobacco users with oral cancer.

Clinical. Oral squamous cell carcinomas arise most frequently in older men. Clinical abnormalities in the affected areas are frequently detected by patients months to years before they seek professional care. There is extensive misinformation about the risk factors and signs of oral cancer; only 25% of adults surveyed could identify one sign of oral cancer.

Oral squamous cell carcinoma appears in a number of different clinical forms. Erythroplakia, erythroleukoplakia, and, less commonly, leukoplakia represent the earliest stage of oral cancer displaying histologic evidence of carcinoma *in situ* or invasive squamous cell carcinoma. Endophytic oral squamous cell carcinomas typically exhibit a central, irregularly shaped ulcer surrounded by a raised, rolled border. Although this presentation is not specific for oral squamous cell carcinoma, when present, it should arouse suspicion of malignancy. Exophytic squamous cell carcinomas are characterized by irregular papillary nodules that extend above the level of normal mucosa (Fig. 5-21). Depending on the amount of hyperkeratosis, the lesion may vary in color, appearing pink, white, or red (Fig. 5-22). Squamous cell carcinomas of the vermilion border of the lip characteristically appear as small, indurated, crusted, nonhealing ulcers (Fig. 5-23). In general, persistent oral ulcerations, nodules, red and white plaques, and indurated lesions should be biopsied to detect early cancers, which are most amenable to therapy. Patients who are alcohol drinkers and cigarette smokers over age 40 should be assessed more frequently. Toluidine blue staining and exfoliative cytologic ex-

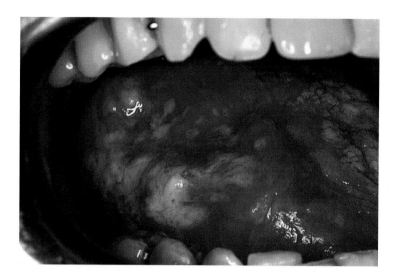

FIG. 5-24   Squamous cell carcinomas arise most commonly on the ventrolateral tongue and typically present as exophytic masses.

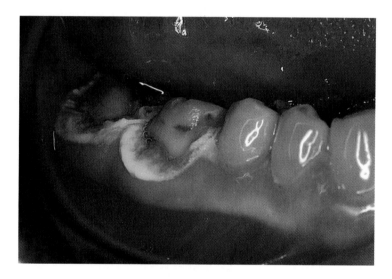

FIG. 5-25   Gingival squamous cell carcinomas develop most frequently in the posterior segment of the mandible.

amination are useful diagnostic adjuncts, particularly as a method of ruling out false-negative clinical impressions. As a mouth rinse, toluidine blue can be used as a guide to improve biopsy yields in high-risk patients and to assess margin status after resection of the cancer.

The most common intraoral sites for squamous cell carcinoma are the posterior lateral and ventral surfaces of the tongue (Fig. 5-24). Less than 5% of tongue carcinomas occur on the dorsal surface. The floor of the mouth is the second most common intraoral site, accounting for more than one third of all cases. In this location the carcinomas most likely arise from a preexisting leukoplakic or erythroplakic lesion. This may account for the high incidence of floor-of-the-mouth cancers in men.

Gingival carcinomas develop most frequently in the posterior segment around the mandibular teeth and are much more frequent in females than in males (Fig. 5-25). Gingival carcinoma commonly mimics other inflammatory and reactive processes observed on the gingiva, often resulting in delayed diagnosis and treatment. Frequently, gingival carcinoma invades the supporting structures of the teeth causing increased tooth mobility. Of all intraoral squamous cell carcinomas, those arising on the gingiva and alveolar mucosa have the least association with cigarette smoking.

Carcinoma of the soft palate and oral pharynx are easily overlooked and frequently undetected by both patients and doctors. Consequently, tumors in this location are typically discovered at an advanced stage when they are large. Their close proximity to regional lymphatics accounts for the high incidence of local and distant metastases present at the time of diagnosis. Symptoms of dysphagia and referred ear pain may be the initial manifestations of these cancers and should not be neglected.

In general, the incidence of metastasis is proportional to both the size and location of the primary lesion. All risk factors being equal, the more posterior the location of the lesion, the higher the likelihood of metastatic disease at the time of diagnosis. Regional metastases to cervical lymph nodes manifest as nontender enlargement with induration. Lymph nodes that are fixed to the underlying tissue and not freely movable imply invasion into adjacent tissue. Distant metastases are uncommon at the time of initial diagnosis, although when present, commonly involve the lungs, liver, and bones. Eventually, 25% to 50% of all oral squamous cell carcinomas metastasize.

Microscopically, oral squamous cell carcinoma encompasses a wide spectrum. This ranges from well-differentiated (low-grade) lesions in which the tumor closely resembles normal epithelium to poorly differentiated or anaplastic (high-grade) lesions in which it becomes exceedingly difficult to morphologically recognize tumor cells as epithelial in origin. Although the histopathologic grading of oral squamous cell carcinoma correlates to some degree with the biologic behavior of the tumor, the clinical staging system is much more predictive of long-term outcomes. An examination of extracellular matrix staining patterns, in addition to the conventional histologic examination, provides objective and practical data to evaluate the invasive and metastatic potential of oral cancers. Stage I disease, defined as tumors less than 2 cm in greatest diameter without nodal involvement or metastasis, has an 85% 5-year survival rate. Patients with larger tumors, 2 to 4 cm (stage II), have a 5-year survival rate of only 66%. The survival rate for stage III, characterized by tumors larger than 4 cm in greatest diameter or ipsilateral lymph node involvement, decreases to 41%. Stage IV disease, which comprises very large tumors, multiple lymph node involvement, or distant metastasis, has a 5-year survival rate of less than 10%. These statistics dramatically illustrate the need for early detection, diagnosis, and treatment. The prognostic significance of loss of heterozygosity at chromosome 3p may help identify patients who should receive more aggressive treatment.

Prevention and therapy. The therapy of intraoral squamous cell carcinomas depends on the stage of the disease. Computed tomography can be accurately used to predict perineural or vascular invasion. The treatment of choice is aggressive surgical intervention, often with postsurgical radiation therapy. One-stage reconstructive procedures, often incorporating osteotomy techniques, miniature bone plating, and free tissue transfer, have greatly diminished the morbidity of oral cancer surgery. Radical neck dissection is performed when there is evidence or suspicion of lymph node involvement. In cases in which the anatomic location of the tumor precludes surgery, radiation therapy alone is frequently used. Chemotherapy is generally not used as primary treatment of oral squamous cell carcinoma, although it is used as adjuvant therapy. Uncomplicated squamous cell carcinoma of the vermilion border of the lower lip treated by wide surgical excision has a 5-year survival rate that approaches 100%. Analogous lesions of the vermilion border of the upper lip have a dramatically different biologic behavior, as one fourth recur, and the 5-year survival rate is less than 60%. Fortunately, upper lip carcinomas are uncommon.

Patients diagnosed with a squamous cell carcinoma of the mouth are at increased risk for both synchronous or metachronous primary lesions in the upper aerodigestive tract including the larynx, esophagus, and lungs. The overall risk of additional primary tumors approximates 10% to 25%, although the incidence increases to 44% in those who continue to smoke tobacco. Metachronous lesions usually develop within 3 years of the initial diagnosis.

Cancer chemoprevention represents an exciting area of intensive research. Retinoids have been demonstrated to induce tumor cell differentiation, inhibit proliferation, and affect cell adhesion and invasion. Clinical studies have shown that retinoids may reverse premalignant lesions and significantly reduce the incidence of second primary tumors in patients with oral cancer who are disease free. Epidemiologic surveys, laboratory and animal studies, and intervention trials in humans have been used to support the role of natural and synthetic antioxidants in oral cancer prevention. The most widely used chemopreventive agents include vitamins A, E, C, and β-carotene, which have been shown to interfere with activation of procarcinogens, inhibit chromosome aberrations, and suppress actions of cancer promoters. Additional human trials are ongoing.

Verrucous Carcinoma

Verrucous carcinoma is a distinctive subtype of squamous cell carcinoma that is locally aggressive and nonmetastasizing. It was initially described nearly 50 years ago in association with the use of smokeless tobacco and, in addition to the oral cavity, characteristically occurs on the foot or glans penis. Human papillomavirus, specifically subtypes 16 and 18, has also been implicated as an etiologic agent.

Verrucous carcinoma comprises fewer than 10% of all oral carcinomas. Its higher prevalence in the southeastern United States reflects the high usage of smokeless tobacco in this region. Despite the fact that only one in five patients with verrucous carcinoma admits to the use of smokeless tobacco, the great majority of these carcinomas occur in tobacco chewers or snuff dippers. Squamous cell carcinomas are still 25 times more likely to develop than verrucous carcinomas in patients who use smokeless tobacco.

Verrucous carcinoma is a neoplasm that develops most commonly during the seventh decade of life. The lesion is usually more common in men, although in the southeastern United States it appears more frequently in women. The mandibular buccal and labial vestibules as well as the mandibular gingiva are the most common oral sites of involvement, corresponding to the areas where smokeless tobacco is held in the mouth. Verrucous carcinomas may also develop on the floor of the mouth, palate, and lip.

Clinically, verrucous carcinoma appears as an exophytic, slow-growing, expanding, well-defined, papillary or verrucous mass (Fig. 5-26). The surface is usually white as a result of hyperkeratosis, although lesions may appear erythematous or pink. The lesions may be small in the initial stages, although commonly, they are quite extensive. This may in part be because of a delay in diagnosis by patients who perceive their slow-growing, asymptomatic lesions as innocuous.

Microscopically, verrucous carcinoma appears relatively indolent. The inferior border, extending deep into the underlying connective tissue, gives the appearance of a pushing margin. Cellular atypia is infrequent, and the individual epithelial cells appear to undergo a normal transition and maturation. For these reasons, incisional biopsies of verrucous carcinoma should include an ample amount of tissue. It is especially important to provide a sufficient sample to evaluate individual

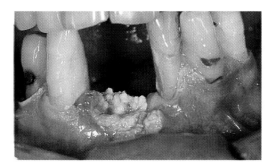

FIG. 5-26 Verrucous carcinomas appear as exophytic, slow-growing, expanding, well-defined papillary or verrucous masses and arise frequently on the gingiva.

cytopathic changes as well as overall histomorphologic patterns of the lesion. Genetic alterations that have been demonstrated in these tumors include the accumulation of p53, suggesting possible mutations of this gene and overexpression of cyclin D1. Multiple biopsies may be required for large lesions because squamous cell carcinomas develop concurrently within verrucous carcinomas in up to 20% of cases.

The treatment of choice for verrucous carcinoma is complete excision. Because the potential for metastasis is low, radical excisions and neck dissections are unnecessary. Conservative excision results in a more than 90% 5-year cure rate, although approximately 10% of patients require additional surgery to remove residual tumor. Treatment failures are most common in individuals who cannot tolerate surgical intervention or who have occult squamous cell carcinoma arising in their verrucous carcinoma. Radiation therapy may be used for local control, although it is less effective than surgery, and the possibility of anaplastic transformation limits its usefulness. Chemotherapy may also be used as an adjunctive modality.

Oral Malignant Melanoma

Cutaneous and noncutaneous melanomas develop from malignant melanocytes. In the United States the incidence of melanoma has almost tripled in the past several decades. Approximately 35,000 new cases in the United States are diagnosed annually, and 7000 die from the disease each year. Projections indicate that by the year 2000, 1 in 90 Americans will develop melanoma.

The precise etiology of melanoma remains obscure, although risk factors include a genetic tendency, exposure to ultraviolet light, and environmental exposures. None of these have been associated with primary melanomas of the oral cavity. For the last 12 years, annual, free, national melanoma screening programs and distributed educational materials have significantly heightened public awareness about the risks and signs of malignant melanoma. These efforts have resulted in early detection, early treatment, and fewer deaths. Unfortunately, oral cavity malignant melanomas, which are extremely conducive to visual screening, have received little attention, as evidenced by the omission of the oral cavity examination during The National Melanoma/Skin Cancer Prevention Campaign. Patient and physician incognizance may, in part, explain why the dismal prognosis for oral melanoma has remained unchanged since the first review of 105 cases in 1958.

Oral melanomas are uncommon and have been reported to constitute a range as broad as 0.1% to 8% of all melanomas. In the United States certain Native American and Latino populations are noted to have a higher incidence of oral melanomas. In Japan and Uganda the oral cavity is a site of predilection for melanoma. The neoplasms develop most frequently in the fourth through seventh decades of life and are exceedingly rare in children and adolescents. Most studies support equal sexual predilection and a relative frequency in African-Americans that is similar to whites.

In more than two thirds of cases, oral melanomas occur on the hard palate and maxillary gingivae. The mandibular gingivae, buccal mucosa, tongue, and lips are other common sites. The presence of asymptomatic oral pigmentation at the site of oral melanoma is detected before diagnosis by approximately one third of patients. These pigmented lesions represent the radial growth phase of the tumor and often go unrecognized by doctors and patients for months or years before tumor invasion.

Oral melanomas may enlarge rapidly, resulting in ulceration, bleeding, pain, and loosening of teeth (Fig. 5-27). More commonly, they persist as asymptomatic pigmented patches or plaques (Fig. 5-28). The absence of symptoms often causes patients to delay seeking medical care. Furthermore, the diagnosis can be complicated because 5% to 15% of all oral melanomas are amelanotic or pink.

Whereas melanomas of the skin are classified into four types (nodular, superficial spreading, lentigo maligna, and acral lentiginous), oral melanomas can be divided into those with a radial growth phase and those exhibiting a vertical growth phase, the former representing superficial melanoma and the latter, nodular melanoma. The determination of the depth of invasion, in millimeters (Breslow depth), has proved to be the single most important prognostic factor for cutaneous melanomas. The

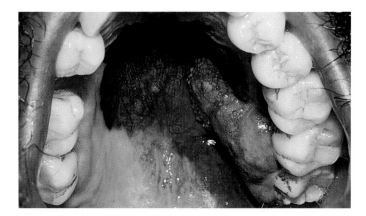

FIG. 5-27   Oral malignant melanomas are generally detected in the advanced stages, as evidenced by the nodular component present at the time of diagnosis in this patient.

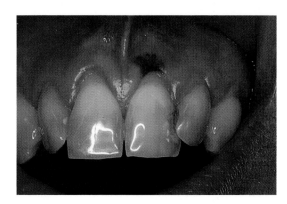

FIG. 5-28   Oral malignant melanomas arise predominantly on the maxillary gingiva and palate, sites that are extremely conducive to visual screening by patients and physicians.

poorer prognosis of oral melanoma compared with cutaneous melanoma is a result of the detection of oral melanomas with advanced Breslow depths. The prognostic value of Clark levels of invasion is inapplicable to oral melanomas because papillary and reticular dermis are absent from oral mucosa.

Histologically, oral melanoma is indistinguishable from its cutaneous counterpart and resembles melanomas on acral skin in its growth pattern. Oral intraepithelial melanomas are comprised of cells with angulated, hyperchromatic nuclei in the basal layer of the epithelium, whereas nodular and invasive lesions consist of spindled melanocytes.

The oral cavity may be the site of metastatic melanoma from the skin. Such lesions are rare and develop most frequently on the tongue and buccal mucosa. Enlarging oral masses, pigmented lesions, and nonhealing extraction sites with masses are common oral presentations for metastatic lesions.

Radical surgery is the treatment of choice whenever feasible. Local recurrence is common, even when adequate surgical margins have been achieved. Radiation therapy and chemotherapy are used as adjuvants with variable success. A new modality that uses excision via an intraoral approach, therapeutic neck dissection, and adjuvant immunochemotherapy may offer a better prognosis than the reported 10% to 20% 5-year survival rate. Because the early detection of oral melanomas results in improved survival, visual screening of the oral cavity, especially the hard palate where the majority of melanomas are found, should be performed regularly by patients and doctors. The detectable radial growth phase of oral melanoma reinforces the need to view all pigmented lesions of the oral cavity with suspicion.

Hodgkin's Disease (Hodgkin's Lymphoma)

Hodgkin's disease is a poorly understood lymphoproliferative disorder characterized by the presence of neoplastic Reed-Sternberg cells. Hodgkin's disease is more common in men than in women and displays a bimodal distribution, with peaks in late adolescence to early adulthood and in geriatric populations. An increased frequency has been noted in patients infected with HIV.

Clinically, Hodgkin's disease most frequently presents with enlarged, nontender, and nonfixed lymphadenopathy. As the disease progresses, the lymph nodes become firm and fixed to the underlying and adjacent tissue. Approximately three fourths of patients display submandibular, cervical, or supraclavicular lymphadenopathy as their initial presenting clinical sign. This feature underscores the need to palpate lymph nodes in the neck as part of the oral cavity screening examination. Other clinical signs and symptoms associated with Hodgkin's disease include fever, night sweats, weight loss, and generalized pruritus. Intraoral lesions of Hodgkin's disease are uncommon and characterized by nondistinctive, persistent ulcerations or erythematous masses.

Histopathologically, Hodgkin's disease is divided into four major subtypes: lymphocyte predominance, nodular sclerosing, lymphocyte depletion, and mixed cellularity, the latter accounting for the majority of cases.

Hodgkin's disease is treated with either radiation therapy or chemotherapy or both, depending on the stage of the disease. Localized disease is generally treated with radiation therapy, and diffuse disease responds more favorably to chemotherapy, often with supplemental radiotherapy. The prognosis for Hodgkin's disease has significantly improved over the last several decades, with 5-year survival rates ranging from 50% to 90% depending on the stage of the disease. Long-term survival is also influenced by the histopathologic subtype, as lymphocyte-predominance and nodular sclerosing Hodgkin's disease have the best prognosis and lymphocyte depletion disease has the poorest.

Non-Hodgkin's Lymphoma

More than 40,000 cases of non-Hodgkin's lymphoma are reported annually in the United States, with approximately 20,000 individuals eventually dying of their disease. Non-Hodgkin's lymphoma is more commonly found in individuals with other immunologic defects including congenital immunodeficiency disease, acquired immunodeficiency syndrome (AIDS), iatrogenic immunosuppression, and autoimmune disease.

Non-Hodgkin's lymphomas comprise a wide array of lymphoreticular malignancies. The majority of non-Hodgkin's lymphomas are of B-lymphocyte origin. T-lymphocyte derived non-Hodgkin's lymphoma is less common, and histiocytic lymphomas are the least common.

The classification of non-Hodgkin's lymphoma is based on histomorphology, immunologic cell surface markers, and molecular genetic analysis. Conceptually, non-Hodgkin's lymphomas can be broadly classified as low-grade, intermediate-grade, and high-grade malignancies. These categories correlate with the biologic behavior of the lesions and their long-term prognosis. The intermediate-grade lymphoma accounts for over half of all cases at the time of diagnosis. Over one third of patients are initially classified as having a low-grade lesion, whereas less than 10% have high-grade disease at the time of their initial diagnosis. Low-grade lesions are well-differentiated tumors and have a better prognosis than the other two types.

The role of viruses as etiologic agents in the development of non-Hodgkin's lymphoma is the subject of intense investigation. Epstein-Barr virus has been implicated in the pathogenesis of certain subtypes of lymphoma, particularly high-grade lymphomas.

Human T-cell lymphotropic virus (HTLV-1) has been linked with adult T-cell lymphoma endemic to Japan, central Africa, and the Caribbean.

Clinically, non-Hodgkin's lymphoma is characterized by nontender regional lymphadenopathy with eventual fixation to adjacent tissues. In addition, non-Hodgkin's lymphomas may have extranodal manifestations. The disease occurs predominantly in adults, although children and adolescents may be affected, especially with the more aggressive subtypes.

Among HIV-positive patients, intraoral lesions account for 5% to 10% of non-Hodgkin's lymphoma. Oral lesions may accompany disseminated disease or on occasion be the initial manifesta-

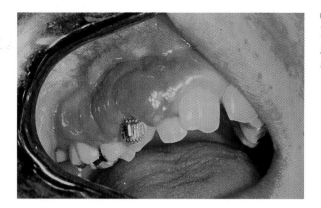

FIG. 5-29   Non-Hodgkin's lymphoma. The posterior gingiva is a common site and the lesion is often firm and indurated.

tion of the disease. Oral mucosal involvement is nonspecific in its clinical presentation and characterized by oral masses or ulceration (Fig. 5-29). The lesions are usually indurated and painless unless they ulcerate. Occasionally, oral non-Hodgkin's lymphoma may appear vascular in nature with secondary ulceration. Oral lesions are most commonly found on the posterior hard palate, tonsillar pillar and oropharynx, buccal vestibule, posterior gingiva, and tongue. The majority of lymphomas that arise in the oral soft tissue are of the high-grade subtypes. Oral reactive processes may occasionally mimic the clinical and histologic features of a malignant lymphoma. Immunohistochemical studies using a panel of lymphoid antibodies may be needed to differentiate reactive and neoplastic lesions. Intraosseous involvement of non-Hodgkin's lymphoma may present as ill-defined jaw pain, which can frequently be confused with a chronic odontogenic infection. Mandibular paresthesia may also be present. Radiographic changes are nondiagnostic and appear as ill-defined, expansile radiolucencies with irregular borders. Left untreated, intraosseous non-Hodgkin's lymphoma may perforate the bone with subsequent soft-tissue involvement.

As with Hodgkin's lymphoma, non-Hodgkin's lymphoma is treated with either radiation therapy or chemotherapy or both, depending on the histologic grade and clinical stage of the disease. Whereas low-grade lymphomas have a relatively indolent clinical course, high-grade lymphomas have less than a 50% 5-year survival rate. The median survival of patients with AIDS-related non-Hodgkin's lymphoma is poor, approximately 5 to 11 months.

Cutaneous T-Cell Lymphoma

Cutaneous T-cell lymphoma (CTCL) comprises a group of malignant proliferations of T-helper (CD4+) lymphocytes and, less commonly, T-suppressor (CD8+) lymphocytes, which exhibit epidermotropism. The incidence of CTCL has been increasing yearly for the last decade and is at least equal to that of Hodgkin's disease. The disease occurs predominantly in middle-aged men but may affect all ages and present even in childhood and adolescence. In the spectrum of CTCL are well-described diseases including mycosis fungoides and Sézary syndrome. The former condition is characterized by the development of patches, plaques, and tumors of the skin, whereas in the latter disease, abnormal CTCL cells circulate in the peripheral blood and result in erythroderma.

The initial patch stage of CTCL resembles dermatitis and is characterized by multiple, scaly, erythematous patches on the skin that can exhibit telangiectasia and atrophy. The plaque stage may follow the patch stage or arise *de novo*. Plaques are characterized by elevated, indurated, sharply demarcated, discoid-shaped lesions that may simulate psoriasis. The tumor stage is characterized by cutaneous red, brown, or purple nodules that are smooth or ulcerated. Visceral involvement is usually present at this stage, most commonly involving the liver, spleen, lung, kidney, and central nervous system; and the disease may involve virtually every organ.

Oral involvement in CTCL is uncommonly reported but probably occurs much more frequently

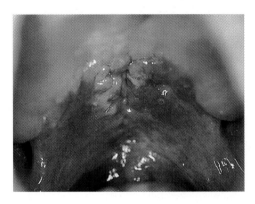

FIG. 5-30   Plaques and tumors of the palate are the most frequent oral manifestation of cutaneous T-cell lymphoma.

than suggested in the literature. The oral manifestations include an ulcerated plaque or tumor most frequently developing on the palate, gingiva, and tongue (Fig. 5-30). Patch stage lesions in the mouth have not been reported and most likely do not occur. The oral lesions develop after skin lesions and usually during the tumor stage or erythrodermic stage. Involvement of the oral cavity is a sign of advanced disease, with most patients dying within 3 years. Local radiation may be used for oral lesions, with few recurrences.

Histologically, a dense, mixed cellular infiltrate with atypical lymphocytes that form microabscesses is noted.

CTCL is most commonly treated by topical and systemic chemotherapy, radiotherapy, and phototherapy with ultraviolet light, depending on the stage of the disease. The prognosis of patients with CTCL depends on a large number of variables including degree of skin involvement, depth of infiltrate, and lymph node and visceral involvement.

Burkitt's Lymphoma

Burkitt's lymphoma, originally described in pediatric African patients, is an undifferentiated lymphoma of lymphocytic origin. The malignancy is strongly associated with Epstein-Barr virus infection, with nearly all patients exhibiting elevated antibody titers to the virus and expression of Epstein-Barr virus nuclear antigen. African Burkitt's lymphoma characteristically affects the jaws, whereas the American Burkitt's lymphoma normally presents as an abdominal mass.

More than two thirds of patients with African Burkitt's lymphoma initially present with swelling of the jaws. The disease most commonly affects preadolescent children in central Africa, although sporadic cases have been described worldwide. The posterior segments of the jaws are more commonly affected, with over two thirds of cases involving the maxilla. An inverse relationship between the patient's age and degree of jaw involvement has been noted.

Clinically, oral lesions manifest as asymptomatic swellings that eventually result in marked destruction of the alveolar bone and increased tooth mobility. The lesions often ulcerate if left untreated. Oral lesions are observed most frequently in the posterior maxillary vestibule and represent direct extension of the tumor into the oral cavity (Fig. 5-31). The radiographic changes seen in Burkitt's lymphoma include poorly outlined bone destruction and loss of lamina dura surrounding the teeth.

Microscopically, Burkitt's lymphoma consists of small, noncleaved, undifferentiated B lymphocytes, with a characteristic "starry-sky" pattern resulting from the presence of macrophages within the tumor.

Burkitt's lymphoma is an aggressive malignancy. Despite the recent advances in chemothera-

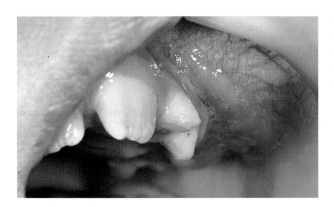

FIG. 5-31 Burkitt's lymphoma. Oral lesions are observed most frequently in the posterior maxillary vestibule and represent direct extension of the tumor into the oral cavity.

peutic regimens that have resulted in improved survival, the disease is ultimately fatal in the majority of patients.

Kaposi's Sarcoma

Kaposi's sarcoma is a malignancy of small blood vessels most likely originating from pluripotential mesenchymal stem cells or from lymphatic or vascular endothelial cells. A number of viral infections have been implicated as etiologic agents in the development of Kaposi's sarcoma. The BK virus, a transforming human papovavirus associated with human tumors, has been consistently detected in Kaposi's sarcoma from classic, endemic, and AIDS-related cases. A new herpesvirus DNA sequence has also been repeatedly identified in Kaposi's sarcoma from AIDS and non-AIDS patients. Other potential etiologies include infection with *Mycoplasma penetrans,* HTLV-1, and cytomegalovirus.

Four patterns of the neoplasm, each affecting relatively distinct populations, have been described. Classic Kaposi's sarcoma affects elderly men of Mediterranean, Eastern European, and Jewish descent. The lesions primarily occur on the skin of the lower extremities. The disease course is indolent, although lymph node and visceral disease may occur.

African-endemic Kaposi's sarcoma occurs in two age groups: (1) young adults who display benign nodular cutaneous lesions mimicking the classic form or aggressive florid lesions with invasion of soft tissue and bone, or visceral involvement, which results in death within 5 years and (2) children with lymphadenopathic disease characterized by rapid dissemination to lymph nodes and visceral organs, which results in death within 2 to 3 years.

Iatrogenic, immunosuppressive, drug-associated Kaposi's sarcoma is characteristically seen in organ transplant recipients, although development of Kaposi's sarcoma may occur in patients receiving immunosuppressive therapy for a variety of other diseases. The lesions appear an average of 13 months after the initiation of therapy, and most lesions resolve with the cessation of immunosuppression.

AIDS-related Kaposi's sarcoma certainly has received the most attention within this group because it was identified as the primary malignancy of AIDS described in the early 1980s.

Although the relative frequency of oral lesions of Kaposi's sarcoma differs among the various patterns, they have been described in all forms of the disease, and all are similar in their clinical presentation. The clinical manifestations and treatment of oral Kaposi's sarcoma are presented in Chapter 13.

Metastatic Neoplasms

Malignancies of all types seldom metastasize to the oral cavity but do so in men more than in women. The metastatic lesions are often the first indication of the existence of an undiagnosed primary malignancy elsewhere. Oral metastatic neoplasms in men originate most frequently from carcinoma of

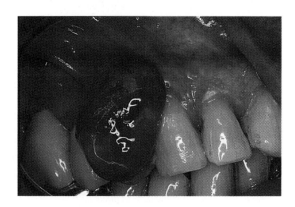

FIG. 5-32 Metastatic lesions to the oral cavity present as sessile or nodular masses that characteristically resemble hyperplastic reactive lesions such as the pyogenic granuloma or peripheral giant cell granuloma.

the lung, kidney, and cutaneous malignant melanoma. In women, breast cancer is the most likely primary site, accounting for approximately one fourth of all oral soft tissue metastases, followed by gynecologic cancers.

The majority of oral mucosal metastases occur on the gingiva and alveolar mucosa, with another 25% involving the tongue. The palate and buccal mucosa are less commonly affected. Clinically, soft tissue metastases typically present as sessile or nodular masses that characteristically resemble hyperplastic reactive lesions such as pyogenic granuloma or peripheral giant cell granuloma (Fig. 5-32). Destruction of underlying alveolar bone frequently results in hypermobility of the teeth. Because the majority of these oral reactive lesions develop in young patients, their presence after age 50 should suggest the possibility of a metastatic lesion.

Osseous metastasis of the jaws is also not common, although when it does occur, more than three fourths of cases involve the mandible rather than the maxilla. The most common primary sites of cancer include the breast, lung, thyroid, prostate, and kidney. Clinically, metastatic disease of the bones manifests as pain, swelling, hypermobility of teeth, and paresthesia. Radiographically, ill-defined destruction of bone is evident; breast, thyroid, and prostate carcinoma may stimulate osteogenesis, resulting in a mixed radiopacity-radiolucency.

The presence of oral metastatic lesions in the soft tissues or bone is indicative of advanced disease. Metastatic lesions may be treated with surgery or radiation therapy, although regardless of the site of the primary tumor, survival beyond 12 months is rare.

SUGGESTED READINGS

Benign lesions

Pyogenic granuloma

Angelopoulos AP: Pyogenic granuloma of the oral cavity: statistical analysis of its clinical features, *J Oral Surg* 29:840, 1971.

Bhaskar SN, Jacoway JR: Pyogenic granuloma—clinical features, incidence, histology, and result of treatment: report of 242 cases, *J Oral Surg* 24:391, 1966.

Butler EJ, Macintyre DR: Oral pyogenic granulomas, *Dent Update* 18:194, 1991.

Daley TD, Nartey NO, Wysocki GP: Pregnancy tumor: an analysis, *Oral Surg Oral Med Oral Pathol* 72:196, 1991.

Lee L et al: Intraoral pyogenic granuloma after allogeneic bone marrow transplant, *Oral Surg Oral Med Oral Pathol* 78:607, 1994.

Vilmann A, Vilmann P, Vilmann H: Pyogenic granuloma: evaluation of oral conditions, *Br J Oral Maxillofac Surg* 24:376, 1986.

Peripheral giant cell granuloma

Carvalho YR et al: Peripheral giant cell granuloma: an immunohistochemical and ultrastructural study, *Oral Dis* 1:20, 1995.

Flanagan AM et al: The multinucleate cells in giant cell granulomas of the jaw are osteoclasts, *Cancer* 62:1139, 1988.

Giansanti JS, Waldron CA: Peripheral giant cell granuloma: review of 720 cases, *J Oral Surg* 17:787, 1969.

Katsikeris N, Kakarantza-Angelopoulou E, Angelopoulos AP: Peripheral giant cell granuloma: clinicopathologic study of 224 new cases and review of 956 reported cases, *Int J Oral Maxillofac Surg* 17:94, 1988.

Mighell AJ, Robinson PA, Hume WJ: Peripheral giant cell granuloma: a clinical study of 77 cases from 62 patients and literature review, *Oral Dis* 1:12, 1995.

Keratoacanthoma

de Visscher JG et al: Giant keratoacanthoma of the lower lip: report of a case of spontaneous regression, *Oral Surg Oral Med Oral Pathol* 81:193, 1996.

Habel G et al: Intra-oral keratoacanthoma: an eruptive variant and review of the literature, *Br Dent J* 170:336, 1991.

Melton JL et al: Treatment of keratoacanthomas with intralesional methotrexate, *J Am Acad Dermatol* 25:1017, 1991.

Netscher D et al: Keratoacanthoma: when to observe and when to operate and the importance of accurate diagnosis, *South Med J* 12:1272, 1994.

Waring AJ et al: Loss of heterozygosity analysis of keratoacanthoma reveals multiple differences from cutaneous squamous cell carcinoma, *Br J Cancer* 73:649, 1996.

Whyte AM, Hansen LS, Lee C: The intraoral keratoacanthoma: a diagnostic problem, *Br J Oral Maxillofac Surg* 6:438, 1986.

Wong WY et al: Treatment of a recurrent keratoacanthoma with oral isotretinoin, *Int J Dermatol* 33:579, 1994.

Amputation neuroma

Appiah-Anane S: Amputation neuroma: a late complication following sagittal split osteotomy of the mandible, *J Oral Maxillofac Surg* 49:1218, 1991.

Gregg JM: Studies of traumatic neuralgias in the maxillofacial region: surgical pathology and neural mechanisms, *J Oral Maxillofac Surg* 48:228, 1990.

Peszkowski MJ, Larsson A: Extraosseous and intraosseous oral traumatic neuromas and their association with tooth extraction, *J Oral Maxillofac Surg* 48:963, 1990.

Sist T, Green G: Traumatic neuroma of the oral cavity, *Oral Surg Oral Med Oral Pathol* 51:394, 1981.

Verruciform xanthoma

Allen CM, Kapoor N: Verruciform xanthoma in a bone marrow transplant recipient, *Oral Surg Oral Med Oral Pathol* 75:591, 1993.

Furue M et al: Colocalization of scavenger receptor in CD68 positive foam cells in verruciform xanthoma, *J Dermatol Sci* 10:213, 1995.

Huang JS et al: Verruciform xanthoma: case report and literature review, *J Periodontol* 67:62, 1996.

Mostafa KA et al: Verruciform xanthoma of the oral mucosa: a clinicopathological study with immunohistochemical findings relating to pathogenesis, *Virchows Arch* 423:243, 1993.

Orchard GE, Wilson Jones E, Russell Jones R: Verruciform xanthoma: an immunocytochemical study, *Br J Biomed Sci* 51:28, 1994.

Takehana S et al: Verruciform xanthoma of the gingiva: report of three cases, *J Oral Maxillofac Surg* 47:1079, 1989.

Fibrous histiocytoma

Fieldman RJ, Morrow TA: Fibrous histiocytomas of the soft palate, *Int J Pediatr Otorhinolaryngol* 18:171, 1989.

Gray PB, Miller AS, Loftus MJ: Benign fibrous histiocytoma of the oral/perioral regions: report of a case and review of 17 additional cases, *J Oral Maxillofac Surg* 50:1239, 1992.

Regezi JA, Nickoloff BJ, Headington JT: Oral submucosal dendrocytes: factor XIIIa+ and CD34+ dendritic cell populations in normal tissue and fibrovascular lesions, *J Cutan Pathol* 5:398, 1992.

Triantafyllou AG, Sklavounou AD, Laskaris GG: Benign fibrous histiocytoma of the oral mucosa, *J Oral Med* 40:36, 1985.

Lipoma

Fujimura N, Enomoto S: Lipoma of the tongue with cartilaginous change: a case report and review of the literature, *J Oral Maxillofac Surg* 50:1015, 1992.

Ghandour K, Issa M: Lipoma of the floor of the mouth, *Oral Surg Oral Med Oral Pathol* 73:59, 1992.

Greer RO, Richardson JF: The nature of lipomas and their significance in the oral cavity, *Oral Surg Oral Med Oral Pathol* 36:551, 1973.

Mentzel T, Fletcher C: Lipomatous tumours of soft tissues: an update, *Virchows Arch* 353:427, 1995.

Seldin HM et al: Lipomas of the oral cavity, *J Oral Surg* 25:270, 1967.

Granular cell tumor

Buley ID et al: Granular cell tumours revisited: an immunohistological and ultrastructural study, *Histopathology* 12:263, 1988.

Collins BM, Jones AC: Multiple granular cell tumors of the oral cavity: report of a case and review of the literature, *J Oral Maxillofac Surg* 53:707, 1995.

Khansur T, Balducci L, Tavassoli M: Granular cell tumor: clinical spectrum of the benign and malignant entity, *Cancer* 60:220, 1987.

Matthews J, Mason G: Oral granular cell myoblastoma: an immunohistochemical study, *J Oral Pathol* 11:343, 1982.

Stewart CM et al: Oral granular cell tumors: a clinicopathologic and immunocytochemical study, *Oral Surg Oral Med Oral Pathol* 65:427, 1988.

Neurilemoma (Schwannoma)

Kun Z, Qi DY, Zhang KH: A comparison between the clinical behavior of neurilemmomas in the neck and oral and maxillofacial region, *J Oral Maxillofac Surg* 51:769, 1993.

López JI, Ballestin C: Intraoral schwannoma: a clinicopathologic and immunohistochemical study of nine cases, *Arch Anat Cytol Pathol* 41:18, 1993.

Williams HK et al: Neurilemmoma of the head and neck, *Br J Oral Maxillofac Surg* 31:32, 1993.

Neurofibroma

Baden E et al: Neurofibromatosis of the tongue: a light and electron-microscopic study with review of the literature from 1849 to 1981, *J Oral Med* 39:157, 1984.

Geist JR, Gander DL, Stefanac SJ: Oral manifestations of neurofibromatosis types I and II, *Oral Surg Oral Med Oral Pathol* 73:376, 1992.

Neville BW et al: Oral neurofibrosarcoma associated with neurofibromatosis type I, *Oral Surg Oral Med Oral Pathol* 72:456, 1991.

Shapiro SD et al: Neurofibromatosis: oral and radiographic manifestations, *Oral Surg Oral Med Oral Pathol* 58:493, 1984.

Zachariades N et al: Benign neurogenic tumors of the oral cavity, *Int J Oral Maxillofac Surg* 16:70, 1987.

Fibrous hyperplasia and other fibrous tumors (fibroma, giant cell fibroma, peripheral ossifying fibroma)

Becker J, Schuppan D, Muller S: Immunohistochemical distribution of collagens type I, III, IV, and VI, of undulin and of tenascin in oral fibrous hyperplasia, *J Oral Pathol Med* 22:463, 1993.

Buchner A, Hansen LS: The histomorphologic spectrum of peripheral ossifying fibroma, *Oral Surg Oral Med Oral Pathol* 63:452, 1987.

Christopoulos P, Sklavounou A, Patrikiou A: True fibroma of the oral mucosa: a case report, *Int J Oral Maxillofac Surg* 23:98, 1994.

Kenney JN, Kaugars GE, Abbey LM: Comparison between the peripheral ossifying fibroma and peripheral odontogenic fibroma, *J Oral Maxillofac Surg* 47:378, 1989.

Magnusson BC, Rasmusson LG: The giant cell fibroma: a review of 103 cases with immunohistochemical findings, *Acta Odontol Scand* 53:293, 1995.

Zain RB, Fei YJ: Fibrous lesions of the gingiva: a histopathologic analysis of 204 cases, *Oral Surg Oral Med Oral Pathol* 70:466, 1990.

Melanotic neuroectodermal tumor of infancy

Irving RM et al: Melanotic neuroectodermal tumour of infancy, *J Laryngol Otol* 107:1045, 1993.

Kapadia SB et al: Melanotic neuroectodermal tumor of infancy: clinicopathological, immunohistochemical, and flow cytometric study, *Am J Surg Pathol* 17:566, 1993.

Kim YG et al: Melanotic neuroectodermal tumor of infancy, *J Oral Maxillofac Surg* 54:517, 1996.

Mirich DR et al: Melanotic neuroectodermal tumor of infancy: clinical, radiologic, and pathologic findings in five cases, *Am J Neuroradiol* 12:689, 1991.

Pettinato et al: Melanotic neuroectodermal tumor of infancy: a reexamination of a histogenetic problem based on immunohistochemical, flow cytometric, and ultrastructural study of 10 cases, *Am J Surg Pathol* 15:233, 1991.

Premalignant lesions

Leukoplakia

Axéll T et al: Oral white lesions with special reference to precancerous and tobacco-related lesions: conclusions of an international symposium held in Uppsala, Sweden, May 18-21 1994, *J Oral Pathol Med* 25:49, 1996.

Bouquot JE: Oral leukoplakia and erythroplakia: a review and update, *Pract Periodontics Aesthet Dent* 6:9, 1994.

Kaugers GE et al: Use of antioxidant supplements in the treatment of human oral leukoplakia, *Oral Surg Oral Med Oral Pathol* 81:5, 1996.

Lippman SM et al: Comparison of low-dose isotretinoin with beta carotene to prevent oral carcinogenesis, *N Engl J Med* 328:15, 1993.

Lummerman H, Freedman P, Kerpel S: Oral epithelial dysplasia and development of invasive squamous cell carcinoma, *Oral Surg Oral Med Oral Pathol* 79:321, 1995.

Palefsky JM et al: Association between proliferative verrucous leukoplakia and infection with human papillomavirus type 16, *J Oral Pathol Med* 24:193, 1995.

Roed-Petersen B: Effect on oral leukoplakia of reducing or ceasing tobacco smoking, *Acta Derm Venereol Suppl (Stockh)* 62:164, 1982.

Roodenburg JLN, Panders AK, Vermey A: Carbon dioxide laser surgery of oral leukoplakia, *Oral Surg Oral Med Oral Pathol* 71:670, 1991.

Sciubba JJ: Oral leukoplakia, *Crit Rev Oral Biol Med* 6:147, 1995.

Silverman S Jr, Gorsky M, Lozada F: Oral leukoplakia and malignant transformation: a follow-up study of 257 patients, *Cancer* 53:563, 1984.

Silverman S Jr, Migliorati C, Barbosa J: Toluidine blue staining in the detection of oral precancerous and malignant lesions, *Oral Surg Oral Med Oral Pathol* 57:379, 1984.

Waldron CA, Shafer WG: Leukoplakia revisited: a clinicopathologic study of 3256 oral leukoplakias, *Cancer* 36:1386, 1975.

WHO Collaborating Center for Oral Precancerous Lesions: Definition of leukoplakia and related lesions: an aid to studies on oral precancer, *Oral Surg Oral Med Oral Pathol* 46:518, 1978.

Erythroplakia (erythroplasia of Queyrat)

Bouquot JE: Oral leukoplakia and erythroplakia: a review and update, *Pract Periodontics Aesthet Dent* 6:9, 1994.

Mashberg A, Samit AM: Early detection, diagnosis, and management of oral and oropharyngeal cancer, *CA Cancer J Clin* 39:67, 1989.

Shafer WG, Waldron CA: Erythroplakia of the oral cavity, *Cancer* 36:1021, 1975.

Smokeless tobacco lesions (snuff dipper's hyperkeratosis; tobacco pouch lesion)

Andersson G, Bjornberg G, Curvall M: Oral mucosal changes and nicotine disposition in users of Swedish smokeless tobacco products: a comparative study, *J Oral Pathol Med* 23:161, 1994.

Creath CJ et al: Oral leukoplakia and adolescent smokeless tobacco use, *Oral Surg Oral Med Oral Pathol* 72:35, 1991.

Hoffmann D et al: Five leading US commercial brands of moist snuff in 1994: assessment of carcinogenic N-nitrosamines, *J Natl Cancer Inst* 87:1862, 1995.

Kaugars GE et al: Evaluation of risk factors in smokeless tobacco associated oral lesions, *Oral Surg Oral Med Oral Pathol* 72:326, 1991.

Kaugars GE et al: The prevalence of oral lesions in smokeless tobacco users and an evaluation of risk factors, *Cancer* 70:2579, 1992.

Kleinman DV, Swango P, Pindborg JJ: Epidemiology of oral mucosal lesions in U.S. school children: 1986-1987, *Community Dent Oral Epidemiol* 22:243, 1994.

Larsson A, Axéll T, Andersson G: Reversibility of snuff dippers' lesion in Swedish moist snuff users: a clinical and histologic follow-up study, *J Oral Pathol Med* 20:258, 1991.

Sterling TD, Rosenbaum WL, Weinkam JJ: Analysis of the relationship between smokeless tobacco and cancer based on data from the National Mortality Followback Survey, *J Clin Epidemiol* 45:223, 1992.

Use of smokeless tobacco among adults—United States, 1991, *Morb Mortal Wkly Rep* 42:263, 1993.

Oral submucous fibrosis

Murti PR et al: Etiology of oral submucous fibrosis with special reference to the role of areca nut chewing, *J Oral Pathol Med* 24:145, 1995.

Pillai R, Balaram P, Reddiar KS: Pathogenesis of oral submucous fibrosis: relationship to risk factors associated with oral cancer, *Cancer* 69:2011, 1992.

Rajendran R: Oral submucous fibrosis: etiology, pathogenesis, and future research, *Bull World Health Organ* 72:985, 1994.

Actinic cheilitis

Johnson TM et al: Carbon dioxide laser treatment of actinic cheilitis: clinicohistopathologic correlation to determine the optimal depth of destruction, *J Am Acad Dermatol* 27:737, 1992.

Kuno Y, Sakakibara S, Mizuno N: Actinic cheilitis granulomatosa, *J Dermatol* 19:556, 1992.

Main JH, Pavone M: Actinic cheilitis and carcinoma of the lip, *J Can Dent Assoc* 60:113, 1994.

Olsen EA et al: A double-blind, vehicle-controlled study evaluating masoprocol cream in the treatment of actinic keratoses on the head and neck, *J Am Acad Dermatol* 24:738, 1991.

Thompson SC, Jolley D, Marks R: Reduction of solar keratoses by regular sunscreen use, *N Engl J Med* 329:1147, 1993.

Malignant neoplasms

Squamous cell carcinoma

Beahrs OH et al, editors: *Manual for staging of cancer,* ed 4, Philadelphia, 1992, JB Lippincott.

Blomqvist G, Hirsch JM, Alberius P: Association between development of lower lip cancer and tobacco habits, *J Oral Maxillofac Surg* 49:1044, 1991.

Boffetta P et al: Carcinogenic effect of tobacco smoking and alcohol drinking on anatomic sites of the oral cavity and oropharynx, *Int J Cancer* 52:530, 1992.

Boring CC et al: Cancer statistics, 1994, *CA Cancer J Clin* 44:7, 1994.

Brennan JA et al: Association between cigarette smoking and mutation of the p53 gene in squamous cell carcinoma of the head and neck, *N Engl J Med* 332:712, 1995.

Centers for Disease Control and Prevention: Examinations for oral cancer—United States, 1992, *Morb Mortal Wkly Rep* 43:198, 1994.

Crissman JD et al: Squamous cell carcinoma of the floor of the mouth, *Head Neck* 3:2, 1980.

Day GI, Blot WJ: Second primary tumors in patients with oral cancer, *Cancer* 70:14, 1992.

Depue RH: Rising mortality from cancer of the tongue in young white males, *N Engl J Med* 315:647, 1989.

Eliezri YD, Israel HA, Pochal WF: Treatment of an oral erythroplastic squamous cell carcinoma with Mohs' micrographic surgery, *Oral Surg Oral Med Oral Pathol* 67:249, 1989.

Epstein JB et al: A clinical trial of bethanechol in patients with xerostomia after radiation therapy, *Oral Surg Oral Med Oral Pathol* 77:610, 1994.

Field JK: Oncogenes and tumour-suppressor genes in squamous cell carcinoma of the head and neck, *Eur J Cancer B Oral Oncol* 28:67, 1992.

Garewal HS, Schantz S: Emerging role of beta-carotene and antioxidant nutrients in prevention of oral cancer, *Arch Otolaryngol Head Neck Surg* 121:141, 1995.

Gnepp DR, editor: *Pathology of the head and neck,* New York, 1988, Churchill Livingstone.

Goldberg H et al: Trends and differentials in mortality from cancers of the oral cavity and pharynx in the United States, 1973-1987, *Cancer* 74:565, 1994.

Gupta PC et al: Effect of cessation of tobacco use on the incidence of oral mucosal lesions in a 10-yr follow-up study of 12,212 users, *Oral Dis* 1:54, 1995.

Gupta PC et al: Primary prevention trial of oral cancer in India: a 10-year follow-up study, *J Oral Pathol Med* 21:433, 1992.

Hong WK et al: Prevention of secondary primary tumors with isotretinoin in squamous cell carcinoma of the head and neck, *N Engl J Med* 323:795, 1990.

Jansma J et al: Protocol for the prevention and treatment of oral sequelae resulting from head and neck radiation therapy, *Cancer* 70:2171, 1992.

Johnson JT et al: Oral pilocarpine for post-irradiation xerostomia in patients with head and neck cancer, *N Engl J Med* 329:390, 1993.

Jones AS et al: Second primary tumors in patients with head and neck squamous cell carcinoma, *Cancer* 75:1343, 1995.

Kleinman DV et al, editors: *Cancer of the oral cavity and pharynx: a statistics review monograph, 1973-1987, NIH Monograph,* Bethesda, Md, 1992, National Institute of Dental Research.

LeVeque FG et al: A multicenter, randomized, double-blind, placebo-controlled, dose-titration study of oral pilocarpine for treatment of radiation-induced xerostomia in head and neck cancer patients, *J Clin Oncol* 11:1124, 1993.

Ng SKC, Kabat GC, Wynder EL: Oral cavity cancer in non-users of tobacco, *J Natl Cancer Inst* 85:743, 1993.

Papac RJ: Distant metastases from head and neck cancer, *Cancer* 53:342, 1984.

Rollo J et al: Squamous carcinoma of the base of the tongue: a clinicopathologic study of 81 cases, *Cancer* 47:333, 1981.

Schwartz LH et al: Synchronous and metachronous head and neck carcinomas, *Cancer* 74:1933, 1994.

Scully C: Viruses and oral squamous carcinoma, *Eur J Cancer B Oral Oncol* 28:57, 1992.

Silverman S Jr, editor: *Oral cancer,* Atlanta, 1990, American Cancer Society.

Silverman S Jr, Gorsky M: Epidemiologic and demographic update in oral cancer: California and national data—1973 to 1985, *J Am Dent Assoc* 120:49, 1990.

Steele C, Shillitoe EJ: Viruses and oral cancer, *Crit Rev Oral Biol Med* 2:153, 1991.

Sundstrom B, Mörnstad H, Axéll T: Oral carcinomas associated with snuff dipping: some clinical and histological characteristics of 23 tumours in Swedish males, *J Oral Pathol* 11:245, 1982.

Toth BB et al: Minimizing complications of cancer treatment, *Oncology* 9:851, 1995.

Vokes EE et al: Head and neck cancer, *N Engl J Med* 328:184, 1993.

Ward-Booth P: Advances in the diagnosis and treatment of oral cancer, *Curr Opin Dent* 1:287, 1991.

Watts SL, Brewer EE, Fry TL: Human papillomavirus DNA types in squamous cell carcinomas of the head and neck, *Oral Surg Oral Med Oral Pathol* 71:701, 1991.

Winn D: Diet and nutrition in the etiology of oral cancer, *Am J Clin Nutr* 61:437, 1995.

Yeudall WA: Human papillomaviruses and oral neoplasia, *Eur J Cancer B Oral Oncol* 28:61, 1992.

Verrucous carcinoma

Ehlinger P, Fossion E, Vrielinck L: Carcinoma of the oral cavity in patients over 75 years of age, *Int J Oral Maxillofac Surg* 22:218, 1993.

Florin EH, Kolbusz RV, Goldberg LH: Verrucous carcinoma of the oral cavity, *Int J Dermatol* 33:618, 1994.

Goldman NC: Verrucous carcinoma, *Otolaryngol Head Neck Surg* 106:108, 1992.

Link JO, Kaugars GE, Burns JC: Comparison of oral carcinomas in smokeless tobacco users and nonusers, *J Oral Maxillofac Surg* 50:452, 1992.

Medina JE, Dichtel W, Luna MA: Verrucous-squamous carcinomas of the oral cavity: a clinicopathologic study of 104 cases, *Arch Otolaryngol* 110:437, 1984.

Shroyer KR et al: Detection of human papillomavirus DNA in oral verrucous carcinoma by polymerase chain reaction, *Mod Pathol* 6:669, 1993.

Oral malignant melanoma

Eisen D, Voorhees JJ: Oral melanoma and other pigmented lesions of the oral cavity, *J Am Acad Dermatol* 24:527, 1991.

Kilpatrick SE, White WL, Browne JD: Desmoplastic malignant melanoma of the oral mucosa: an underrecognized diagnostic pitfall, *Cancer* 78:383, 1996.

Manganaro AM et al: Oral melanoma: case reports and review of the literature, *Oral Surg Oral Med Oral Pathol* 80:670, 1995.

Rapini RP et al: Primary malignant melanoma of the oral cavity: a review of 177 cases, *Cancer* 55:1543, 1985.

Strauss JE, Strauss SI: Oral malignant melanoma: a case report and review of literature, *J Oral Maxillofac Surg* 52:972, 1994.

Umeda M, Shimada K: Primary malignant melanoma of the oral cavity—its histological classification and treatment, *Br J Oral Maxillofac Surg* 32:39, 1994.

Hodgkin's disease (Hodgkin's lymphoma)

Baden E et al: Hodgkin's lymphoma of the oropharyngeal region: report of four cases and diagnostic value of monoclonal antibodies in detecting antigens associated with Reed-Sternberg cells, *Oral Surg Oral Med Oral Pathol* 64:88, 1987.

Jacobs P: Hodgkin's disease and the malignant lymphomas, *Dis Mon 39:213, 1993.*

Non-Hodgkin's lymphoma

Bellome J, Meyers JF, McGregor DH: Non-Hodgkin's lymphoma presenting as submandibular swelling and palatal ulceration, *J Oral Maxillofac Surg* 51:1278, 1993.

Eisenbud L et al: Oral presentations in non-Hodgkin's lymphoma: a review of thirty-one cases. Part III. Six cases in children, *Oral Surg Oral Med Oral Pathol* 59:44, 1985.

Gulley ML et al: Lymphomas of the oral soft tissues are not preferentially associated with latent or replicative Epstein-Barr virus, *Oral Surg Oral Med Oral Pathol* 80:425, 1995.

Hicks MJ et al: Intraoral presentation of anaplastic large-cell Ki-1 lymphoma in association with HIV infection, *Oral Surg Oral Med Oral Pathol* 76:73, 1993.

Howell RE et al: Extranodal oral lymphoma. Part II. Relationships between clinical features and the Lukes-Collins classification of 34 cases, *Oral Surg Oral Med Oral Pathol* 64:597, 1987.

Langford A et al: Oral manifestations of AIDS-associated non-Hodgkin's lymphomas, *Int J Oral Maxillofac Surg* 20:136, 1991.

Cutaneous T-cell lymphoma

Barnett ML, Cole RJ: Mycosis fungoides with multiple oral mucosal lesions: a case report, *J Periodontol* 56:690, 1985.

Evans GE, Dalziel KL: Mycosis fungoides with oral involvement: a case report and literature review, *Int J Oral Maxillofac Surg* 16:634, 1987.

Quarterman MJ et al: Rapidly progressive CD8-positive cutaneous T-cell lymphoma with tongue involvement, *Am J Dermatopathol* 17:287, 1995.

Sirois DA et al: Oral manifestations of cutaneous T-cell lymphoma: a report of eight cases, *Oral Surg Oral Med Oral Pathol* 75:700, 1993.

Vicente A et al: Mycosis fungoides with oral involvement, *Int J Dermatol* 30:864, 1991.

Yao ZY, Xu C, Wang C: Mycosis fungoides with oral involvement, *Chin Med J Engl* 105:260, 1992.

Burkitt's lymphoma

Anavi Y et al: Head, neck, and maxillofacial childhood Burkitt's lymphoma: a retrospective analysis of 31 patients, *J Oral Maxillofac Surg* 48:708, 1990.

Arotiba GT: A study of orofacial tumors in Nigerian children, *J Oral Maxillofac Surg* 54:34, 1996.

Sariban E, Donahue A, Magrath IT: Jaw involvement in American Burkitt's lymphoma, *Cancer* 53:1777, 1984.

van Sickels JE et al: Nonendemic American Burkitt's lymphoma, *J Oral Maxillofac Surg* 43:453, 1985.

Kaposi's sarcoma

Beckstead JH: Oral presentation of Kaposi's sarcoma in a patient without severe immunodeficiency, *Arch Pathol Lab Med* 116:543, 1992.

DiGiovanna IJ, Safai B: Kaposi's sarcoma: retrospective study of 90 cases with particular emphasis on the familial occurrence, ethnic background and prevalence of other diseases, *Am J Med* 71:779, 1981.

Farman AG, Uys PB: Oral Kaposi's sarcoma, *Oral Surg Oral Med Oral Pathol* 39:288, 1975.

Friedman-Kien AE, Saltzman BR: Clinical manifestations of classical, endemic African, and epidemic AIDS-associated Kaposi's sarcoma, *J Am Acad Dermatol* 22:1237, 1990.

Metastatic neoplasms

Clark JL: Metastatic carcinoma of the jaws: report of a case, *Henry Ford Hosp Med J* 38:36, 1990.

Hirshberg A, Leibovich P, Buchner A: Metastatic tumors to the jawbones: analysis of 390 cases, *J Oral Pathol Med* 23:337, 1994.

Thompson CC, Bartley MH, Woolley LH: Metastatic tumors of the head and neck: a 20-year oral tumor registry report, *J Oral Med* 41:175, 1986.

Zachariades N: Neoplasms metastatic to the mouth, jaws and surrounding tissues, *J Craniomaxillofac Surg* 17:283, 1989.

CHAPTER 6

Oral Bacterial Infections

Two of the most common bacterial diseases that afflict humans are dental caries (Fig. 6-1) and periodontal disease. *Streptococcus mutans,* the etiologic pathogen of dental caries, and *Porphyromonas gingivalis,* the bacterial species most strongly associated with adult periodontitis, are inhabitants of the normal oral flora. In fact, more than 300 different bacteria, including *Staphylococcus aureus,* coliform bacteria, *Klebsiella,* and *Pseudomonas,* reside in the oral cavity and comprise what is regarded as normal oral flora. When a species of bacteria increases in number or when the host defense threshold is exceeded, disease arises. In immunocompromised patients, these bacteria may be the source of serious oral infections that usually manifest clinically as chronic and painful ulcerations or nodules. Life-threatening systemic infections may also be caused by the hematogenous spread of these oral bacteria through ulcerated or inflamed epithelium. Additionally, dental plaque and the oral mucosa are colonized heavily with bacteria that cause nosocomial pneumonia and may be important reservoirs of these pathogens. Even in immunocompetent hosts the potential spread of oral bacteria in patients with endoprostheses, congenital cardiac malformations, and valvular damage necessitates the prophylactic use of antibiotics before dental or oral surgical procedures. A regimen for adults effective against *Streptococcus viridans,* the most common oral infectious agent of subacute bacterial endocarditis, is amoxicillin, 2 g, administered 1 hour before a dental procedure. The oral cavity is also the site of a number of primary bacterial infections and systemic bacterial infections.

GINGIVITIS AND PERIODONTITIS

Periodontal disease is a term used to describe disorders of the soft and hard tissues that support the teeth. The bacterially induced inflammatory conditions may involve the gingiva (gingivitis) and the supporting structures including the connective tissue, periodontal ligament, and alveolar bone (periodontitis).

Gingivitis is initiated by the accumulation of dental plaque (the diverse microbial complex on teeth surfaces embedded in a matrix of polymers of bacterial and salivary origin) adjacent to the gingival tissues. The colonization of specific bacteria, primarily the gram-positive cocci *Streptococcus sanguis* and *Streptococcus mitis,* occurs initially. If dental plaque control is inadequate, numerous other bacteria including *Actinomyces* species and gram-negative organisms colonize the area, resulting in gingival disease. Clinically, gingivitis is characterized by erythema, edema, gingival alterations in form and position, and bleeding, especially when the gingiva is brushed or probed (Fig. 6-2). Gingivitis may be a manifestation of a number of systemic diseases including blood dyscrasias (leukemia), viral infections (acute herpetic gingivostomatitis), and mucocutaneous diseases (lichen planus, pemphigus, and pemphigoid). Additionally, gingivitis is influenced by hormonal disturbances as evidenced by its increased incidence during pregnancy and puberty. Systemic medications such as phenytoin, cyclosporine, and nifedipine may result in gingival hyperplasia and inflammation,

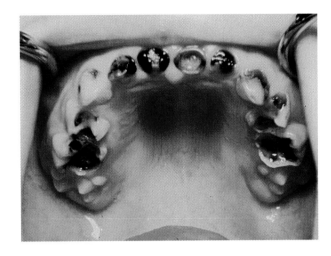

FIG. 6-1   Severe caries resulting in destruction of the teeth.

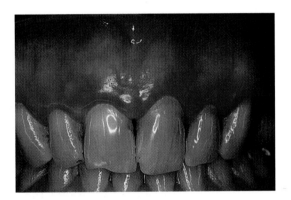

FIG. 6-2   Gingivitis characterized by erythema and edema of the marginal and attached gingiva.

whereas anticholinergic and antidepressant agents that alter salivary flow may precipitate painful gingivitis. The dramatic clinical presentation of necrotizing ulcerative gingivitis and linear gingival erythema in human immunodeficiency virus (HIV)-positive patients with reduced systemic resistance underscores the importance of the immune system in regulating the disease process.

Periodontitis, the most common cause of tooth loss in adults, comprises a diverse group of related but distinct diseases that differ in etiology, natural history, progression, and response to therapy. In all forms, periodontitis is characterized by loss of connective tissue, resorption of alveolar bone, and periodontal pockets. The disease is usually painless and the gingivae commonly appear healthy, not revealing the destruction of the underlying supporting structures. Although the disease may be preceded or accompanied by severe gingivitis, its presence is not indicative of periodontal disease (Fig. 6-3). The detection and diagnosis of periodontitis are based on the abnormal findings of a careful dental examination and radiographs.

Adult periodontitis, arising after age 35, accounts for the majority of cases. Although the disease is episodic, advancing at different rates at various sites, if left untreated, it is progressive with eventual destruction of the tissues. Plaque and calculus (mineralized plaque) that are present on the teeth and subgingivally are the prime etiologic agents of periodontitis (Fig. 6-4). They enhance gingival inflammation, limit natural self-cleansing mechanisms, restrict optimal oral hygiene, retain toxic substances, and reduce drainage from gingival crevicular areas. The role of *Porphyromonas gingivalis* as an etiologic agent of periodontitis is supported by numerous studies that have demonstrated elevated numbers of organisms in diseased lesions, clinical improvement by their elimination, and elevated serum antibody levels in patients with periodontitis. The overgrowth of *Treponema denticola, Prevotella intermedia,* and *Bacteroides forsythus* may also be responsible for the destruction observed clinically. Microbial enzymes from these bacteria may damage connective tissue directly or indirectly by activating a host-mediated response via complement activation and the release of lysosomal enzymes and connective tissue matrix metalloproteinases. The role of the neutrophil-antibody complement system in the pathogenesis of periodontitis is evidenced by the presence of severe disease in patients with impaired neutrophil function.

Juvenile periodontitis occurs at puberty and is a highly destructive disease. Overwhelming evidence suggests that the bacteria *Actinobacillus actinomycetemcomitans* is the etiologic agent. Unlike other forms of periodontitis, juvenile periodontitis is characterized by minimal plaque and inflammation. The disease has a genetic tendency, and abnormalities in leukocyte chemotaxis and bactericidal activity are present.

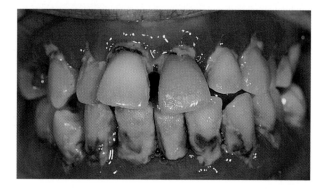

FIG. 6-3   Severe gingival inflammation and destruction resulting from poor oral hygiene in a patient with periodontitis.

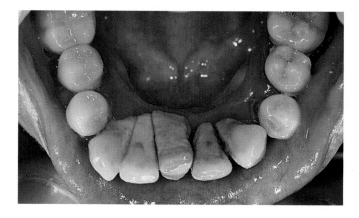

FIG. 6-4   The lingual aspect of the lower mandibular teeth is the most frequent site of calculus accumulation.

As with gingivitis, systemic diseases may influence the nature of periodontal disease. Patients with Down syndrome, diabetes, and HIV infection are predisposed to aggressive forms of periodontitis.

The mechanical removal of dental plaque by tooth-brushing and flossing, thereby decreasing the number of etiologic bacteria, is the single most important treatment. Plaque removal rinses may be of value in aiding this process. Supplementation with professional tooth and root cleaning can often result in the resolution of gingivitis and mild periodontitis. Systemic antibiotics including tetracycline and metronidazole, antimicrobial rinses such as chlorhexidine, and periodontal surgery are often used when the disease is in an advanced state or refractory to conservative therapy.

NECROTIZING GINGIVOSTOMATITIS

Acute necrotizing ulcerative gingivitis, necrotizing ulcerative periodontitis, and necrotizing stomatitis, formerly known as Vincent's infection and now collectively termed *necrotizing gingivostomatitis,* is an uncommon oral infection with characteristic clinical findings. The disease is most commonly observed in young white adults between 18 and 21 years of age and may be precipitated by poor oral hygiene, emotional stress, inadequate nutrition, and alcohol or tobacco use. Although it occurs frequently in epidemic proportions in closed communities such as in the military or on college campuses, it is not considered to be communicable. Patients with impaired immunity, primarily those infected with HIV, are especially predisposed toward the development of necrotizing gingivostomatitis.

Clinically, the characteristic lesion begins as a cratered ulceration involving the gingival surfaces between adjacent teeth (interdental papillae) (Fig. 6-5). Necrosis of the gingival tissues, as evidenced by a white pseudomembrane, is observed in the majority of cases. Gingival bleeding, severe pain, and a foul, fetid odor are almost always present. Patients may also be noted to have fever and lymphadenopathy. The lesions may remain localized to the interdental papillae or even spontaneously regress. More commonly, the inflammation is diffuse, extending along the marginal gingiva (Fig. 6-6). In less than 10% of cases the disease is progressive, resulting in severe destruction of the gingiva and exposure of the alveolar bone.

The role of bacteria in the etiology of necrotizing gingivostomatitis is well documented. Species of *Treponema, Selenomonas, Fusobacterium,* and *Prevotella intermedia* can be consistently demon-

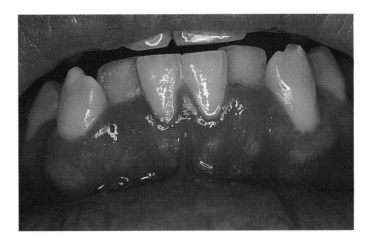

FIG. 6-5   Early manifestations of necrotizing gingivostomatitis are inflammation and blunting of the interdental papillae.

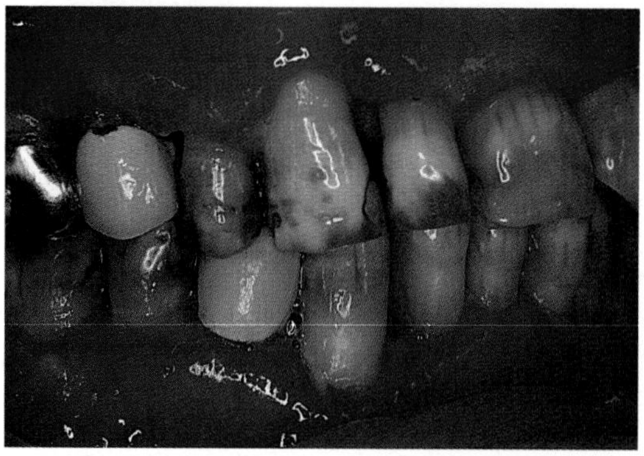

FIG. 6-6   In the advanced stages of necrotizing gingivostomatitis, erythema and ulcerations result in gingival destruction.

strated by culture, although their presence is not diagnostic. Electron microscopic data also reveal the invasion of ulcerated lesions by spirochetes. Although these specific bacteria may account for all of the clinical findings, they may not be responsible for initiating the disease and may be opportunistic, proliferating in an impaired immunologic state. The latter theory is supported by numerous investigations that have uncovered altered immunologic defects in patients with necrotizing gingivostomatitis.

The diagnosis can usually be established by the unique clinical findings including cratered gingival papillae, pain, and bleeding. Histologic features are nondiagnostic and include a mixed inflammatory infiltrate. Necrotizing gingivostomatitis is most readily confused with primary herpetic gingivostomatitis; however, in the latter condition, vesicles, widespread oral involvement, and systemic symptoms are invariably present, and interdental papilla ulcerations are lacking. Necrotizing gingivostomatitis may also appear identical to HIV-associated gingivitis and periodontitis; as such, all newly diagnosed patients should be tested for HIV infection.

Treatment consists of optimizing oral hygiene measures by instructing patients in methods of tooth-brushing and flossing, by professionally scaling and removing plaque, and by using antiseptic rinses. Systemic antibiotics, specifically metronidazole and penicillin, have been shown to reduce bacterial colonization and hasten resolution of the disease.

TUBERCULOSIS

The incidence of intraoral involvement of tuberculosis is low and approximates 1% to 2% of all infected patients. Almost all patients with oral tuberculosis have coexisting pulmonary disease. The rare patient with primary oral tuberculosis usually has accompanying cervical lymphadenopathy. Oral cavity involvement is thought to occur as a result of self-inoculation with infected sputum, hematogenous spread, or, rarely, direct inoculation. Patients with systemic tuberculosis who have poor oral hygiene, fresh extraction wounds, or leukoplakia are considered to be predisposed to developing oral lesions. Primary oral lesions occur in younger patients, whereas secondary lesions are most prevalent in the fifth decade of life.

The oral lesions of tuberculosis may be single or multiple and most commonly appear as an irregular ulcer with surrounding erythema (Fig. 6-7). Pain is usually present, especially when the ulcers are deep and result in bone destruction. Induration is typically absent; however, satellite lesions and simultaneous involvement of the oropharynx are frequently observed. The tongue and gingiva are the most frequent sites of involvement followed by the soft palate, lips, and floor of the mouth.

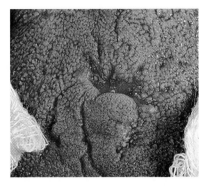

FIG. 6-7   Deep, painful, and irregular ulcerations are the most frequent oral finding of tuberculosis.

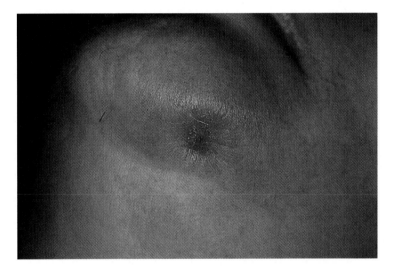

FIG. 6-8   The oral-cutaneous fistula represents a sinus tract from an infected tooth that spreads through the bone and eventually to the skin.

Oral lesions may also appear as nodules, patches, plaques, or vesicles, necessitating a high index of suspicion in patients with chronic oral lesions and pulmonary symptoms.

Patients with lupus vulgaris, a chronic and progressive form of cutaneous tuberculosis occurring in previously sensitized individuals, may display oral lesions characterized by coalescing vegetative nodules and ulcerations.

A biopsy, usually obtained because the lesions clinically resemble oral cancer, demonstrates granulomatous inflammation with multinucleated giant cells and caseous necrosis. Chest radiographs and skin tests should be performed in all patients. The oral lesions respond well to therapy administered for pulmonary disease.

ORAL-CUTANEOUS FISTULAS

Cutaneous-draining sinus tracts of the face and neck are infrequent manifestations of chronic bacterial infections of the oral cavity. The suppurative skin lesions are usually fixed to the underlying tissue as nontender, erythematous, nodulocystic, or ulcerative lesions (Fig. 6-8). Misdiagnosis and the administration of ineffective treatments, including antibiotics and excision, are common because patients lack oral symptoms and the lesions resemble neoplasms. The source of these sinus tracts is dental infection, which may be caused by tooth decay, trauma, or thermal or chemical injury. The dental abscess spreads from a necrotic tooth pulp through the apical foramen into alveolar bone, dissecting along fascial planes distal to muscular attachments and eventually to the skin. The sites of the cutaneous fistulas are usually anatomically close to the infected tooth. The majority arise from infected mandibular anterior teeth, with fistulas developing on the chin and neck. Dental fistulas from maxillary teeth appear at distant sites such as intranasally, in the nasal sinuses, or adjacent to the orbit.

All chronic suppurative lesions on the middle or lower portion of the face should be investigated for possible dental infections. Intraoral findings include a cordlike sinus tract that can be palpated, and the diagnosis is supported by evidence of carious teeth, poor oral hygiene and periodontal disease, fractured or discolored teeth, and tenderness to percussion or thermal stimulation. The source of the infection can best be demonstrated by radiographs, preferably with a radiopaque, dental gutta-percha cone inserted into the sinus tract. After the infected tooth is properly identified, it can be treated with root canal therapy or extraction if it cannot be properly restored. Complete resolution of the fistula occurs in 5 to 14 days.

GONORRHEA

More than 1 million cases of gonorrhea are reported yearly in the United States. The disease is caused by the gram-negative intracellular diplococcus, *Neisseria gonorrhoeae,* and is sexually transmitted with an incubation period of 3 to 7 days. Men most often present with a purulent urethral discharge accompanied by burning on urination and erythema of the urethral meatus. Women are commonly asymptomatic but can also display a vaginal discharge and swelling of the vulva. Pelvic inflammatory disease may develop in untreated women, and reproductive complications include infertility and ectopic pregnancy. Disseminated disease in both sexes can cause septic arthritis, tenosynovitis, bursitis, meningitis, and pericarditis.

The oral lesions of gonorrhea result from fellatio (not cunnilingus) and occur more frequently in homosexuals and prostitutes. The oropharynx is the most frequent site of involvement, characterized by diffuse erythema, with or without small pustules on the tonsillar pillars (Fig. 6-9). The in-

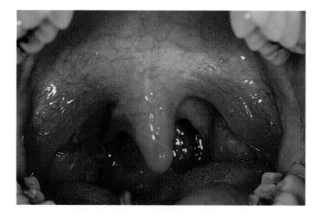

FIG. 6-9   Oropharyngeal gonorrhea is transmitted by fellatio and is characterized by diffuse erythema, ulceration, and pseudomembrane formation.

tensity of the pharyngitis is variable, with some displaying mild erythema without regional lymphadenopathy and others exhibiting severe mucopurulent discharge and cervical lymphadenitis. Most cases of gonococcal pharyngitis are asymptomatic and occur concomitantly with urethritis, cervicitis, or proctitis.

Less frequently, other oral sites may be involved, often causing stinging, burning, and repulsive fetid breath. The intraoral lesions are inconsistent in appearance and consist of swelling and erosions of the lips, desquamation and edema of the gingiva, and diffuse ulcerations and erythema. In all cases a pseudomembrane covering the lesions is evident and oral pain is pronounced. The oral infection may serve as a reservoir of *N. gonorrhoeae* in the transmission of this infectious disease and may be a source of gonococcemia resulting in dissemination.

Because the oral lesions are nondiagnostic, a high index of suspicion is required to establish the correct diagnosis. High-risk patients, including those sexually exposed to persons infected with *N. gonorrhoeae* and exhibiting pharyngitis or unexplained oral erosions, should be cultured in media that selectively permit the growth of *N. gonorrhoeae*. Gram stains, routinely performed from the genital area, are not advisable from the oral cavity, as the oral cavity harbors many *Neisseria* species. Confirmation of isolates by biochemical, enzyme substrate, serologic, or nucleic acid testing is recommended when there is uncertainty.

Among the many antimicrobial agents available for the treatment of uncomplicated gonococcal infections, ceftriaxone, cefixime, ciprofloxacin, and ofloxacin have proven to be efficacious and safe. Oropharyngeal infections have been shown to be statistically more resistant to therapy, often necessitating multiple agents.

SYPHILIS

Syphilis is a sexually transmitted disease caused by the spirochete *Treponema pallidum*. During the 1980s the rate of reported cases increased dramatically in part because of drugs, prostitution, and HIV infection. Oral lesions are a prominent feature in all stages of syphilis and may be the first manifestation of the disease.

Primary syphilis is characterized by the presence of a chancre appearing at the site of inoculation approximately 2 to 3 weeks after exposure. The genitalia are common sites of involvement, although the lips are the most frequent site of extragenital chancres. Painless ulcerations with firm indurated borders occur equally in frequency on the upper lip (Fig. 6-10) and lower lip followed by the

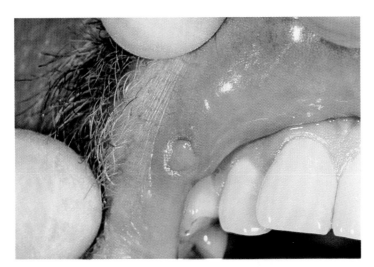

FIG. 6-10   The lips are the most frequent extragenital site for primary chancres.

tongue, buccal mucosa, and oropharynx. Nontender anterior and cervical lymphadenopathy is almost always present and should alert the clinician to the possibility of syphilis. When the lesions occur on the tongue, enlargement of the folate papillae and displacement of the uvula and anterior tonsillar pillar are commonly observed. The demonstration of *T. pallidum* by darkfield examination establishes the diagnosis of genital syphilis. Because a number of spirochetes normally inhabit the oral cavity, the test should not be performed from an oral cavity lesion but rather from a regional lymph node. The rapid plasma reagin test, the Venereal Disease Research Laboratory test, and the fluorescent treponemal antibody absorption test may be used to diagnose the disease. Histologic examination of the oral chancre reveals a dense, chronic, inflammatory infiltrate consisting of plasma cells, lymphocytes, and macrophages accompanied by thickening of the arterioles. The oral chancres heal within 2 to 4 weeks, often with minimal scaring.

Secondary syphilis occurs 2 to 10 weeks after the primary lesion has healed. Generalized adenopathy accompanies a widespread eruption, alopecia, and protean systemic symptoms including headaches, arthralgias, lacrimation, and sore throat. The oral lesions appear concurrently with the cutaneous lesions, and their recognition can result in an early diagnosis. The oral mucous membrane lesions, referred to as *mucous patches,* are predominantly located on the tongue and appear as slightly elevated plaques or, occasionally, ulcerations that are usually oval and covered with a white or gray pseudomembrane (Figs. 6-11 and 6-12). Lesions described as painful, red, firm plaques occur on the

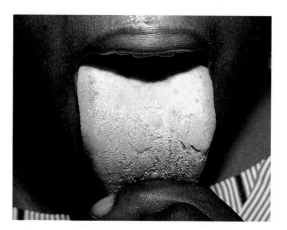

FIG. 6-11   Secondary syphilis of the oral cavity is characterized by mucous patches that develop on the tongue and appear as oval, painless plaques.

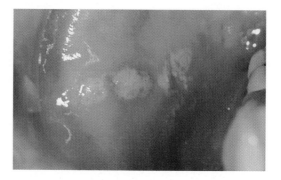

FIG. 6-12   Secondary syphilis lesions of the oral cavity may also consist of chronic ulcerations. (From Anneroth G, Anneroth I, Lynch DP: *J Oral Maxillofac Surg* 44:956, 1986.)

palate less frequently. The two types may heal spontaneously but often recur over a period of months. Split, moist, flat papules known as *condylomata lata* may occur at the lip commissures. Both the oral chancres of primary syphilis and the mucous patches of secondary syphilis are highly contagious by contact through kissing or sexual exposure. The reaginic and treponemal tests are positive in secondary syphilis and should be performed in all suspected cases.

The tertiary stage develops in approximately one third of untreated patients with syphilis, usually 5 to 10 years after the initial infection. Oral lesions occur most commonly during this stage and are characterized by a chronic interstitial glossitis (Fig. 6-13). Marked atrophy of the filiform and fungiform papillae with deep fissuring results in a large and lobulated tongue. Areas of leukoplakia may be present and should be subjected to biopsy to exclude malignant transformation into squamous cell carcinoma. The hard and soft palates may be the site for gummatous formation, which begins as a firm, infiltrated plaque and may eventually result in perforation. Fortunately, gummas in the oral cavity occur less frequently than they do in the skin and bone.

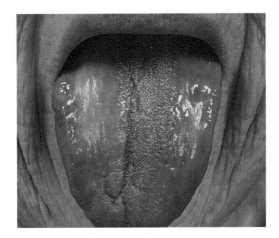

FIG. 6-13   Interstitial glossitis of tertiary syphilis characterized by atrophy of the fungiform and filiform papillae.

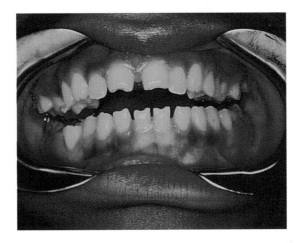

FIG. 6-14   Crescentic notching of central incisors is characteristic of Hutchinson's teeth in congenital syphilis.

Congenital syphilis occurs when spirochetes pass from the placenta to the fetal circulation. During the early stage, usually in the first 3 months of life, oral lesions resembling those of acquired secondary syphilis are evident. In the late stage approximately half will exhibit Hutchinson's teeth. These maxillary central incisors or, less commonly, mandibular incisors, display either a distinct crescentic notch at the incisal edge or a depression on the labial gingival aspect of the tooth and are screw-driver or peg shaped (Fig. 6-14). Hutchinson's teeth, interstitial keratitis, and eighth nerve deafness constitute Hutchinson's triad, which is pathognomonic for congenital syphilis. Mulberry molars, also known as *Moon's molars,* are characterized by first molar teeth with a larger than normal number of poorly defined (rounded, rather than pointed) occlusal cusps and are present in approximately one fourth of patients with congenital syphilis. Hypocalcification of the enamel predisposes these teeth to caries. Both Hutchinson's teeth and Mulberry molars affect only the permanent dentition.

The treatment of syphilis consists of intramuscularly administered depot preparations of penicillin.

ACTINOMYCOSIS

Actinomycetes are commensal organisms of the oral cavity that can be isolated from dental plaque and dental caries. Additionally, they are occasionally discovered inadvertently by histologic examination of dental pulps, oral cysts, and periodontal bony defects. Only rarely do they act as pathogens and cause actinomycosis. Of the several strains identified, *Actinomyces israelii* has been implicated most frequently as the infecting organism, although others may cause the disease. The oral actinomyces are anaerobes and appear most frequently as gram-positive, nonacid-fast, branching mycelia.

Cervicofacial actinomycosis, or "lumpy jaw," is the most common form of the disease. It occurs most often in young adults and affects men more often than women.

Undoubtedly, the infection is initiated by an oral pathologic condition such as dental extractions, periodontal abscesses, oral trauma, oral abrasions or erosions, and oral surgery. These portals of entry allow the infection to spread to adjacent tissues, resulting in persistent swelling that occurs most often in the submandibular and cervical regions. The disease may infrequently appear in the submental, parotid, or maxillary area. The overlying skin is indurated and exhibits a characteristic purple-red color (Fig. 6-15). Multiple abscesses and extraoral sinus tracts develop and drain purulent material containing 0.25 to 2.5 mm yellow "sulfur granules" consisting of colonies of *Actino-*

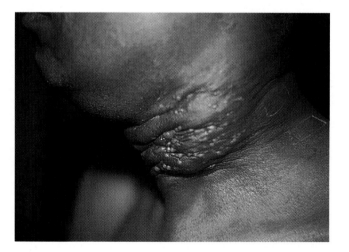

FIG. 6-15   Cervicofacial actinomycosis is usually the result of a dental infection; multiple abscesses and sinus tracts develop with a characteristic red-purple color of the overlying skin.

myces species cemented together by host phosphatase activity. These granules require definitive identification because a number of other infections, including fungal infections caused by *Nocardia* and *Streptomyces,* result in granule formation. In the acute presentation of actinomycosis the disease resembles a dental abscess with pain and fever. The cause is usually an infection of dental origin, and extraction of the offending tooth combined with antibiotics results in resolution. In the more common chronic and protracted form of the disease, pain, systemic symptoms, and regional lymphadenopathy may be absent. Fibrosis, suppuration, and scar formation at the site of recurrent abscess formation resemble a malignancy. The infection may result in extensive bone destruction and osteomyelitis, usually of the mandible.

The diagnosis of actinomycosis can be elusive unless the proper diagnostic studies are performed. These include anaerobic cultures of homogenized tissue or granules, histologic examination of the granules demonstrating a basophilic mass with eosinophils radiating outward and surrounded by neutrophils, and fluorescent antibody stains. Treatment consists of a prolonged course of a high-dose penicillin. Erythromycin, cephalothin, minocycline, clindamycin, and chloramphenicol are effective as alternative agents. In some instances patients require surgical débridement of fibrotic tissue, abscesses, and persistent sinus tracts.

PARULIS

An abscess that develops in the alveolar bone may originate from an infected tooth or an infected periodontal pocket. Occasionally, such an infection may spread through the cortical bone and result in a soft-tissue fistula on the alveolar mucosa. This opening is covered by a small hyperplastic nodule called a *parulis* or *gum boil* (Fig. 6-16). Although the lesion is most commonly observed on the maxillary buccal gingiva, any labial or lingual alveolar site may be involved. It is usually painless and drains spontaneously. The diagnosis of a parulis can readily be confirmed by the presence of pus when incision and drainage are performed. The parulis usually regresses after the tooth or periodontal infection is adequately treated.

MISCELLANEOUS INFECTIONS
Scarlet Fever

This infection, caused by group B *Streptococci,* displays prominent oral manifestations. In the early stage, the hard palate is congested and red. The tongue is coated white, and the fungiform papillae

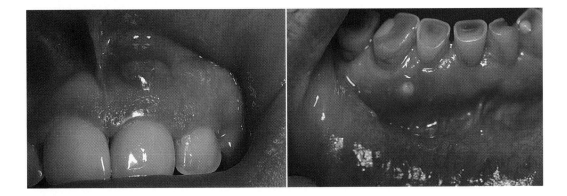

FIG. 6-16   These *parulides* represent fistulas through the alveolar bone from either an infected tooth or a periodontal abscess.

are hyperemic and project above the dorsal surface, giving it the appearance of a "strawberry tongue" (Fig. 6-17). In the late stage the edematous papillae persist, but the white tongue coating is replaced by a deeply erythematous hue that has been termed *raspberry tongue.*

Diphtheria

Diphtheria is caused by the gram-positive bacillus *Corynebacterium diphtheriae.* Oral mucous membranes may be involved, usually through direct extension of the disease from the tonsils, pharynx, and larynx. The characteristic membranous exudate that covers these areas appears as a thick grayish film with well-demarcated borders and an erythematous halo (Fig. 6-18). This membrane, which may also be observed on the gingiva and even on the buccal mucosa and tongue, can be wiped away, revealing bloody erosions. Unlike tonsillitis, diphtheria is rapidly progressive and patients are often acutely ill. Treatment with diphtheria antitoxin should be instituted promptly before confirmation by culture and polymerase chain reaction assay if the disease is suspected.

Tularemia

Francisella tularensis, the organism responsible for tularemia, is usually acquired by contact with infected animals—most frequently rabbits and cats. The manifestations of oropharyngeal tularemia,

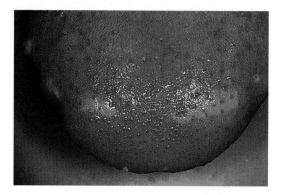

FIG. 6-17   Strawberry tongue of scarlet fever. The tongue is coated white, and the fungiform papillae are hyperemic.

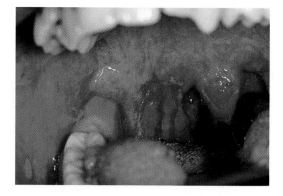

FIG. 6-18   Diphtheria of the oral cavity most frequently affects the oropharynx and is characterized by erythema covered by a gray, membranous exudate.

presumably acquired by direct inoculation, include a severely painful necrotic and indurated oral ulcer or a diffuse stomatitis. Painful regional lymphadenopathy is usually prominent and is accompanied by fever, chills, and headache.

Granuloma Inguinale

Granuloma inguinale is a rare sexually transmitted disease that is caused by *Calymmatobacterium granulomatis.* Oral lesions are the most frequent extragenital form of granuloma inguinale and, like genital lesions, can appear in several morphologic variants. Painful, bloody, oral ulcerations are most frequently encountered, and vegetative and proliferative nodules are less common. A characteristic finding is the severe cicatrization that may be extensive and limit mouth movements. The oral lesions usually follow genital involvement.

Leprosy

Leprosy affects more than 5 million people worldwide and is caused by the acid-fast bacillus *Mycobacterium leprae.* Oral lesions are not uncommon and appear predominantly in the lepromatous form and occasionally in the borderline and reactional tuberculoid leprosy forms. Oral tumorlike lesions called *lepromas* begin as firm, pink-yellow nodules that eventually ulcerate. Scar formation and tissue destruction are usually evident after the ulcerations heal. The lesions appear most frequently on the palate and tongue, and multiple sites of involvement are usual. The tongue is also a common site for lepromatous infiltration, which results in macroglossia. Reddening of the upper teeth ("pink spots") may be observed in lepromatous leprosy and is caused by direct infection of the dental pulp by mycobacteria.

Suppurative Infection of the Salivary Glands

The intraoral duct openings of the parotid gland and, less commonly, the submandibular gland may be the sites of a suppurative infection. Erythema is evident around the orifice of the infected gland's duct, and pus is discharged either spontaneously or with pressure on the gland. The infection is usually caused by *S. aureus, S. viridans,* or *Escherichia coli,* although other bacteria may induce the infection. The disease usually afflicts debilitated patients with multiple medical problems and occurs either during infancy or more commonly in elderly persons. The diagnosis should be suspected in patients with unilateral pain, swelling, and induration of a salivary gland accompanied by an intraoral purulent discharge from the duct orifice. Cultures should be obtained to determine antibiotic sensitivity.

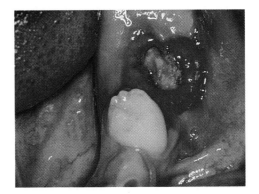

FIG. 6-19   Noma, caused by a mixed infection, characteristically starts focally, destroying gingiva and teeth, and rapidly progresses to involve the entire oral cavity and face.

Noma

Also known as *cancrum oris,* this rare gangrenous disease originates in the oral cavity and is characterized by the rapid necrotizing and mutilating destruction of the oral tissues and underlying bone. Noma occurs in Africa, Asia, and South America and usually in children whose socioeconomically depressed status has resulted in malnutrition, poor oral hygiene, debilitation, and generalized illnesses. Adults who are immunocompromised with HIV infection may also be predisposed. The disease is caused by a mixed infection of oral bacterial pathogens, predominantly *Fusobacterium necrophorum.* Clinically, the disease starts as a painful ulcerative gingivitis, which results in bone destruction and tooth loss. Gangrenous and disfiguring ulcerations develop rapidly within hours and result in massive destruction of the oral cavity and facial skin (Fig. 6-19). Treatment consists of antibiotics and correcting the underlying predisposing factor, most frequently malnutrition.

SUGGESTED READINGS

General

Asikainen S, Alaluusua S: Bacteriology of dental infections, *Eur Heart J* 14:43, 1993.

Dahlen G et al: A retrospective study of microbiologic samples from oral mucosal lesions, *Oral Surg Oral Med Oral Pathol* 53:250, 1982.

Dajani AS et al: Prevention of bacterial endocarditis: recommendations by the American Heart Association, *J Am Med Assoc* 272:1794, 1997.

Durack DT: Prevention of infective endocarditis, *N Engl J Med* 332:38, 1995.

Gill Y, Scully C: Orofacial odontogenic infections: review of microbiology and current treatment, *Oral Surg Oral Med Oral Pathol* 70:155, 1990.

Scannapieco FA, Stewart EM, Mylotte JM: Colonization of dental plaque by respiratory pathogens in medical intensive care patients, *Crit Care Med* 20:740, 1992.

Gingivitis and periodontitis

Adams D, Addy M: Mouthrinses, *Adv Dent Res* 8:291, 1994.

Genco RJ: Host responses in periodontal diseases, *J Periodontol* 63:338, 1992.

Lang NP, Bragger U: Periodontal diagnosis in the 1990s, *J Clin Periodontol* 18:370, 1991.

Mandel ID: Calculus update: prevalence, pathogenicity and prevention, *J Am Dent Assoc* 126:573, 1995.

Moore LVH et al: Bacteriology of human gingivitis, *J Dent Res* 66:989, 1987.

Smalley JW: Pathogenic mechanisms in periodontal disease, *Adv Dent Res* 8:320, 1994.

Socransky SS, Haffajee AD: The bacterial etiology of destructive periodontal disease: current concepts, *J Periodontol* 63:322, 1992.

Tanner A, Stillman N: Oral and dental infections with anaerobic bacteria: clinical features, predominant pathogens, and treatment, *Clin Infect Dis* 16:304, 1993.

Williams RC: Periodontal diseases: gingivitis, juvenile periodontitis, adult periodontitis, *Curr Clin Top Infect Dis* 13:146, 1993.

Necrotizing gingivostomatitis

Glick M et al: Necrotizing ulcerative periodontitis: a marker for immune deterioration and a predictor for the diagnosis of AIDS, *J Periodontol* 65:393, 1994.

Horning GM, Cohen ME: Necrotizing ulcerative gingivitis, periodontitis, and stomatitis: clinical staging and predisposing factors, *J Periodontol* 66:990, 1995.

Johnson BD, Engel D: Acute necrotizing ulcerative gingivitis: a review of diagnosis, etiology and treatment, *J Periodontol* 57:141, 1986.

Melnick SL et al: Epidemiology of acute necrotizing ulcerative gingivitis, *Epidemiol Rev* 10:191, 1988.

Tuberculosis

Eng HL et al: Oral tuberculosis, *Oral Surg Oral Med Oral Pathol* 81:415, 1996.

Mani NJ: Tuberculosis initially diagnosed by asymptomatic oral lesions: report of three cases, *J Oral Med* 40:39, 1985.

Smith WHR et al: Intraoral and pulmonary tuberculosis following dental manipulation, *Lancet* 1:842, 1982.

Oral-cutaneous fistulas

Foster KH, Primack PD, Lkulid JC: Odontogenic cutaneous sinus tract, *J Endod* 18:6, 1992.

Hodges TP, Cohen DA, Deck D: Odontogenic sinus tracts, *Am Fam Physician* 40:113, 1989.

Marasco PV Jr et al: Dentocutaneous fistula, *Ann Plast Surg* 29:205, 1992.

McWalter GM et al: Cutaneous sinus tracts of dental etiology, *Oral Surg Oral Med Oral Pathol* 66:608, 1988.

Gonorrhea

Chue PWY: Gonorrhea: its natural history, oral manifestations, diagnosis, treatment, and prevention, *J Am Dent Assoc* 90:1297, 1975.

Giunta JL, Fiumara NJ: Facts about gonorrhea and dentistry, *Oral Surg Oral Med Oral Pathol* 62:529, 1986.

Jamsky RJ, Christen AG: Oral gonococcal infections: report of two cases, *Oral Surg Oral Med Oral Pathol* 53:358, 1982.

Moran JS, Levine WC: Drugs of choice for the treatment of uncomplicated gonococcal infections, *Clin Infect Dis* 20:S47, 1995.

Syphilis

Junkins-Hopkins JM: Multiple painful oral ulcerations: secondary syphilis, *Arch Dermatol* 131:833, 1995.

Manton SL et al: Oral presentation of secondary syphilis, *Br Dent J* 160:237, 1986.

Meyer I, Shklar G: The oral manifestations of acquired syphilis: a study of eighty-one cases, *Oral Surg Oral Med Oral Pathol* 23:45, 1967.

Putkonen T: Dental changes in congenital syphilis, *Acta Derm Venereol* 42:44, 1962.

Shklar G: Oral reflections of infectious diseases, *Postgrad Med* 68:147, 1971.

Terezhalmy GT: Oral manifestations of sexually related diseases, *Ear Nose Throat J* 62:5, 1983.

Actinomycosis

Bennhoff DF: Actinomycosis: diagnostic and therapeutic considerations and a review of 32 cases, *Laryngoscope* 94:1198, 1984.

Lerner PI: The lumpy jaw: cervicofacial actinomycosis, *Infect Dis Clin North Am* 2:203, 1988.

Stenhouse D: Intraoral actinomycosis: report of five cases, *Oral Surg* 39:547, 1975.

Stenhouse D, MacDonald DG, MacFarlane TW: Cervico-facial and intra-oral actinomycosis: a 5-year retrospective study, *Br J Oral Surg* 13:172, 1975.

Miscellaneous infections

Enwonwu CO: Noma: a neglected scourge of children in sub-Saharan Africa, *Bull World Health Organ* 73:541, 1995.

Krippachne W, Hunt TK, Dunphy J: Acute suppurative parotitis: study of 161 cases, *Ann Surg* 156:251, 1962.

Pallen MJ et al: Polymerase chain reaction for screening clinical isolates of corynebacteria for the production of diphtheria toxin, *J Clin Pathol* 47:353, 1994.

Reichart P: Facial and oral manifestations in leprosy: an evaluation of seventy cases, *Oral Surg* 41:385, 1976.

Rendall JR, McDougall AC: Reddening of the upper central incisors associated with periapical granuloma in lepromatous leprosy, *Br J Oral Surg* 13:271, 1976.

Scully C, Williams G: Oral manifestations of communicable diseases, *Dent Update* July/August:295, 1978.

CHAPTER 7

Viral Infections

HUMAN HERPESVIRUSES

Human herpesviruses (HHVs) are comprised of a family of deoxyribonucleic acid (DNA) viruses that characteristically result in primary infection followed by latent infection with reactivation at various intervals, particularly in the setting of immunosuppression. The clinical manifestations of primary and recurrent infections are usually distinctive from one another. The diseases that result from the eight classified HHVs are listed in Table 7-1.

Herpes Simplex Virus Type 1 (HHV-1)

Herpes simplex virus type 1 (HSV-1) is one of the most common viral infections of humans and classically affects oral mucosa and perioral skin. Worldwide, more than 85% of adults from both urban and rural locations display serologic evidence of prior HSV-1 exposure, with the highest rates detected in lower socioeconomic communities. The primary infection (acute herpetic gingivostomatitis), defined as the first viral exposure in a seronegative individual, occurs primarily by direct exposure through mucocutaneous contact with another infected patient. The vast majority of infections occur subclinically, with only 15% of cases manifesting clinical signs and symptoms. The infection occurs most frequently in children and young adults, with a peak incidence between ages 2 and 5 years. Its occurrence in adults is uncommon and even more rare before the age of 6 months because of passive protection from maternal antibodies.

In those patients with symptoms, acute herpetic gingivostomatitis results in fever, sore throat, malaise, and swollen, tender cervical lymphadenopathy. Symptoms develop 3 to 14 days after exposure to the virus. The initial oral lesions are characterized by painful vesicles that rapidly ulcerate and often coalesce. The lesions, which can resemble recurrent aphthous stomatitis, may develop on any or all of the oral mucous membranes, with frequent diffuse involvement of the gingiva (Fig. 7-1). The attached gingivae surrounding the teeth are often strikingly reddened and may be covered with a pseudomembrane or studded with ulcerations (Fig. 7-2). This finding is useful in differentiating acute herpetic gingivostomatitis from recurrent aphthous stomatitis. Perioral lesions are commonly present and pharyngeal ulcerations may also be noted, especially in young adults. Healing occurs spontaneously in 14 to 21 days.

Recurrent HSV-1 infections occur when the latent virus is reactivated from the nerve root ganglion. Approximately 30% to 50% of all HSV-infected patients develop recurrences, with an average of three to four episodes per year. The onset of a recurrence, also known as a *fever blister* or *cold sore,* is heralded by dysesthesia of the vermilion border of the lip and perioral skin. A cluster of erythematous macules progresses to painful vesicles, which ulcerate and become crusted (Fig. 7-3). Constitutional symptoms are generally absent. Although exposure to sunlight has been demonstrated to be a consistent precipitating factor of recurrent HSV infections, trauma, stress, hormonal imbalance, and a variety of triggering events have also been implicated. Complete resolution occurs in 7 to 10 days.

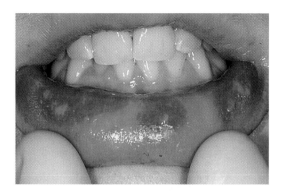

FIG. 7-1   Primary herpetic gingivostomatitis presents with widespread ulcerations resembling aphthous stomatitis.

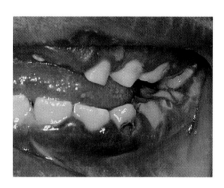

FIG. 7-2   The gingiva is typically inflamed and hemorrhagic and may be studded with ulcerations in primary herpetic gingivostomatitis.

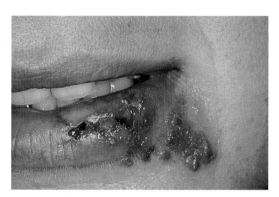

FIG. 7-3   Fever blisters represent reactivated herpes simplex virus type 1 infection typically precipitated by sunlight.

Table 7-1   Human Herpesviruses (HHVs)

HHV TYPE	COMMON NAME AND DISEASE
1	Herpes simplex virus type 1: herpes labialis
2	Herpes simplex virus type 2: genital herpes
3	Varicella-zoster virus: chickenpox, herpes zoster
4	Epstein-Barr virus: infectious mononucleosis, Burkitt's lymphoma, oral hairy leukoplakia
5	Cytomegalovirus: mononucleosis, retinitis, pneumonitis, encephalitis, oral ulcerations
6	Roseola infantum
7	Undefined; viral exanthem
8	Kaposi's sarcoma-associated herpesvirus

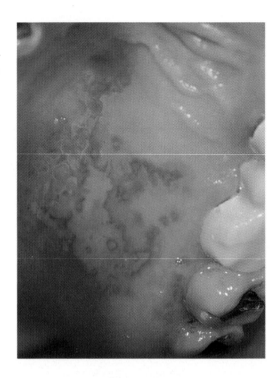

FIG. 7-4   Recurrent oral herpes simplex virus type 1 infection typically occurs on keratinized mucosa, most often on the palate and attached gingiva.

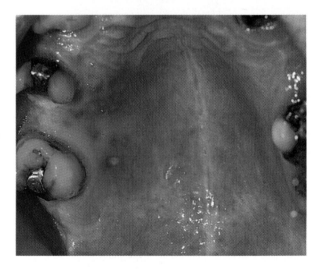

FIG. 7-5   Recurrent oral herpes simplex virus type 1 (HSV-1). Grouped vesicles on an erythematous base identical to recurrent (HSV-1) lesions on the skin.

Recurrent HSV-1 infections may occur intraorally, although this is uncommon. Unlike the primary HSV-1 infection, which may affect all of the oral mucosa, intraoral recurrent HSV-1 infections are generally limited to the attached gingiva and hard palate, which are keratinized. Intact oral vesicles are not commonly observed because they are traumatized by mastication and rupture shortly after development. Typically, intraoral recurrent HSV-1 manifests as a cluster of shallow ulcers covered by a pseudomembrane on an erythematous base (Figs. 7-4 and 7-5). Recurrences commonly follow trauma such as a dental procedure. Like their cutaneous counterparts, intraoral lesions heal without scarring after 7 to 14 days.

In patients who are severely immunocompromised, the primary infection is generally more severe, with increased tissue destruction and the potential for dissemination (Fig. 7-6). Recurrent HSV-1 infections of the mouth may appear atypical and occur on nonkeratinized mucosa. The pres-

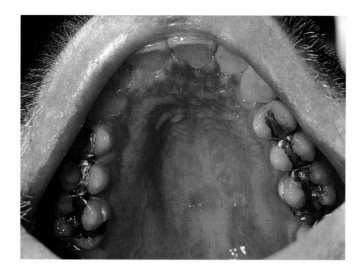

FIG. 7-6   In immunocompromised patients, recurrent oral herpes simplex virus type 1 infections are common and more extensive, with potential for dissemination. (From Weinert M, Grimes RM, Lynch DP: *Ann Intern Med* 125:485, 1996.)

ence of multiple or grouped oral ulcerations in immunocompromised patients should suggest the possibility of reactivated herpesvirus infection and prompt a viral culture. A unique form of recurrent HSV-1 infection described in immunocompromised patients, termed *herpetic geometric glossitis,* is characterized by extremely painful, cross-hatched, branched, or linear fissures on the dorsal aspect of the tongue.

The diagnosis of HSV-1 infections is primarily clinical, although definitive confirmation may be obtained by culturing the virus from a vesicle or early ulceration. The presence of multinucleated giant cells with 2 to 15 nuclei in a Tzanck preparation obtained from the base of a lesion is a rapid and valuable approach in establishing the diagnosis. Infection may also be confirmed within hours by visualization of HSV-1 antigens in cells of smears from secretions using rapid immunofluorescent or enzyme-linked immunosorbent assay (ELISA)-based diagnostic methods. The recent development of polymerase chain reaction technique allows the isolation and duplication of specific herpesvirus DNA segments. A fourfold rise in antibody titers between acute and convalescent sera is indicative of an HSV-1 infection.

The treatment of choice for primary and orofacial HSV-1 infections is acyclovir. Although its use for primary oral infections in immunocompetent hosts does not decrease the incidence of recurrences, it ameliorates the symptoms and shortens the duration of the disease. Episodic treatment of recurrent orofacial HSV-1 infections with acyclovir is acceptable for the majority of patients. In immunocompromised patients or in immunocompetent patients who develop multiple recurrences, orofacial HSV-1 infections may be prevented by the chronic administration of acyclovir safely and without significant toxicity. Acyclovir-resistant HSV-1 disease has emerged predominantly in patients infected with human immunodeficiency virus (HIV) and has prompted investigations for alternative antiviral agents. Foscarnet is currently the treatment of choice in such cases.

A variety of mouth rinses may be used palliatively for primary and recurrent oral herpes infections. These include topical anesthetics, which are useful in alleviating pain, and chlorhexidine, which may decrease viral load and promote healing.

Herpes Simplex Virus Type 2 (HHV-2)

Herpes simplex virus type 2 (HSV-2) is the most common cause of genital herpes. The major glycoproteins of HSV-1 and HSV-2 are similar, with 80% homology. Neutralizing antibodies to the virus

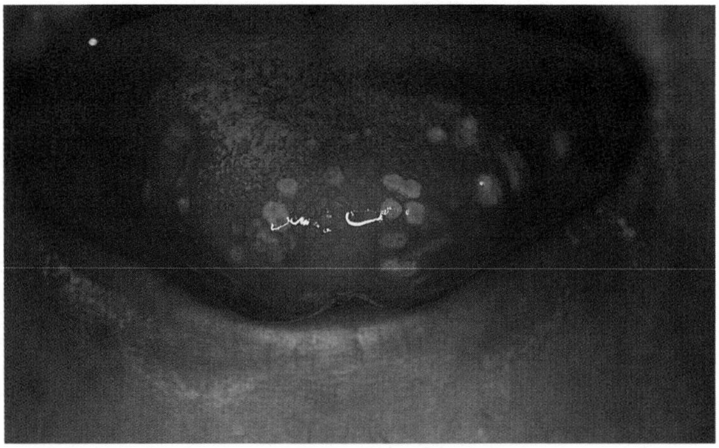

FIG. 7-7   Primary herpes simplex virus type 2 infection of the tongue caused by herpes simplex virus type 2 acquired after oral sex. (From Weinert M, Grimes RM, Lynch DP: *Ann Intern Med* 125:485, 1996.)

are induced by these glycoproteins and cross-react between the two types. In recent years an increasing number of oral HSV-2 infections have been recognized, as have genital HSV-1 infections. The oral manifestations of HSV-2 infection are identical to those observed in HSV-1 infections (Fig. 7-7). The frequency of recurrence is low for orofacial HSV-2 infections.

Varicella-Zoster Virus (HHV-3)

Varicella-zoster virus (VZV) causes two distinct clinical entities: varicella (chickenpox) and varicella-zoster (shingles). The primary infection, varicella, occurs in the nasopharynx and is transmitted via the respiratory route. The vast majority of individuals in the United States demonstrate serologic evidence of previous VZV infection.

After a 10- to 20-day incubation period, infected patients develop symptoms of fever, malaise, and pharyngitis, followed by an intensely pruritic exanthem. The characteristic skin rash initially manifests as maculopapules that progress to vesicles on an erythematous base and then to pustules. Lesions at all stages characteristically develop simultaneously. The resultant pustules become crusted and eventually resolve without scarring.

Oral lesions are commonly observed in varicella and are characterized by small, 1- to 3-mm vesicles. The lesions rupture shortly after they develop, resulting in superficial erosions surrounded by erythema (Fig. 7-8). Although any oral surface may be involved, the lesions occur most frequently on the palate, gingiva, and buccal mucosa. The small erosions are usually asymptomatic. In immunocompromised patients oral lesions are more severe and widely distributed.

After the primary varicella infection, the virus remains dormant in the nerve ganglion. Reactivation of the virus occurs in over 10% of the general population at any age but is most common after age 50. The incidence of herpes zoster and its severity are increased in immunocompromised patients.

Herpes zoster is characterized by a distinctive eruption, which is localized, unilateral, and limited to the area of skin innervated by a single sensory ganglion. The skin eruption is preceded by radicular pain and is accompanied by fever and malaise. The individual lesions of varicella and herpes zoster are identical, although in the latter condition, they are often closely grouped as opposed to the random distribution observed in varicella. The vesicles develop into pustules and eventually crust before resolving 2 to 3 weeks later.

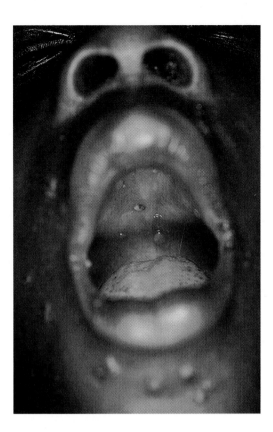

FIG. 7-8   Patient with chickenpox and oral lesions, which characteristically start as blisters that rapidly rupture.

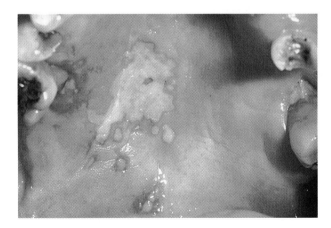

FIG. 7-9   Herpes zoster in the oral cavity most often affects the hard palate and is characterized by unilateral ulcerations accompanying skin lesions.

When herpes zoster affects the second or third divisions of the trigeminal nerve, oral lesions commonly develop. These may be the predominant feature of the disease with relatively few skin lesions, or they may accompany a unilateral facial rash. Clusters of vesicles, which ulcerate and form on an erythematous base, develop most commonly on the hard palate and maxillary gingiva when the second division of the trigeminal nerve is involved (Fig. 7-9). Herpes zoster of the third division may result in ulcerations of the tongue, floor of the mouth, mandibular gingiva, and buccal mucosa. Oral lesions outside the affected dermatome, resulting from hematogenous spread, occur in im-

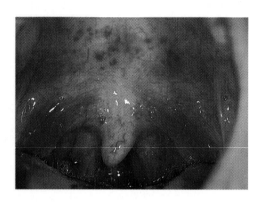

FIG. 7-10 Infectious mononucleosis demonstrating palatal petechiae and erythema of the oropharynx.

munocompromised patients. In rare instances oral herpes zoster may result in necrosis of the underlying bone or devitalization of the affected teeth. The Ramsay Hunt syndrome, characterized by involvement of cranial nerves VI and VII, manifests as herpes zoster of the ear and tympanic membrane and results in facial palsy, vertigo, tinnitus, and deafness. Unilateral oral lesions develop on the tongue, buccal mucosa, and labial vestibule.

Both varicella- and herpes zoster viruses are diagnosed clinically on the basis of the physical findings. Confirmation may be achieved by a Tzanck smear, culture, or biopsy specimens, which may be stained with monoclonal antibodies for VZV antigen.

Uncomplicated varicella in children is treated palliatively, whereas herpes zoster is managed with acyclovir or with one of the newer antiviral agents, famciclovir or valacyclovir. These agents have been demonstrated to increase healing, decrease pain, and reduce the incidence of postherpetic neuralgia. Oral lesions may be palliatively treated with topical anesthetics and heal rapidly, which may account for the absence of postherpetic neuralgia in the mouth.

Epstein-Barr Virus (HHV-4)

The Epstein-Barr virus (EBV) is unique within the herpesvirus family in that it establishes a latent state in infected B lymphocytes. The virus is trophic for salivary gland epithelial cells and, in infected individuals, is shed in oropharyngeal secretions. EBV is the etiologic agent of infectious mononucleosis and has been associated with a variety of other clinical diseases including hairy leukoplakia (see Chapter 13), Burkitt's lymphoma (see Chapter 5), and nasopharyngeal carcinoma.

Infectious mononucleosis is a highly contagious disease transmitted by interpersonal contact, usually through intimate oral contact. The disease is more prevalent in lower socioeconomic groups, although over 90% of adults develop antibodies to EBV.

The primary infection in children is usually asymptomatic or characterized by a mild upper respiratory infection and pharyngitis. In young adults, fever, pharyngitis, and cervical lymphadenopathy are the most frequent manifestations and are preceded by a prodrome of anorexia, fatigue, and malaise. Skin eruptions, hepatitis, splenic rupture, and neurologic abnormalities are uncommon. The oral manifestations of infectious mononucleosis include diffuse palatal petechiae and erythema of the oropharynx developing in up to one fourth of all infected individuals (Fig. 7-10). The petechiae arise between days 5 and 17 and usually fade within days of their appearance. Tonsillar enlargement, often covered with an exudate, and uvular edema are also characteristic of pharyngeal EBV infection. Diffuse and severe gingival inflammation resembling acute necrotizing ulcerative gingivitis (see Chapter 6) is a less frequent oral finding.

Reactivation of EBV occurs in immunocompromised patients and results in EBV lymphoproliferative disorders including B- and T-cell lymphomas, oral hairy leukoplakia, and a syndrome characterized by recurrent oral and facial necrotizing nodules.

The clinical suspicion of EBV infection may be confirmed by the presence of heterophil anti-

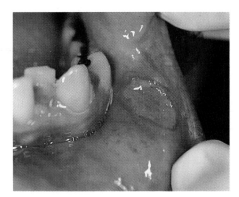

FIG. 7-11   Cytomegalovirus ulcerations in the oral cavity appear identical to recurrent aphthous stomatitis.

bodies. Infected individuals display leukocytosis characterized by lymphocytosis with atypical lymphocytes. The presence of the virus can also be demonstrated through indirect immunofluorescence and ELISA techniques.

In the vast majority of cases infectious mononucleosis resolves spontaneously in 4 to 6 weeks. Treatment primarily consists of supportive therapy. Nonsteroidal antiinflammatory medications may relieve generalized discomfort associated with the infection. Systemic antiviral medications have been used with variable success but do not affect symptoms. Systemic corticosteroids reduce the duration of fever and pharyngitis, but their use in the treatment of mononucleosis has not yet gained acceptance.

Cytomegalovirus (HHV-5)

Cytomegalovirus (CMV) infection is common worldwide, with most asymptomatic primary infections dominating. The incidence of CMV infection exposure increases with age. Approximately 2% of infants display serologic evidence of CMV infection, whereas 50% demonstrate CMV infection antibodies by mid-adulthood. The incidence increases to nearly 100% in elderly persons.

CMV inclusion disease is the most common congenital viral infection and develops in infants born to mothers who become infected during pregnancy. Infected infants may develop psychomotor, hearing, and ocular abnormalities. Over one third of cases are characterized by defective odontogenesis, which clinically manifests as yellow, discolored dentin and hypoplastic pitted enamel. CMV infection in the neonatal period may result in diverse physical and laboratory abnormalities similar to other viral infections.

Adults who experience CMV infection develop clinical manifestations similar to those seen with infectious mononucleosis. The heterophil-antibody test is negative, and oral manifestations are much less common. CMV infections in immunosuppressed patients result in a wide spectrum of disease and are discussed in the chapter on oral manifestations of HIV infection (see Chapter 13). Oral lesions resemble recurrent aphthous stomatitis (Fig. 7-11).

The diagnosis of CMV infection requires correlation of clinical features and confirmatory laboratory tests including viral culture and serology. Characteristic morphologic changes manifested by large intranuclear inclusion bodies (owl's-eye cells) can be found in biopsy specimens. Virus can also be detected in tissue sections through various immunohistochemical methods.

CMV infection is most often a self-limiting disease that does not require treatment. Ganciclovir or foscarnet is used in treating immunocompromised patients with active disease.

ENTEROVIRUSES

Three dozen enteroviruses (single-stranded, unenveloped ribonucleic acid [RNA] viruses) have been identified, many of which cause viral exanthems. Enterovirus infections with prominent oral man-

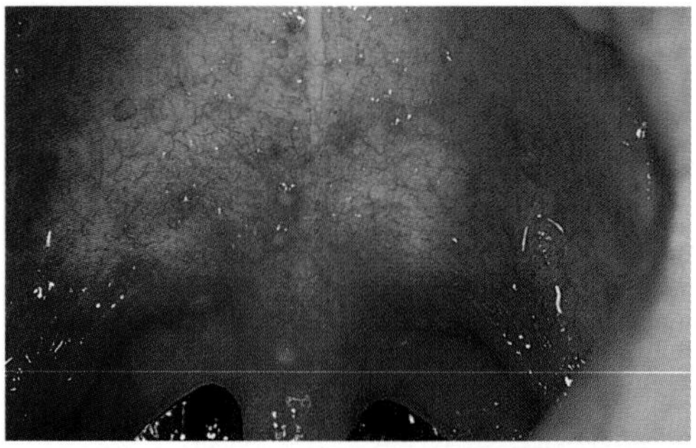

FIG. 7-12   Herpangina displaying characteristic small ulcerations with surrounding erythema on the palate and uvula.

ifestations include herpangina, hand-foot-and-mouth disease, and acute lymphonodular pharyngitis. The oral lesions that develop in these infections result in significant pain, which can be palliatively treated with topical anesthetics. All of the enterovirus infections generally occur more commonly in the late summer or early fall and develop in those with crowded living conditions and poor hygiene.

Herpangina

Herpangina is an acute febrile disease involving the oral mucosa, predominantly affecting young children. Group A coxsackieviruses are the most consistent etiologic agents, although group B coxsackie viruses and echoviruses have been implicated sporadically. The incubation period averages 3 to 10 days and the disease starts with fever, anorexia, and sore throat. Clinically, herpangina is characterized by the development of small, 1- to 2-mm erythematous macules, which subsequently develop into vesicles that ulcerate rapidly. The superficial ulcers are surrounded by erythema and the pharyngeal mucosa is diffusely reddened (Fig. 7-12). The lesions most commonly appear on the soft palate, uvula, and tonsillar pillar areas. Occasionally, buccal mucosal and tongue ulcerations may be noted. The oropharyngeal lesions heal spontaneously in 7 to 10 days. Repeated attacks of herpangina may occur because immunity is only virus-type specific.

Hand-Foot-and-Mouth Disease

Hand-foot-and-mouth disease is highly contagious and often epidemic, spreading by oral-oral and fecal-oral routes. The disease results most commonly from coxsackie A16 virus, but many other enteroviruses have been implicated. Hand-foot-and-mouth disease affects children and young adults most frequently. After an incubation period of 3 to 6 days, a short prodrome, characterized by fever, malaise, and abdominal pain, develops in most patients.

The initial manifestation is ulcerative oral lesions that result in a painful mouth and inability to eat. The number of oral lesions may be as few as 5 or as many as 50, but their presence is the hallmark of the disease and is required to establish the diagnosis. Oral papules, ranging from 1 to 10 mm, progress into vesicles that rupture and form shallow ulcerations with surrounding erythema (Fig. 7-13). Although they may be distributed on any oral mucosal site, they are most frequent on the tongue, buccal mucosa, and palate. In contrast to herpangina, the oral lesions of hand-foot-and-mouth disease are more numerous and larger.

The cutaneous lesions develop concomitantly or, more commonly, shortly after the appearance of oral lesions. They are characterized by small papules and vesicles, often surrounded by erythema. The most common locations involved are the dorsal aspects of the hands and feet, although the volar

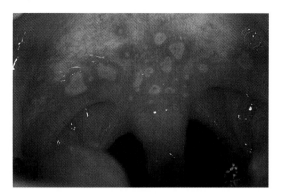

FIG. 7-13   Patients with hand-foot-and-mouth disease develop oral vesicles that rupture, revealing superficial ulcerations. The ulcers are typically larger than those of herpangina.

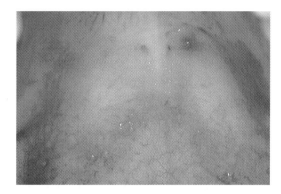

FIG. 7-14   Acute lymphonodular pharyngitis is characterized by the absence of vesicles and the presence of small papules surrounded by erythema on the posterior palate.

surfaces of the hands and feet and the buttocks may less frequently be affected. The oral and cutaneous lesions resolve without treatment in approximately 7 to 10 days.

Acute Lymphonodular Pharyngitis

Acute lymphonodular pharyngitis is an acute and distinct febrile disease resulting predominantly from group A coxsackieviruses that occurs mostly in children with the onset of headache, malaise, and painful sore throat. The oral lesions are characteristic and develop on the uvula, anterior pillars, and oropharynx. Unlike the oral lesions observed in herpangina and hand-foot-and-mouth disease, those of acute lymphonodular pharyngitis do not result in vesicle formation. Rather, the lesions are 3- to 6-mm white or yellow solid papules surrounded by erythema (Fig. 7-14). Microscopically, the nodules represent hyperplastic lymphoid aggregates. Acute lymphonodular pharyngitis is self-limiting and resolves in 10 to 14 days.

RUBEOLA (MEASLES)

Measles represents an acute infection by a paramyxovirus that characteristically develops in winter and spring. Although the incidence has declined significantly since the introduction of vaccines,

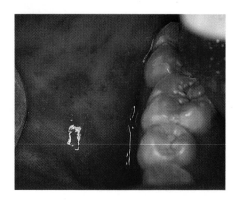

FIG. 7-15   Koplik's spots in rubeola develop on the buccal mucosa opposite lower posterior teeth and are characterized by bright red macules with white-blue centers.

measles continues to be a major health concern in developing nations and occurs sporadically as epidemics in the United States, especially in children of low socioeconomic status who have not been vaccinated. Additionally, the disease occurs in young adults who have been ineffectively vaccinated.

Rubeola is transmitted primarily through the spread of infected respiratory droplets. After a 10- to 14-day incubation period, patients develop fever, malaise, coryza, conjunctivitis, and respiratory symptoms. During this prodrome, pathognomonic oral Koplik's spots develop on the buccal mucosa, adjacent to the posterior teeth. The lesions consist of brightly erythematous macules with a white or blue pinpoint papule in the center (Fig. 7-15). Histologically, the lesions consist of giant cells with nuclear and cytoplasmic inclusions. Koplik's spots generally resolve shortly after the appearance of the cutaneous eruption.

Within several days after the prodrome, an exanthem appears and is characterized by erythematous papules that gradually coalesce. The eruption spreads centripetally from head to foot. Nonspecific oral lesions may accompany the rash and consist of single or coalescing red macules and vesicles on the palate and pharynx. Rubeola infections may also affect odontogenesis and result in enamel hypoplasia and pitting.

The diagnosis of measles is generally made by the characteristic clinical findings, although the virus may be isolated from blood or other tissues, and may be demonstrated in serologic samples in atypical cases.

Uncomplicated measles is self-limiting and lasts approximately 10 days. Infection in immunosuppressed patients may result in complications including pneumonia, encephalitis, and pericarditis.

RUBELLA (GERMAN MEASLES)

Rubella is a mild viral illness caused by a togavirus that is transmitted via respiratory droplets. Like rubeola, the incidence of the disease has declined dramatically as a result of vaccinations. Epidemics still occur, especially in developing countries and usually in the spring. After a 2- to 3-week incubation period, patients develop a prodrome of malaise, fever, anorexia, and nausea. Generalized lymphadenopathy is evident, most frequently affecting the suboccipital, postauricular, and cervical nodes. An exanthem, consisting of red or pink macules and papules, develops on the face and subsequently on the trunk and extremities. The facial lesions resolve first followed by the remainder within 2 to 3 days after their appearance. Intraorally, patients with rubella may exhibit Forscheimer's spots, which consist of tiny dusky-red macules involving the posterior hard palate and soft palate (Fig.

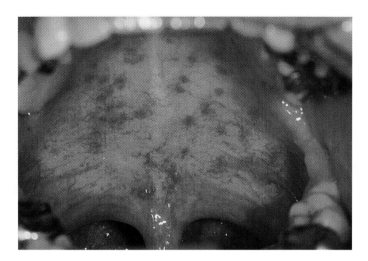

FIG. 7-16   Forsheimer's spots in rubella are characterized by red macules diffusely scattered on the palate.

7-16). These lesions develop at the end of the prodromal stage or at the beginning of the cutaneous eruption.

Congenital rubella may result in numerous abnormalities including hepatitis, encephalitis, heart disease, retinopathy, and osteomyelitis. Oral lesions are usually absent.

The diagnosis may be confused with other viral exanthems. Virus may be isolated from various sources, including blood. Hemagglutination inhibition and serology may be confirmatory. The disease is self-limiting and treatment is palliative. In older patients arthritis may be a complication of rubella.

HUMAN PAPILLOMAVIRUS INFECTIONS

The human papillomaviruses (HPVs) are the causative agents for a large spectrum of epithelial disorders including cutaneous, genital, and mucosal warts. The various types of HPVs can be classified based on the differences in the specific order of their nucleotides. More than 70 different HPV genotypes have been isolated, accounting for the diverse disease patterns resulting from their infection. Patients infected with HIV often develop multiple warts of the oral cavity with unusual HPV types. Specifically, HPV 7, found typically in butcher's warts, and two new HPV types, 72 and 73, have been identified in oral warts from HIV-infected patients, the latter types associated with histologic atypia. HPV has also been associated with the development of epithelial cancers including oral squamous cell carcinomas.

Squamous Papilloma

Squamous papillomas of the oral mucosa are common, comprising 3% of all oral cavity lesions subjected to biopsy. These oral lesions are analogous to papillomas of the esophagus, both having multifactorial origins. HPV types 6 and 11 have been isolated from these lesions, although trauma has also been implicated as an important etiologic factor, especially in cases that fail to identify HPV as a cause.

Squamous papillomas typically arise in adults and occur equally in males and females. Clinically, they are exophytic, sessile, or pedunculated lesions that often display verrucous, fingerlike projections. The lesions may range in color from red to white depending on the degree of surface kera-

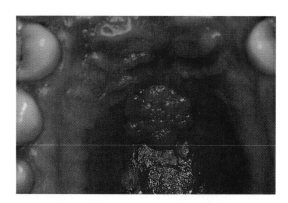

FIG. 7-17 Squamous papilloma of the hard palate resembles a wart but is not always caused by human papillomavirus infection.

tinization (Fig. 7-17). The squamous papilloma is the most common soft-tissue lesion of the tongue and palate and arises on these sites most frequently. The initial growth rate of papillomas is rapid; however, once a size of 0.5 cm is reached, growth generally ceases. Oral squamous papillomas are clinically identical to oral warts, and in many instances the two lesions probably represent the same entity. Although they occur typically as solitary lesions, multiple squamous papillomas may develop and simulate many diseases that display cobblestoning including focal dermal hypoplasia, tuberous sclerosis, and Crohn's disease.

Microscopically, the squamous papilloma consists of a central connective tissue core covered by hyperkeratotic squamous epithelium. The lesion may exhibit increased mitotic activity, which can be mistaken for early dysplasia, especially in incompletely excised lesions.

Squamous papillomas are best treated by surgical excision or by destructive modalities including cryosurgery and electrodesiccation. The recurrence rate is low.

Verruca Vulgaris (Common Wart)

Oral verruca vulgaris is an epithelial hyperplasia that is always virally induced and associated most frequently with HPV types 2, 4, 40, and 57. Although verruca vulgaris is common on the skin, oral mucosal lesions develop much less frequently. Most oral lesions result from autoinoculation from hands and fingers.

Oral verruca vulgaris arises in children much more frequently than in adults invariably because of the high incidence of cutaneous warts on hands and fingers in this age group. The lesions develop at sites of autoinoculation, most commonly the labial mucosa, tongue, and gingiva. Clinically, oral warts are solitary or multiple, asymptomatic, exophytic growths with a roughened or verrucous surface identical to cutaneous warts (Figs. 7-18 and 7-19). The lesions may be pedunculated or sessile and range in color from pink to white. Like squamous papillomas, oral verruca vulgaris grows rapidly and achieves an average size of 0.5 to 1 cm.

Microscopically, verruca vulgaris is characterized by a converging or "cupping" arrangement of the peripheral rete ridges. The stratum granulosum is pronounced, and significant koilocytic changes are present as evidenced by pyknotic nuclei with perinuclear vacuoles and enlarged keratohyaline granules. Viral particles may be detected by electron microscopy, immunoperoxidase staining, or in situ hybridization.

In addition to surgical excision, oral warts respond well to treatments used for cutaneous lesions. These include cryosurgery, electrosurgery, and laser. Multiple treatments may be needed and recurrences are common. Like cutaneous warts, oral lesions will often spontaneously resolve.

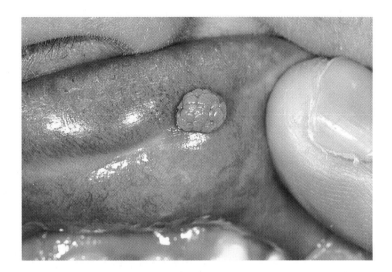

FIG. 7-18   Common verruca vulgaris of the lip.

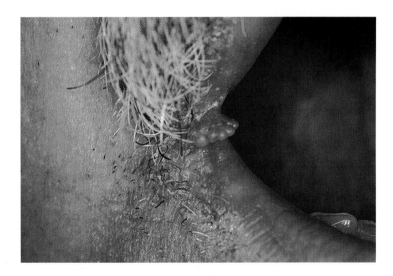

FIG. 7-19   Warts at the lip commissure are generally acquired by autoinoculation from the hands.

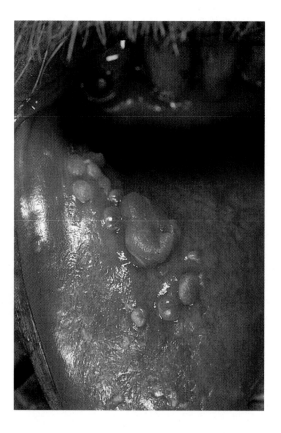

FIG. 7-20   Venereal warts in the oral cavity are most frequently detected on the lower lip and are generally larger than common warts.

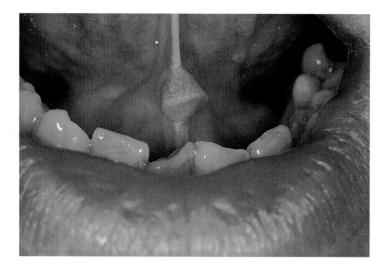

FIG. 7-21   Condyloma accuminatum in the oral cavity frequently develops on the lingual frenulum after oral-genital contact.

Condyloma Acuminatum (Venereal Wart)

Condyloma acuminatum, or genital wart, is the most common sexually transmitted disease. Its occurrence in the oral cavity by autoinoculation or, more commonly, by orogenital sexual transmission has been reported with increasing frequency. Condyloma acuminatum has been associated most often with HPV types 6, 11, 16, and 18.

Condyloma acuminatum develops most frequently in young adults, although it has been reported in all age groups. The presence of oral condyloma acuminatum in an infant or child mandates further investigation to exclude sexual abuse. Oral lesions arise most frequently on the labial mucosa (Fig. 7-20) followed by lingual frenum (Fig. 7-21), soft palate, and gingiva. They present as asymptomatic, pink, pedunculated, or, more frequently, sessile, exophytic cauliflower-like growths. The lesions are frequently multiple rather than solitary. Oral condylomata are typically larger than squamous papillomas or verruca vulgaris, ranging from 1 to 3 cm.

The microscopic features of condyloma acuminatum are the same as other HPV-induced oral lesions with prominent koilocytic changes.

Oral condyloma acuminatum can be treated by surgical excision as well as with cryosurgery, electrosurgery, and laser. The topical application of podophyllin as a 20% solution in tincture of benzoin has been used with variable success. This agent is teratogenic and toxic to the kidneys, the brain, and the myocardium when absorbed in sufficient quantities. As is true of genital warts, the recurrence rate of oral condyloma acuminatum is high; however, by contrast, oral lesions have not been reported to undergo malignant transformation.

Multifocal Papillomavirus Epithelial Hyperplasia (Heck's Disease)

Originally termed *focal epithelial hyperplasia,* the newly suggested name, *multifocal papilloma virus epithelial hyperplasia,* reflects a more accurate description of this distinct clinical entity. The disease represents an infection of the oral mucosa caused by HPV types 13 and 32, both of which occur only in the oral cavity but not exclusively in this disease. Additional HPV types including 6, 11, and 16 have infrequently been identified. Other important etiologic factors include a genetic predisposition, which has been demonstrated by several investigators, and malnutrition, poor hygiene, and crowded living conditions, which may predispose toward infection with viruses. The disease was first described in adult Eskimos and Native American children, but it is now apparent that its occurrence is worldwide.

Multifocal papillomavirus epithelial hyperplasia develops in all groups but predominantly affects children and young adults and females more than males. Oral lesions occur on the lips, buccal

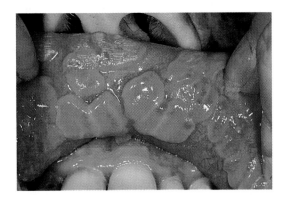

FIG. 7-22   Multiple and confluent fleshy papules of the upper lip in a child with Heck's disease.

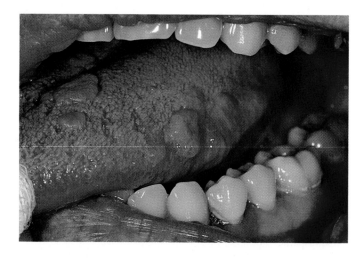

FIG. 7-23 Multifocal papillomavirus epithelial hyperplasia with characteristic display of numerous papules and plaques caused by human papillomavirus infection.

mucosa, and lateral borders of the tongue and rarely elsewhere. The lesions typically manifest as asymptomatic, soft, fleshy papules and plaques and range in color from pink to white. Multiple and confluent lesions are almost always present, and the surface of the lesions may be smooth or papillary (Figs. 7-22 and 7-23). The individual lesions are small, ranging from 2 to 4 mm, but are frequently clustered together, resulting in a cobblestone or fissured appearance of the tissue.

Microscopically, multifocal papillomavirus epithelial hyperplasia is characterized by acanthosis with lateral anastomosing rete ridges. Keratinocyte nuclear abnormalities reflect changes of HPV infection and are diagnostic.

Treatment by excision or other destructive modalities may be performed to improve the cosmetic appearance of visible lesions. Typically, the lesions may be left untreated because diffuse oral involvement makes total eradication difficult, and in most instances multifocal papillomavirus epithelial hyperplasia spontaneously and completely resolves.

SUGGESTED READINGS

General

Laskaris G: Oral manifestations of infectious diseases, *Dent Clin North Am* 40:395, 1996.

Schubert MM: Oral manifestations of viral infections in immunocompromised patients, *Curr Opin Dent* 1:384, 1991.

Scully C et al: Viruses and chronic disorders involving the human oral mucosa, *Oral Surg Oral Med Oral Pathol* 72:537, 1991.

Human herpesviruses

Herpes simplex virus type 1 (HHV-1)

Axéll T, Liedholm R: Occurrence of recurrent herpes labialis in an adult Swedish population, *Acta Odontol Scand* 48:119, 1990.

Epstein JB et al: Clinical study of herpes simplex virus infection in leukemia, *Oral Surg Oral Med Oral Pathol* 70:38, 1990.

Gangarosa LP et al: Iontophoresis for enhancing penetration of dermatologic and antiviral drugs, *J Dermatol* 22:865, 1995.

Gunbay T, Gunbay S, Kandemir S: Herpetic whitlow, *Quintessence Int* 24:363, 1993.

Malouf DJ, Oates RK: Herpes simplex virus infections in the neonate, *J Paediatr Child Health* 31:332, 1995.

Nesbit SP, Gobetti JP: Multiple recurrence of oral erythema multiforme after secondary herpes simplex: report of case and review of literature, *J Am Dent Assoc* 112:348, 1986.

O'Brien JJ, Campoli-Richards DM: Acyclovir: an updated review of its antiviral activity, pharmacokinetic properties and therapeutic efficacy, *Drugs* 37:233, 1989.

Redding SW: Role of herpes simplex virus reactivation in chemotherapy-induced oral mucositis, *NCI Monogr* 9:103, 1990.

Scully C: Orofacial herpes simplex virus infections: current concepts in the epidemiology, pathogenesis, and treatment, and disorders in which the virus may be implicated, *Oral Surg Oral Med Oral Pathol* 68:701, 1989.

Spruance SL: Pathogenesis of herpes simplex labialis: excretion of virus in the oral cavity, *J Clin Microbiol* 19:675, 1984.

Spruance SL et al: The natural history of ultraviolet radiation-induced herpes simplex labialis and response to therapy with perioral and topical formulations of acyclovir, *J Infect Dis* 163:728, 1991.

Taieb A et al: Clinical epidemiology of symptomatic primary herpetic infection in children: a study of 50 cases, *Acta Paediatr Scand* 76:128, 1987.

Weathers DR, Griffin JW: Intraoral ulcerations of recurrent herpes simplex and recurrent aphthae: two distinct clinical entities, *J Am Dent Assoc* 81:81, 1970.

Woo SB, Sonis ST, Sonis AL: The role of herpes simplex virus in the development of oral mucositis in bone marrow transplant recipients, *Cancer* 66:2375, 1990.

Yura Y et al: Recurrent intraoral herpes simplex virus infection, *Int J Oral Maxillofac Surg* 15:457, 1986.

Herpes simplex virus type 2 (HHV-2)

Docherty JJ et al: Lack of oral HSV-2 in a college student population, *J Med Virol* 16:283, 1985.

MacPhail LA et al: Acyclovir-resistant, foscarnet-sensitive oral herpes simplex type 2 lesion in a patient with AIDS, *Oral Surg Oral Med Oral Pathol* 67:427, 1989.

Miller RG et al: Acquisition of concomitant oral and genital infection with herpes simplex virus type 2, *Sex Transm Dis* 14:41, 1987.

Yura Y et al: Herpes simplex virus type 1 and type 2 infection in human oral mucosa in culture, *J Oral Pathol Med* 20:68, 1991.

Varicella-zoster virus (HHV-3)

Arbeter AM et al: Combination measles, mumps, rubella, and varicella vaccine, *Pediatrics* 78:742, 1986.

Badger GR: Oral signs of chickenpox (varicella): report of two cases, *J Dent Child* 47:349, 1980.

Balfour HH Jr et al: Acyclovir halts progression of herpes zoster in immunocompromised patients, *N Engl J Med* 308:1448, 1983.

Barrett AP et al: Zoster sine herpete of the trigeminal nerve, *Oral Surg Oral Med Oral Pathol* 75:173, 1993.

Feldman SR, Ford MJ, Briggaman RA: Herpes zoster and facial paralysis, *Cutis* 42:523, 1988.

McKenzie CD, Gobetti JP: Diagnosis and treatment of orofacial herpes zoster: report of cases, *J Am Dent Assoc* 120:679, 1990.

Mintz SM, Anavi K: Maxillary osteomyelitis and spontaneous tooth exfoliation after herpes zoster, *Oral Surg Oral Med Oral Pathol* 73:664, 1992.

Straus SE et al: Varicella-zoster virus infections: biology, natural history, treatment and prevention, *Ann Intern Med* 108:221, 1988.

Whitley RJ et al: Acyclovir with and without prednisone for the treatment of herpes zoster: a randomized, placebo-controlled trial, *Ann Intern Med* 125:376, 1996.

Epstein-Barr virus (HHV-4)

Felix DH et al: Detection of Epstein-Barr virus and human papilloma virus type 16 in hairy leukoplakia by in situ hybridization and the polymerase chain reaction, *J Oral Pathol Med* 22:277, 1993.

Green TL, Eversole LR: Oral lymphomas in HIV-infected patients: association with Epstein-Barr virus DNA, *Oral Surg Oral Med Oral Pathol* 67:437, 1989.

Murray PG et al: In situ detection of the Epstein-Barr virus-encoded nuclear antigen 1 in oral hairy leukoplakia and virus-associated carcinomas, *J Pathol* 178:44, 1996.

Schmidt-Westhausen A et al: Epstein-Barr virus in lingual epithelium of liver transplant patients, *J Oral Pathol Med* 22:274, 1993.

Cytomegalovirus (HHV-5)

Berman S, Jensen J: Cytomegalovirus-induced osteomyelitis in a patient with the acquired immunodeficiency syndrome, *South Med J* 83:1231, 1990.

Epstein JB, Scully C: Cytomegalovirus: a virus of increasing relevance to oral medicine and pathology, *J Oral Pathol Med* 22:348, 1993.

Epstein JB, Sherlock CH, Wolber RA: Oral manifestations of cytomegalovirus infection, *Oral Surg Oral Med Oral Pathol* 75:443, 1993.

French PD, Birchall MA, Harris JRW: Cytomegalovirus ulceration of the oropharynx, *J Laryngol Otol* 105:739, 1991.

Greenberg MS et al: Relationship of oral disease to the presence of cytomegalovirus DNA in the saliva of AIDS patients, *Oral Surg Oral Med Oral Pathol* 79:175, 1995.

Jones AC et al: Cytomegalovirus infections of the oral cavity: a report of six cases and review of the literature, *Oral Surg Oral Med Oral Pathol* 75:76, 1993.

Kanas RJ et al: Oral mucosal cytomegalovirus as a manifestation of the acquired immune deficiency syndrome, *Oral Surg Oral Med Oral Pathol* 64:183, 1987.

Langford A et al: Cytomegalovirus associated oral ulcerations in HIV-infected patients, *J Oral Pathol Med* 19:71, 1990.

Leimola-Virtanen R, Happonen RP, Syrjanen S: Cytomegalovirus (CMV) and *Helicobacter pylori* (HP) found in oral mucosal ulcers, *J Oral Pathol Med* 24:14, 1995.

Liang GS et al: An evaluation of oral ulcers in patients with AIDS and AIDS-related complex, *J Am Acad Dermatol* 29:563, 1993.

Schubert MM et al: Oral infections due to cytomegalovirus in immunocompromised patients, *J Oral Pathol Med* 22:268, 1993.

Stagno S et al: Congenital and perinatal cytomegalovirus infections: clinical characteristics and pathogenic factors, *Birth Defects* 20:65, 1984.

Enteroviruses

Asano Y, Yoshikawa T: Enterovirus infections in children, *Curr Opin Pediatr* 7:24, 1995.

Cherry JD, Nelson DB: Enterovirus infections: their epidemiology and pathogenesis, *Clin Pediatr* 5:659, 1966.

Herpangina

Yamadera S et al: Herpangina surveillance in Japan, 1982-1989, *Jpn J Med Sci Biol* 44:29, 1991.

Hand-foot-and-mouth disease

Bendig JW, Fleming DM: Epidemiological, virological, and clinical features of an epidemic of hand, foot, and mouth disease in England and Wales, *Commun Dis Rep CDR Rev* 6:81, 1996.

Buchner A: Hand, foot, and mouth disease, *Oral Surg Oral Med Oral Pathol* 41:333, 1976.

Higgins PG, Warin RP: Hand, foot, and mouth disease: a clinically recognizable virus infection seen mainly in children, *Clin Pediatr* 6:373, 1967.

Thomas I, Janniger CK: Hand, foot, and mouth disease, *Cutis* 52:265, 1993.

Tindall JP, Callaway JL: Hand-foot-mouth disease—it's more common than you think, *Am J Dis Child* 124:372, 1972.

Acute lymphonodular pharyngitis

Steigman AJ, Lipton MM, Braspennickx H: Acute lymphonodular pharyngitis: a newly described condition due to coxsackie virus, *J Pediatr* 61:331, 1962.

Rubeola (measles)

Markel H, Koplik H: The Good Samaritan Dispensary of New York City, and the description of Koplik's spots, *Arch Pediatr Adolesc Med* 150:535, 1996.

Rubella (German measles)

Arbeter AM et al: Combination measles, mumps, rubella, and varicella vaccine, *Pediatrics* 78:742, 1986.

Human papillomavirus infections

Garlick JA, Taichman LB: Human papillomavirus infection of the oral mucosa, *Am J Dermatopathol* 13:386, 1991.

Squamous papilloma

Abbey LM, Page DG, Sawyer DR: The clinical and histopathologic features of a series of 464 oral squamous cell papillomas, *Oral Surg Oral Med Oral Pathol* 49:419, 1980.

Batsakis JG, Raymond AK, Rice DH: The pathology of head and neck tumors: papillomas of the upper aerodigestive tract, part 18, *Head Neck* 5:332, 1983.

Bouquot JE, Gundlach KKH: Oral exophytic lesions in 23,616 white Americans over 35 years of age, *Oral Surg Oral Med Oral Pathol* 62:284, 1986.

Verruca vulgaris (common wart)

Adler-Storthz K et al: Identification of human papillomavirus types in oral verruca vulgaris, *J Oral Pathol* 15:230, 1986.

Eversole LR, Laipis PJ, Green TL: Human papillomavirus type 2 DNA in oral and labial verruca vulgaris, *J Cutan Pathol* 14:319, 1987.

Green TL, Eversole LR, Leider AS: Oral and labial verruca vulgaris: clinical, histologic, and immunohistochemical evaluation, *Oral Surg Oral Med Oral Pathol* 62:410, 1986.

Premoli-de-Percoco G et al: Detection of human papillomavirus-related oral verruca vulgaris among Venezuelans, *J Oral Pathol Med* 22:113, 1993.

Condyloma acuminatum (venereal wart)

Barone R et al: Prevalence of oral lesions among HIV-infected intravenous drug abusers and other risk groups, *Oral Surg Oral Med Oral Pathol* 69:169, 1990.

Butler S et al: Condyloma acuminatum in the oral cavity: four cases and a review, *Rev Infect Dis* 10:544, 1988.

Emmanouil DE, Post AC: Oral condyloma acuminatum in a child: case report, *Pediatr Dent* 9:232, 1987.

Greenspan D et al: Unusual HPV types in oral warts in association with HIV infection, *J Oral Pathol* 17:482, 1988.

Malik PA et al: Condyloma acuminatum of the tongue, *Ann Plast Surg* 10:417, 1983.

Panici PB et al: Oral condyloma lesions in patients with extensive genital human papillomavirus infection, *Am J Obstet Gynecol* 167:451, 1992.

Silverman S Jr et al: Oral findings in people with or at high risk for AIDS: a study of 375 homosexual males, *J Am Dent Assoc* 112:187, 1986.

Zunt SL, Tomich CE: Oral condyloma acuminatum, *J Dermatol Surg* 15:591, 1989.

Multifocal papillomavirus epithelial hyperplasia (Heck's disease)

Bon A, Eichmann A, Grob R: Focal epithelial hyperplasia, *Dermatology* 184:294, 1992.

Carlos R, Sedano HO: Multifocal papilloma virus epithelial hyperplasia, *Oral Surg Oral Med Oral Pathol* 77:631, 1994.

Cohen PR, Hebert AA, Adler-Storthz K: Focal epithelial hyperplasia: Heck disease, *Pediatr Dermatol* 10:245, 1993.

Harris AM, van Wyk CW: Heck's disease (focal epithelial hyperplasia): a longitudinal study, *Community Dent Oral Epidemiol* 21:82, 1993.

Morrow DJ, Sandhu HS, Daley TD: Focal epithelial hyperplasia (Heck's disease) with generalized lesions of the gingiva: a case report, *J Periodontol* 64:63, 1993.

Padayachee A, van Wyk CW: Human papillomavirus (HPV) DNA in focal epithelial hyperplasia by *in situ* hybridization, *J Oral Pathol Med* 20:210, 1991.

Tan AK et al: Focal epithelial hyperplasia, *Otolaryngol Head Neck Surg* 112:316, 1995.

Vilmer C et al: Focal epithelial hyperplasia and multifocal human papillomavirus infection in an HIV-seropositive man, *J Am Acad Dermatol* 30:497, 1994.

CHAPTER 8

Fungal Infections

CANDIDIASIS

Candidiasis, synonymously termed *candidosis*, is the most common infection of the oral cavity with the exception of dental caries and periodontal disease. *Moniliasis* is an old and inaccurate term that has been abandoned. Most cases of oral candidiasis are caused by *Candida albicans*, although a large number of species of yeasts may be found intraorally. These include *C. tropicalis, C. krusei, C. parapsilosis,* and *C. guilliermondii,* which are occasionally associated with oral infections, especially in immunocompromised patients.

Candida is a component of the normal oral microflora, which can be isolated in up to one half of otherwise asymptomatic, healthy individuals. The development of an oral infection caused by *Candida* species depends on a complex interaction between the pathogenicity of the organism and the defense mechanism of the host. Cytologic, biochemical, and genetic assessments of oral clinical isolates have revealed that *C. albicans* switches frequently and reversibly between a number of general phenotypes that may affect pathogenicity. The change from budding yeast phase to hyphal form generally implies ensuing infection. Tissue invasion may also be assisted by secreted hydrolytic enzymes and contact sensing displayed by candidal hyphae. The adherence of *Candida* to epithelial cells of the oral cavity may also be a function of host-cell–related and yeast-related factors. Oral candidiasis results from yeast overgrowth and penetration of the oral tissues when the physical and immunologic defenses of the host have been compromised. Predisposing factors for colonization and infection by these opportunistic pathogens include systemic infections; diabetes and other endocrine dysfunctions; congenital or acquired defective immunity (especially patients with acquired immunodeficiency syndrome [AIDS], leukemia, and organ and bone marrow transplants); malignancy; infancy; pregnancy; vitamin deficiencies and malnourishment; denture wearing; antibiotic, corticosteroid, and immunosuppressive use; and radiotherapy. Undoubtedly, *C. albicans* is responsible for the majority of all fungal infections among immunocompromised patients and is the most common cause of septicemia. Although certain *Candida* strains exhibit resistance to host-clearing mechanisms, it is the host's immune competence that ultimately determines whether infection occurs.

Oral candidiasis can manifest in a variety of clinical forms, and the wide diversity can make diagnosis difficult. The most widely recognized pattern is acute pseudomembranous candidiasis or thrush. Although classically observed in infants, patients taking broad-spectrum antibiotics, and debilitated geriatric individuals, pseudomembranous candidiasis is currently detected with great frequency in individuals who are severely immunosuppressed as a result of human immunodeficiency virus (HIV) infection, leukemia, and systemic chemotherapy. The oral infection is characterized by the development of localized or generalized, loosely adherent white patches and plaques resembling cottage cheese or curdled milk on any or all mucosal surfaces (Figs. 8-1 to 8-3). The white lesions are composed of fungal hyphae, yeasts, desquamated epithelial cells, and debris. Typically, pseudomembranous candidiasis can be removed by scraping the mucosa with a blunt instrument or rubbing with gauze, revealing, in most cases, an erythematous base. A bleeding or ulcerated base is distinctly uncommon. Patients may complain of generalized stomatopyrosis and stomatodynia as

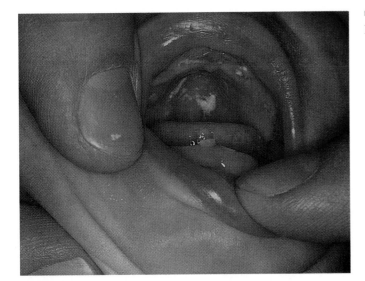

FIG. 8-1 Thrush on the palate of a newborn.

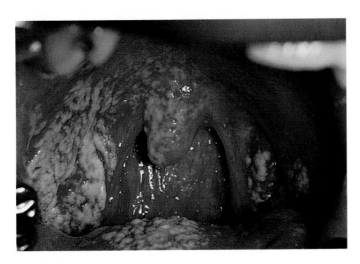

FIG. 8-2 Extensive pseudomembranous candidiasis commonly observed in immunocompromised patients.

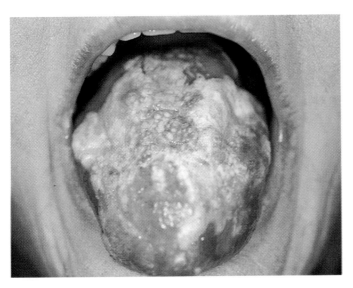

FIG. 8-3 Pseudomembranous candidiasis developing in a diabetic patient.

well as dysgeusia. Frequently the breath of infected individuals has a characteristic "yeasty" odor.

Erythematous candidiasis refers to a general category of oral candidiasis that encompasses a variety of clinical forms including acute atrophic candidiasis, median rhomboid glossitis, chronic multifocal candidiasis, angular cheilitis, and chronic atrophic candidiasis. All of these variants share the absence of superficial, white, curdlike colonies on the oral mucosa and the presence of focal or diffuse areas of erythema with variable symptomatology.

Acute atrophic candidiasis (antibiotic sore mouth) is a frequent complication of broad-spectrum antibiotic use (Fig. 8-4). Patients display diffuse erythema of the oral mucosa, often accompanied by atrophy of the filiform papillae on the dorsal surface of the tongue. The lesions are painful and burning.

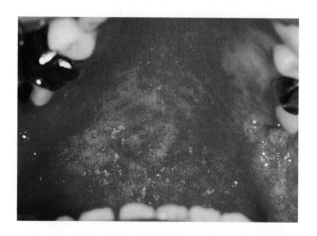

FIG. 8-4 Erythematous candidiasis of the palate developing after a course of antibiotics.

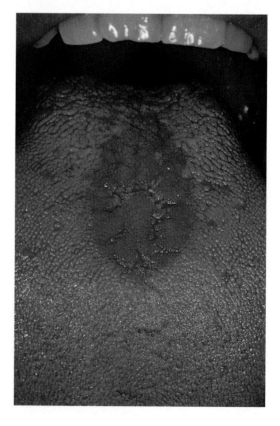

FIG. 8-5 Median rhomboid glossitis characterized by an erythematous, smooth plaque on the dorsal surface of the tongue.

Median rhomboid glossitis was previously thought to result from faulty involution of the tuberculum impar at the junction of the anterior two thirds and posterior one third of the tongue. Because this lesion has never been reported in children, the developmental defect theory seems unlikely. Furthermore, *C. albicans* can be consistently demonstrated microscopically from biopsied lesions. This form of localized chronic atrophic candidiasis also occurs more frequently in patients with AIDS. Median rhomboid glossitis clinically appears as a diamond- or oval-shaped, erythematous, depapillated area on the posterior dorsal tongue, always arising anterior to the circumvallate papillae (Fig. 8-5). The surface of the lesion may be smooth or lobulated. Without therapy the lesion frequently resolves spontaneously, but in most cases it remains unchanged and asymptomatic.

Chronic multifocal candidiasis represents a variant of median rhomboid glossitis. Multiple areas of atrophic candidiasis, characterized by red patches and plaques, develop most frequently on the posterior dorsal tongue, at the junction of the hard and soft palates, and in the corners of the mouth. The palatal lesions may result from inoculation from the dorsal surface of the tongue.

Angular cheilitis or perlèche may develop as a result of multiple causes including vitamin deficiencies (see Chapter 12) and candidal infections. When angular cheilitis is caused by *Candida,* it usually occurs in patients with ill-fitting dentures who have lost facial vertical dimension or who habitually lick the corners of their lips. These predisposing conditions allow saliva to collect in the creases and corners of the mouth. As *Candida* proliferates in the constantly moist environment, maceration, fissuring, erythema, and erosions develop at the commissures (Fig. 8-6). Frequently, patients with angular cheilitis have a superimposed bacterial infection, usually *Staphylococcus aureus.*

Chronic atrophic candidiasis may be the most frequently occurring form of oral candidiasis. Affected individuals present with varying degrees of erythema restricted to the denture-bearing areas of the mucosa (Fig. 8-7). In almost all cases the reddened lesions are asymptomatic and result from the continuous wearing of dentures without removing them while sleeping. In addition, patients who exhibit poor denture hygiene are predisposed toward the development of candidiasis. In the majority of cases denture stomatitis (see Chapter 3) is caused by *Candida* and represents chronic atrophic candidiasis, although it may also result from a hypersensitivity reaction to a component of the denture acrylic or acrylic monomer released from poorly processed dentures. In contrast to chronic atrophic candidiasis, these reactive processes cause pain and acute inflammation of the adjacent mucosa.

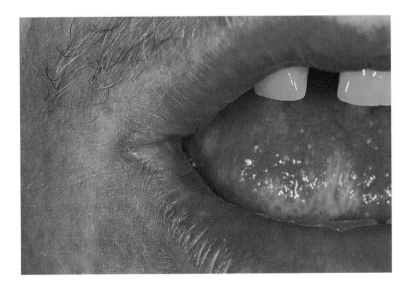

FIG. 8-6   Angular cheilitis with erythema, maceration, and fissuring at the lip commissure.

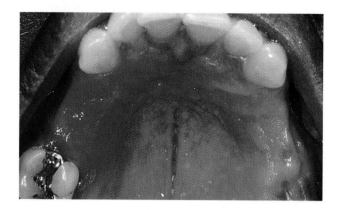

FIG. 8-7   Chronic atrophic candidiasis developing on the denture-bearing oral mucosa.

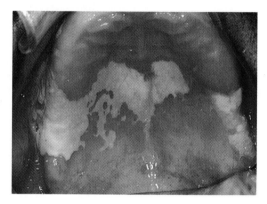

FIG. 8-8   Well-demarcated, thick plaques of candidal leukoplakia.

Chronic hyperplastic candidiasis or candidal leukoplakia is unique among the forms of oral candidiasis in that the plaques cannot be easily scraped or rubbed off. The lesions are generally well-demarcated, white, thick, or verrucous plaques that develop most frequently on the anterior buccal mucosa and palate (Fig. 8-8). Clinically they resemble leukoplakia and often reveal atypia histologically, especially when accompanied by areas of erythema. There is controversy as to whether the dysplastic changes observed in chronic hyperplastic candidiasis are caused by *Candida* colonizing and infecting a preexisting plaque of leukoplakia or *Candida* inducing the development of leukoplakia. Even when *Candida* is isolated from such plaques, care must be taken to ensure the complete resolution of these lesions with therapy.

Chronic mucocutaneous candidiasis encompasses a heterogenous group of clinical diseases that are characterized by chronic candidal infections of the skin, nails, and mucous membranes. In the majority of patients, immunologic abnormalities may be demonstrated, although the magnitude and pathogenesis of the immunologic defect vary considerably. Several types of chronic mucocutaneous candidiasis may be familial and present during early childhood. A diverse group of abnormalities may accompany chronic mucocutaneous candidiasis including significant viral, bacterial, and other fungal infections as well as ectodermal, gastrointestinal, and hematologic disorders. In general, the oral signs and symptoms of candidal infections parallel the severity of the immunologic defect. Early lesions resemble pseudomembranous plaques, whereas chronic lesions are more verrucous and extensive, similar to hyperplastic candidiasis, but cover much of the oral cavity surfaces (Fig. 8-9). Cutaneous crusted lesions appear on the face and scalp, and nail involvement is characterized by severe

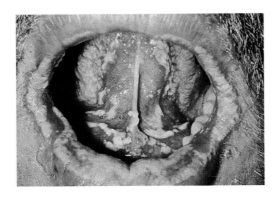

FIG. 8-9   Thick, verrucous, and widespread candidal plaques are typically observed in patients with chronic mucocutaneous candidiasis.

Table 8-1   Chronic Mucocutaneous Candidiasis (CMC)

TYPE	INHERITANCE	ORAL INVOLVEMENT	ASSOCIATED FINDINGS
Localized CMC	Sporadic	Mild and patchy	Pulmonary infections, esophagitis
Diffuse CMC	Autosomal recessive	Severe and diffuse, perlèche	Candidal blepharitis, pharyngitis, laryngitis, cutaneous granulomas
	Sporadic	Severe and diffuse, perlèche	Above features and bacterial infections, iron deficiency anemia
CMC with endocrinopathy	Autosomal recessive	Severe and diffuse, degree of endocrine abnormalities; enamel hypoplasia	Numerous autoimmune diseases; pernicious anemia, gonadal failure, diabetes, thyroid disease, vitiligo, Addison's disease
CMC with thymoma	Sporadic	Mild to moderate	Myasthenia gravis, polymyositis, hypogammaglobulinemia, aplastic anemia

dystrophy and thickening with paronychial infections. Dental abnormalities and enamel hypoplasia are a result of the defect in ectodermal development. Candidiasis endocrinopathy syndrome is a distinct form of chronic mucocutaneous candidiasis that occurs in association with hypofunction of multiple organs including the thyroid, parathyroid, adrenal cortex, and pancreas. Chronic candidal infection of the oral cavity is often the initial presenting feature of many of these disorders, and endocrinopathies may not manifest for many years, although the sequence may also be reversed. Table 8-1 summarizes the features of some of the chronic mucocutaneous candidiasis syndromes and their related oral abnormalities.

The clinical diagnosis of oral candidiasis should be confirmed by laboratory tests and can be accomplished by one of several methods. The most common procedure involves digestion of an exfoliative cytologic preparation with 10% potassium hydroxide (KOH). The demonstration of pseudo-hyphae or budding cells provides evidence that fungi consistent with the morphology of *Candida* are present. Rapid latex agglutination-based tests, developed and approved for use in vulvovaginal candidiasis, are useful in confirming oral candidal infections. Definitive identification of the organism is accomplished by culture grown on Sabouraud's dextrose agar. Species identification requires subculturing the yeast to identify morphologic and biochemical characteristics. Speciation can also be accomplished through the use of kits that differentiate species on the basis of carbohydrate fermentation. The clinical diagnosis of candidal leukoplakia often requires a biopsy for confirmation, which can be stained with periodic acid-Schiff (PAS) for visualizing *Candida* species.

In immunocompetent patients the main treatments for oral candidiasis are topical preparations of nystatin, amphotericin B, miconazole, and clotrimazole. Topical therapy necessitates sufficient contact between the drug and oral mucosa. Nystatin, a polyene antibiotic that has been in use for more than 40 years, is available as a suspension (100,000 units/ml) or licorice-flavored pastille (200,000 units/ml) for the treatment of oral candidiasis. Nystatin has an inherently bitter taste, which is masked with sucrose. As such, the suspension, which contains 50% sucrose, should not be selected for use in diabetics or those at high risk for dental caries. Dermatologic and gynecologic formulations of nystatin do not contain appreciable amounts of sugar, although they too have objectionable tastes and may be administered with sugar-free gum. Nystatin creams or ointments may be used for the treatment of angular cheilitis, and the powder form may be applied to the trauma-bearing surfaces of dentures. Because nystatin is not well absorbed from the gastrointestinal tract, side effects are unusual. Amphotericin B, as cream or lotion intended for cutaneous use, may be applied topically or as a swish using a diluted systemic intravenous solution. Clotrimazole troches, 10 mg, may be dissolved five times a day in the oral cavity. Nausea and vomiting are infrequent complications, and absorbed clotrimazole loses efficacy with continued administration because of induction of liver microsomal enzymes. Clotrimazole also contains dextrose, which is cariogenic. Miconazole oral gel is available in Europe but not in the United States. Chlorhexidine, an antibacterial mouth rinse, may be used as a prophylactic agent in the prevention of oral candidiasis in patients undergoing bone marrow transplantation.

Systemic therapy with the azole compounds may be required in patients who do not respond to topical therapy or those with widespread infection. Ketoconazole, 200 mg a day for 2 weeks, is generally effective, although higher doses are required for immunocompromised patients. Fluconazole produces a more rapid response at daily doses of 100 mg for 1 week. Similarly, itraconazole at doses of 100 mg daily for 1 to 3 weeks results in clinical improvement, although the response is slower than that achieved by fluconazole. Fluconazole- and ketoconazole-resistant *Candida* isolates are increasing in AIDS patients, presumably as a result of the chronic administration of these drugs as prophylactic agents against oral candidiasis. Although factors such as diminishing cellular immunity, drug interactions, or decreased drug absorption may account for some treatment failures, it is likely that *Candida* organisms are developing drug resistance. Continuous prophylactic therapy with topical or systemic antifungal agents for oral candidiasis in HIV-positive patients should be substituted with intermittent therapy for active infections. A careful drug history should be obtained before administering azole antifungal medications because of numerous potential drug interactions with these agents. In addition to systemic therapy, patients with chronic mucocutaneous candidiasis may be treated with *Candida*-specific transfer factor, which may induce long periods of remission.

The use of topical antifungal agents in the prevention of candidiasis in patients undergoing chemotherapy or bone marrow transplantation is controversial because they may be ineffective. However, the use of systemic agents in this population group is justified in preventing septicemia. In general, correction of the predisposing factors that resulted in oral infection is as important as the specific therapeutic agent. For example, replacement of poorly fitting dentures, control of elevated blood glucose levels in diabetics, and altering antibiotic therapy may all have a significant impact on therapeutic outcome. Persistent or unexplained relapses of candidiasis should prompt an evaluation for systemic diseases that result in immunosuppression.

OPPORTUNISTIC FUNGAL INFECTIONS

The emergence of newly identified fungal pathogens and the reemergence of previously uncommon fungal infections are primarily the result of the increased number of susceptible individuals. HIV-infected patients, bone marrow and organ transplant recipients, cancer patients treated with chemotherapy, and very low–birth-weight infants constitute an immunosuppressed population that is extremely vulnerable to opportunistic fungal infections. The oral cavity is a frequent site of involvement and commonly represents the initial or primary manifestation of a fungal infection. Fungi, once believed to represent contamination or harmless colonization when isolated from the oral cavity of immunosuppressed patients, are now considered pathogenic and a significant cause of morbidity and mortality. Specifically, fungi such as *Fusarium* species, *Trichosporon* species, and *Torulopsis* species are emerging pathogens that may invade the oral mucosa during periods of immunosuppression. Dissemination of opportunistic fungal infections to the oral cavity is common in diseases such as zygomycosis, aspergillosis, and cryptococcosis. Furthermore, immunocompromised patients are at risk for infections with pathogens that usually infect otherwise healthy individuals not previously exposed to endemic fungi such as *Histoplasma capsulatum, Paracoccidioides brasiliensis,* and *Blastomyces dermatitidis.* In general, the oral infections are clinically characterized by irregularly large, persistent, verrucous, and necrotic ulcerations often covered by black or necrotic debris (Figs. 8-10 and 8-11). The presence of oral cavity lesions indicates dissemination of the infection, which

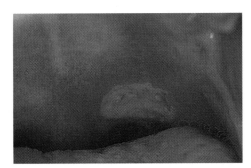

FIG. 8-10   Chronic ulceration of the palate caused by *Fusarium* in a bone marrow transplant patient.

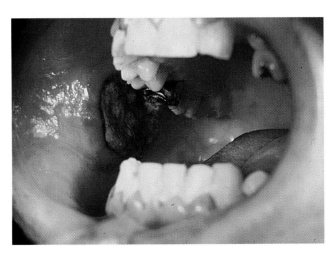

FIG. 8-11   Large, irregular necrotic ulceration caused by *Trichosporon,* an emerging pathogen in immunosuppressed patients.

necessitates early diagnosis and institution of aggressive antifungal therapy. The oral azole drugs, namely, ketoconazole, fluconazole, and itraconazole, represent a major advance in systemic antifungal therapy and are effective alternatives to amphotericin B and flucytosine for selected systemic mycoses. Ketoconazole and itraconazole may be used to treat blastomycosis, coccidioidomycosis, and histoplasmosis; and fluconazole can be used to treat cryptococcosis and serious candida syndromes. Itraconazole is the most effective azole-based drug for treating aspergillosis. Despite these advances, mortality rates in affected patients are still high.

Histoplasmosis

H. capsulatum is the causative agent of histoplasmosis, the most common systemic fungal infection in the United States. Like *C. albicans, H. capsulatum* is dimorphic, growing as a yeast in humans and as a mold in the environment living in soil, particularly in association with bird droppings and bat guano. Histoplasmosis has a worldwide distribution and is endemic in the Ohio and Mississippi River valleys in the United States, where inhaled spores germinate in the lungs. Epidemiology studies in endemic areas indicate that up to 90% of the population has been exposed to the organism and display positive histoplasmin skin tests.

In most cases, primary pulmonary histoplasmosis is either subclinical or resembles a mild, nonspecific flulike illness. In healthy individuals the severity of symptoms is proportional to the number of spores inhaled. Individuals who inhale a large inoculum experience acute histoplasmosis characterized by fever, headache, anorexia, and cough. These flulike symptoms are self-limiting. Chronic histoplasmosis develops in patients who have underlying pulmonary disease, such as emphysema, and in geriatric and immunosuppressed individuals. The clinical manifestations of chronic histoplasmosis are similar to those observed in tuberculosis and include fever, weight loss, weakness, fatigue, dyspnea, cough, and hemoptysis. Pulmonary radiographs reveal superior lobe infiltrates, often with cavitation. Disseminated histoplasmosis is a rare complication of both acute and chronic infections. It is most commonly seen in extremely debilitated or immunosuppressed patients, occurring in up to 10% of patients with AIDS. Disseminated histoplasmosis may affect the liver, spleen, lymph nodes, adrenal glands, central nervous system, and kidneys and is an AIDS-defining infection.

The oral mucosa is a frequent site of involvement and becomes infected in approximately 30% to 50% of patients with disseminated histoplasmosis. The oral lesions may be the primary or solitary manifestation of the disease, especially in patients with AIDS. The lesions have no distinctive features and may appear as nodules, papules, or, most commonly, persistent, deep, and vegetative ulcerations (Fig. 8-12). On palpation the ulcers are consistently indurated and often have rolled bor-

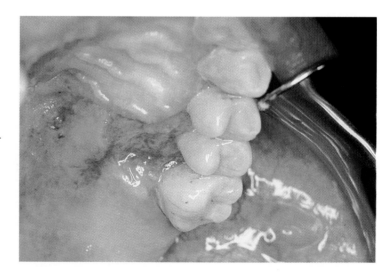

FIG. 8-12   Histoplasmosis of the palate characterized by an irregular, deep ulceration.

ders, which can lead to confusion with squamous cell carcinoma. The lesions have been reported in all oral sites but arise most frequently on the tongue, palate, and buccal mucosa. Focal or multiple sites may be involved.

Microscopically, oral lesions of histoplasmosis exhibit multinucleated giant cells and granulomatous inflammation. The organisms may be more apparent with either PAS or Gomori's methenamine-silver stains. *H. capsulatum* can also be cultured, although growth may take 6 weeks. Exposure to the organism can be confirmed serologically using complement fixation antibodies and immunodiffusion tests.

Acute histoplasmosis requires only palliative care. Untreated chronic histoplasmosis may result in significant pulmonary damage with a 20% fatality rate. Disseminated histoplasmosis, despite aggressive antifungal therapy, has a mortality rate approximating 25%. Ketoconazole, itraconazole, and intravenous amphotericin B are the drugs of choice for chronic and disseminated forms of the disease.

Zygomycosis (Mucormycosis, Phycomycosis)

Zygomycosis is an acute and often lethal opportunistic fungal infection caused by a number of organisms, most commonly *Absidia, Mucor, Cunninghamella,* and *Rhizopus.* These organisms are ubiquitous and can be cultured from the oral cavity in healthy persons. Poorly controlled insulin-dependent diabetics and immunocompromised individuals, especially patients with hematologic malignancies and AIDS, are predisposed toward infection with these organisms.

Zygomycosis may involve a number of anatomic sites. The rhinocerebral form is the most common presentation and occurs predominantly in patients with diabetic ketoacidosis. Infected patients often exhibit nasal obstruction, headache, facial pain and swelling, cellulitis, bloody nasal discharge, and proptosis with visual impairment. Frequently there is involvement of the maxillary sinus with concomitant intraoral swelling. Almost all cases of oral zygomycosis display palatal ulceration with the formation of an oral-antral fistula (Fig. 8-13). Occasionally the infection may involve other oral structures including the mandibular gingiva, buccal mucosa, and lips and may occur as ulcerated nodules. Untreated disease frequently spreads to the orbit and brain, resulting in death.

The microscopic appearance of the organisms that cause zygomycosis is characterized by broad, nonseptate hyphae that exhibit obtuse or right-angle branching. These distinctive hyphae can be visualized in biopsy sections with PAS or methenamine-silver stains. The pathologic hallmark of infection is hyphal invasion of blood vessels resulting in vascular thrombosis, infarction of tissues, and ischemic necrosis.

Early diagnosis and improved therapy of zygomycosis have resulted in improved survival. Treat-

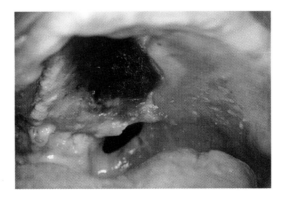

FIG. 8-13   Palatal necrotic ulceration and perforation are the most common oral presentations of zygomycosis.

ment consists of extensive surgical débridement combined with intravenous amphotericin B and correction of the underlying immunosuppression. When the disease occurs in healthy patients without predisposing factors, the lesions are often limited and the infection is more readily controlled.

Paracoccidioidomycosis (South American Blastomycosis)

Paracoccidioidomycosis is an opportunistic systemic mycosis that occurs predominantly in Colombia, Venezuela, Uruguay, Argentina, and particularly in Brazil. The disease is caused by *P. brasiliensis,* a saprophyte of soil or decaying vegetation. The disease usually affects adult Hispanic men with low income occupations who work outdoors. The infection is acquired through the respiratory tract and spreads hematogenously. The oral cavity is probably the most frequent initial site of involvement and often the first manifestation of the disease. Skin lesions on the face, characterized by pustules and subcutaneous abscesses, are also common at presentation. Oral lesions are painful, chronic, proliferative nodules or ulcerations that sometimes display a characteristic mulberry-like appearance with pinpoint hemorrhages. The majority of patients exhibit multiple lesions that develop most frequently on the alveolar mucosa, gingiva, and palate (Fig. 8-14). Lesions on the tongue or floor of the mouth are uncommon. Oral lesions spread to cervical lymphatics, resulting in characteristic massively enlarged lymph nodes. Pulmonary involvement can usually be detected radiographically at the time of diagnosis of the oral infection. Dissemination to bone, adrenal glands, central nervous system, and spleen can result in serious complications.

Histologically, oral lesions display a suppurative granuloma with giant cells accompanied by prominent acanthosis and occasionally, pseudoepitheliomatous hyperplasia. The fungus blastospores appear as double contoured buds, often surrounded by daughter spores, which can be visualized in- side giant cells with the aid of PAS or methenamine-silver stains. Detection of the fungus from di- rect smears of oral lesions with serologic investigations including immunodiffusion, counterimmunoelectrophoresis, and immunoblot may preclude the need for biopsy in diagnosing paracoccidioidomycosis. The diagnosis can also be established by the isolation and identification of the causative organism, although *P. brasiliensis* grows extremely slowly.

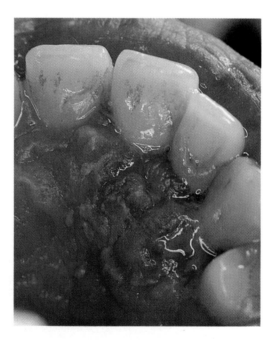

FIG. 8-14   Chronic, proliferative ulceration with pinpoint hemorrhages of the alveolar mucosa and palate is the most common presentation of paracoccidioidomycosis.

Mortality from paracoccidioidomycosis has been greatly diminished with early treatment using a number of antimicrobial agents including amphotericin B, ketoconazole, and itraconazole.

Aspergillosis

Aspergillus species are ubiquitous and can be detected in soil, water, and decaying vegetation. Infection occurs predominantly in the respiratory route, although numerous other locations including the cornea, auditory canal, gastrointestinal tract, nasopharynx, and skin may be the primary site of infection. Invasive fungal disease develops in predisposed patients who exhibit immunosuppression. Profound neutropenia and corticosteroid therapy, especially in leukemia and bone marrow transplant patients, are the greatest risk factors, although a dramatic increase in the number of cases has been recorded in AIDS patients.

The most common clinical manifestation of the disease is pneumonia that is unresponsive to antibiotics. Hemoptysis is common, as the organism tends to invade blood vessels. Other presentations include sinusitis, which can progress to adjacent structures including the brain. Aspergillosis is the second most frequent orofacial fungal infection in patients receiving chemotherapy exceeded only by candidiasis. The oral infection may be primary or, less commonly, secondary through dissemination. Oral lesions may appear in one of several forms. In the early stage the isolated oral mucosal surfaces affected may be violaceous and consist of degenerated epithelium and connective tissue. In advanced lesions, large and necrotic ulcerations, which are often covered by black eschars as a result of thrombotic vascular infarction, may be observed (Fig. 8-15). Destruction of the underlying alveolar bone and surrounding facial muscles is typical of the late stages of invasive oral aspergillosis. The gingiva is the most frequent site of involvement followed by the palate.

Definitive diagnosis of invasive aspergillosis requires the demonstration of the organism in tissue by histopathology in addition to a positive culture. Special stains such as Gridley, methenamine-silver, or PAS may be required to visualize the fungi, which appear as septate hyphae, dichotomously branched at acute angles. Potassium hydroxide preparations, which indicate the presence of a large number of organisms, may be obtained from oral lesions.

The treatment of choice for aspergillosis is early aggressive systemic antifungal therapy with amphotericin B and surgical resection of the involved tissue. Itraconazole and liposomal amphotericin preparations are promising new treatments, although resolution of the underlying neutropenia or predisposing factors may be as important in eradicating the infection. Because the majority of oral aspergillosis begins with the gingiva, improvement of oral hygiene may prevent infection.

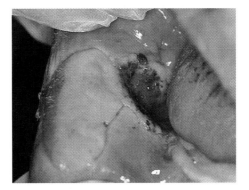

FIG. 8-15   Aspergillosis. A typical, large ulceration partially covered by a black eschar, which develops as a result of vascular infarction.

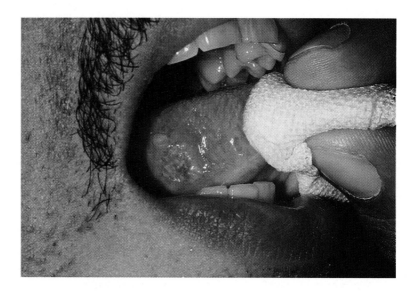

FIG. 8-16   Cryptococcosis of the tongue appears most frequently as a persistent, ulcerated nodule and resembles squamous cell carcinoma. (From Lynch DP, Naftolin LZ: *Oral Surg Oral Med Oral Pathol* 64:449, 1987.)

Cryptococcosis

Cryptococcosis is an opportunistic systemic disease caused by the yeast *Cryptococcus neoformans.* Cryptococcosis is the most common life-threatening fungal infection in AIDS, developing in approximately 10% of patients. It is especially common among AIDS patients who are black, male, or injecting drug users. The organism is acquired by the respiratory route, resulting in an asymptomatic and self-limited primary pulmonary infection. Dissemination involves the central nervous system in the form of meningitis with common symptoms of fever, headache, cervical rigidity, and vomiting. Cutaneous lesions, most often on the head and neck, develop in up to 20% of patients with disseminated disease and are characterized by a diverse group including erythematous papules, pustules, plaques, abscesses, granulomas, ulcers, and nodules. Oral lesions are relatively uncommon. They present as nonhealing nodules of granulation tissue, masses, and most commonly indurated ulcerations that mimic squamous cell carcinoma (Fig. 8-16). Typical affected locations include the tongue, gingiva, and palate.

Microscopically, the characteristic ovoid yeast and surrounding clear capsule can be readily identified with PAS or methenamine-silver stains. The surrounding mucopolysaccharide capsule stains with mucicarmine, methylene blue, and alcian blue. Cryptococcosis may be diagnosed by culture and confirmed by the cryptococcal latex agglutination test, which detects capsular antigen.

Treatment of cryptococcosis is with amphotericin B with or without flucytosine. Fluconazole and itraconazole have also been used for systemic infections, although they are generally administered as suppressive agents to prevent relapses.

Blastomycosis (North American Blastomycosis)

Blastomycosis is caused by *B. dermatitidis* and occurs predominantly in the south central and midwestern United States. Epidemics affect patients of all ages and both sexes, although endemic cases usually develop in young adult men. The incidence and severity of blastomycosis are increased in immunocompromised patients, who suffer a high mortality rate.

Pneumonia is the most common manifestation of this fungal disease, and the lungs are almost

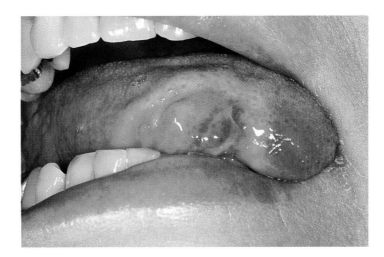

FIG. 8-17   Irregular, ulcerated masses are frequently observed in patients with blastomycosis.

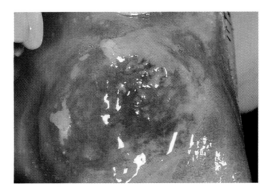

FIG. 8-18   Disseminated coccidioidomycosis of the oral cavity presents as a chronic, irregularly shaped, and malignant-appearing ulceration.

always the organ initially infected. Pulmonary disease may become chronic and resemble malignancy. The majority of patients display cutaneous lesions characterized by verrucous plaques with peripheral microabscesses. Bone involvement in the form of osteomyelitis and joint and genitourinary disease occur in approximately 50% of patients. Oral lesions in patients with blastomycosis are common and develop in approximately 25% of patients. The lesions may be similar to cutaneous verrucous plaques, or they may appear as irregular ulcerations with firm borders (Fig. 8-17). In many instances cutaneous facial plaques extend beyond the vermilion border into the oral cavity, spreading along the buccal mucosa or labial vestibule.

B. dermatitidis has a double-contoured refractile wall and displays broad-based, single budding. KOH preparations from oral lesions may reveal the yeast, although confirmation requires culture of the organism.

Ketoconazole and itraconazole may be administered to immunocompetent patients with blastomycosis. In those with meningeal involvement or in immunocompromised patients, amphotericin B is the treatment of choice.

Coccidioidomycosis

Coccidioides immitis is a dimorphic fungus and the causative agent of coccidioidomycosis. The disease is endemic to the desert regions of the southwestern United States, Mexico, and South America. Inhaled arthrospores are responsible for human infection, and it is estimated that over 100,000 individuals are infected annually with *C. immitis.*

A nonspecific, flulike illness develops within several weeks after exposure, although many patients remain totally asymptomatic. Accompanying the pulmonary infection are skin lesions that may appear as erythema multiforme, erythema nodosum, or a morbilliform eruption. Chronic coccidioidomycosis, like chronic histoplasmosis, resembles tuberculosis with persistent low-grade fever, weight loss, cough, and hemoptysis. Disseminated coccidioidomycosis occurs in less than 1% of all reported cases, usually in individuals who are immunosuppressed or otherwise debilitated. Coccidioidomycosis is an uncommon AIDS-defining illness. Common sites for dissemination include the skin, bones, joints, and meninges. The oral manifestations of disseminated coccidioidomycosis consist of large ulcerations and nodules that resemble malignancy (Fig. 8-18).

Microscopically, characteristic spherules may be demonstrated by PAS and methenamine silver stains. These endospores are found within a suppurative and granulomatous inflammatory infiltrate. The organisms may also be identified in sputum, in bronchial swabs, and in oral lesions by KOH preparations and by culture. Routine serologic testing is helpful in establishing the diagnosis, although it is less sensitive when used for patients who are not infected with HIV.

Uncomplicated cases of coccidioidomycosis do not require treatment. Individuals who are immunosuppressed or debilitated or who have preexisting pulmonary or disseminated disease are treated with either intravenous amphotericin B or fluconazole.

SUGGESTED READINGS

Candidiasis

Allen CM: Diagnosing and managing oral candidiasis, *J Am Dent Assoc* 123:77, 1992.

Baughman RA: Median rhomboid glossitis: a developmental anomaly? *Oral Surg Oral Med Oral Pathol* 31:56, 1971.

Bergendal T, Isacsson G: A combined clinical, mycological and histological study of denture stomatitis, *Acta Odontol Scand* 41:33, 1983.

Budtz-Jorgensen E: Etiology, pathogenesis, therapy, and prophylaxis of oral yeast infections, *Acta Odontol Scand* 48:61, 1990.

Cannon RD et al: Oral candida: clearance, colonization, or candidiasis? *J Dent Res* 74:1152, 1990.

Challacombe SJ: Immunologic aspects of oral candidiasis, *Oral Surg Oral Med Oral Pathol* 78:202, 1994.

Como JA, Dismukes WE: Oral azole drugs as systemic antifungal therapy, *N Engl J Med* 330:263, 1994.

Fetter A et al: Asymptomatic oral *Candida albicans* carriage in HIV-infection: frequency and predisposing factors, *J Oral Pathol Med* 22:57, 1993.

Fotos PG, Vincent SD, Hellstein JW: Oral candidosis: clinical historical and therapeutic features of 100 cases, *Oral Surg Oral Med Oral Pathol* 74:41, 1992.

Garber GE: Treatment of oral Candida mucositis infections, *Drugs* 47:734, 1994.

Heimdahl A, Nord CE: Oral yeast infections in immunocompromised and seriously diseased patients, *Acta Odontol Scand* 48:77, 1990.

Holmstrup P, Axell T: Classification and clinical manifestations of oral yeast infections, *Acta Odontol Scand* 48:57, 1990.

Iacopino AM, Wathen WF: Oral candidal infection and denture stomatitis: a comprehensive review, *J Am Dent Assoc* 123:46, 1992.

Jeganathan S, Chan YC: Immunodiagnosis in oral candidiasis: a review, *Oral Surg Oral Med Oral Pathol* 74:451, 1992.

Konsberg R, Axell T: Denture stomatitis—a review of the aetiology, diagnosis and management, *Surg Oral Med Oral Pathol* 78:306, 1994.

Lewis MAO, Samaranayake LP, Lamey PJ: Diagnosis and treatment of oral candidosis, *J Oral Maxillofac Surg* 49:996, 1991.

Lynch DP: Oral candidiasis: history, classification, and clinical presentation, *Oral Surg Oral Med Oral Pathol* 78:189, 1994.

Odds FC, Rinaldi MG: Nomenclature of fungal disease, *Curr Top Med Mycol* 6:33, 1995.

Oühman SC et al: Angular cheilitis: a clinical and microbial study, *J Oral Pathol* 15:213, 1986.

Redding S et al: Resistance of *Candida albicans* to fluconazole during treatment of oropharyngeal candidiasis in a patient with AIDS: documentation by in vitro susceptibility testing and DNA subtype analysis, *Clin Infect Dis* 18:240, 1994.

Rossie KM et al: Influence of radiation therapy on oral *Candida albicans* colonization: a quantitative assessment, *Oral Surg Oral Med Oral Pathol* 64:698, 1987.

Samaranayake LP: Superficial oral fungal infections, *Curr Opin Dent* 1:415, 1991.

Samaranayake LP, Holmstrup P: Oral candidiasis and human immunodeficiency virus, *J Oral Pathol Med* 18:554, 1989.

Scully C, el-Kabir M, Samaranayake LP: Candida and oral candidosis: a review, *Crit Rev Oral Biol Med* 5:125, 1994.

Opportunistic fungal infections

Dixon DM et al: Fungal infections: a growing threat, *Public Health Rep* 111:226, 1996.

Dreizen S, Keating MJ, Beran M: Orofacial fungal infections: nine pathogens that may invade during chemotherapy, *Postgrad Med* 91:349, 1992.

Samaranayake LP: Oral mycoses in HIV infection, *Oral Surg Oral Med Oral Pathol* 73:171, 1992.

Scully C, de Almeida OP: Orofacial manifestations of the systemic mycoses, *J Oral Pathol Med* 21:289, 1992.

Vartivarian SE, Anaissie EJ, Bodey GP: Emerging fungal pathogens in immunocompromised patients: classification, diagnosis, and management, *Clin Infect Dis* 17:487, 1993.

Zegarelli DJ: Fungal infections of the oral cavity, *Otolaryngol Clin North Am* 26:1069, 1993.

Histoplasmosis

Chinn H et al: Oral histoplasmosis in HIV-infected patients: a report of two cases, *Oral Surg Oral Med Oral Pathol* 79:710, 1995.

Heinic GS et al: Oral *Histoplasma capsulatum* infection in association with HIV infection: a case report, *J Oral Pathol Med* 21:85, 1992.

Ng KH, Siar CH: Review of oral histoplasmosis in Malaysians, *Oral Surg Oral Med Oral Pathol* 81:303, 1996.

Oda D et al: Oral histoplasmosis as a presenting disease in acquired immunodeficiency syndrome, *Oral Surg Oral Med Oral Pathol* 70:631, 1990.

Wheat W: Diagnosis and management of histoplasmosis, *Eur J Clin Microbiol Infect Dis* 8:480, 1989.

Zygomycosis

Economopoulou P et al: Rhinocerebral mucormycosis with severe oral lesions: a case report, *J Oral Maxillofac Surg* 53:215, 1995.

Jones AC, Bentsen TY, Freedman PD: Mucormycosis of the oral cavity, *Oral Surg Oral Med Oral Pathol* 75:455, 1993.

Rinaldi MG: Zygomycosis, *Infect Dis Clin North Am* 3:19, 1989.

Rosenberg SW, Lepley JB: Mucormycosis in leukemia, *Oral Surg Oral Med Oral Pathol* 54:26, 1982.

Sugar AM: Mucormycosis, *Clin Infect Dis* 14:S126, 1992.

Van der Westhuijzen AJ et al: A rapidly fatal palatal ulcer: rhinocerebral mucormycosis, *Oral Surg Oral Med Oral Pathol* 68:32, 1989.

Paracoccidioidomycosis

Sposto MR et al: Oral paracoccidioidomycosis: a study of 36 South American patients, *Oral Surg Oral Med Oral Pathol* 75:461, 1993.

Sposto MR et al: Paracoccidioidomycosis manifesting as oral lesions: clinical, cytological and serological investigation, *J Oral Pathol Med* 23:85, 1994.

Aspergillosis

Chambers MS et al: Oral complications associated with aspergillosis in patients with a hematologic malignancy: presentation and treatment, *Oral Surg Oral Med Oral Pathol* 79:559, 1995.

Dreizen S et al: Orofacial aspergillosis in acute leukemia, *Oral Surg Oral Med Oral Pathol* 59:499, 1985.

Meunier-Carpentier F, Cruciani M, Klastersky J: Oral prophylaxis with miconazole or ketoconazole of invasive fungal disease in neutropenic cancer patients, *Eur J Cancer Clin Oncol* 19:43, 1983.

Myoken Y et al: Pathologic features of invasive oral aspergillosis in patients with hematologic malignancies, *J Oral Maxillofac Surg* 54:263, 1996.

Cryptococcosis

de Almeida OP, Scully C: Oral lesions in the systemic mycoses, *Curr Opin Dent* 1:423, 1991.

Glick M et al: Oral manifestations of disseminated *Cryptococcus neoformans* in a patient with acquired immunodeficiency syndrome, *Oral Surg Oral Med Oral Pathol* 64:454, 1987.

Levitz SM: The ecology of *Cryptococcus neoformans* and the epidemiology of cryptococcosis, *Rev Infect Dis* 13:1163, 1991.

Lynch DP, Naftolin LZ: Oral *Cryptococcus neoformans* infection in AIDS, *Oral Surg Oral Med Oral Pathol* 64:449, 1987.

Pinner RW, Hajjeh RA, Powderly WG: Prospects for preventing cryptococcosis in persons infected with human immunodeficiency virus, *Clin Infect Dis* 21:103, 1995.

Schmidt-Westhausen A et al: Oral cryptococcosis in a patient with AIDS: a case report, *Oral Dis* 1:77, 1995.

Blastomycosis

Bradsher RW: Blastomycosis, *Clin Infect Dis* 14:82, 1992.

Pappas PG et al: Blastomycosis in immunocompromised patients, *Medicine* 72:311, 1993.

Reder PA, Neel HB: Blastomycosis in otolaryngology: review of a large series, *Laryngoscope* 103:53, 1993.

Coccidioidomycosis

Cardone JS, Vinson R, Anderson LL: Coccidioidomycosis: the other great imitator, *Cutis* 56:33, 1995.

Einstein HE, Johnson RH: Coccidioidomycosis: new aspects of epidemiology and therapy, *Clin Infect Dis* 16:349, 1993.

Galgiani JN: Coccidioidomycosis: changes in clinical expression serological diagnosis, and therapeutic options, *Clin Infect Dis* 14:100, 1992.

Jones JL et al: Coccidioidomycosis among persons with AIDS in the United States, *J Infect Dis* 171:961, 1995.

Stevens DA: Coccidioidomycosis, *N Engl J Med* 332:1077, 1995.

CHAPTER 9

Vesiculoerosive Diseases

RECURRENT APHTHOUS STOMATITIS

Recurrent aphthous stomatitis (RAS), also known as canker sores, is the most common cause of oral ulcerations in children and adults, affecting an estimated 25% of the world's population. Although the onset of the disease is during childhood or young adolescence, the frequency and severity of episodes usually decrease after the fifth decade of life. Clinically, RAS is characterized by the recurrent development of one or more painful ulcerations and classified into one of three types (Table 9-1). Minor aphthae (recurrent aphthae of Mikulicz) are the most common form, accounting for 85% of cases. Episodes of one or many discrete ulcerations, with a yellow cratered base surrounded by an erythematous halo, develop recurrently (Figs. 9-1 and 9-2). The lesions are usually less than 1 cm, cause minimal to moderate pain, and heal in 7 to 10 days without scarring. Major aphthae (Sutton's disease or periadenitis mucosa necrotica recurrens), which comprise 10% of cases, are characterized by fewer but significantly larger, deeper, and more painful ulcerations, often 2 to 3 cm in size (Fig. 9-3). Scarring is frequently observed, especially at sites of ulcerations, and persists for 6 weeks or longer. Herpetiform aphthous ulcerations are the rarest variety and morphologically resemble lesions of primary cutaneous and oral human herpesvirus type 1 infection. Multiple 1- to 2-mm ulcerations develop in clusters, often on an erythematous base, and resolve in 7 to 10 days without scarring (Fig. 9-4). Considerable overlapping of clinical features of these types are found among patients with recurrent aphthous ulcerations.

RAS occurs on the nonkeratinized oral mucosa. Minor and herpetiform aphthae develop most frequently on the labial and buccal mucosa, lateral tongue, and floor of the mouth. Major aphthous ulcers have a predilection for the soft palate, oropharynx, and lips.

The severity of aphthous ulcerations is extremely variable, with some patients encountering occasional episodes and others enduring continuous disease. Multiple etiologies have been proposed; however, the cause remains obscure. Mechanical trauma to the oral soft tissues, as well as emotional stress, can precipitate an episode in some patients. Food allergies, when identified by patch testing, or sensitivity to sodium lauryl sulfate, commonly found in dentifrices, can result in exacerbations of the disease. An infectious etiology involving herpes simplex virus, varicella zoster virus, or cytomegalovirus infection has been fervently pursued, but no studies have conclusively demonstrated any of these viruses as the cause. Specific haplotypes (HLA-B12 and HLA-B51) are sometimes associated with patients who develop aphthae, and there is an increased prevalence in those with a positive family history of RAS. An immunologically mediated process is supported by numerous immunologic abnormalities reported in patients with recurrent aphthous ulceration and by the response of this disease to immunosuppressive agents.

Recurrent ulcerations may be a manifestation of a large and diverse group of systemic diseases. A comprehensive hematologic investigation including serum iron, total iron binding capacity, folate, and vitamin B_{12} levels may reveal deficiencies that can result in aphthae; if corrected, the aphthous ulcerations improve. Patients with inflammatory bowel disease and systemic lupus erythematosus

Table 9-1   Characteristics of Recurrent Aphthous Stomatitis

	MINOR APHTHAE	MAJOR APHTHAE	HERPETIFORM APHTHAE
Number of lesions	1-10	1-5	5-100
Incidence	Common	Uncommon	Rare
Pain	None-moderate	Moderate-severe	Mild-moderate
Size of ulcers	<1 cm	1-3 cm	1-4 mm
Duration	7-14 days	30-60 days	7-14 days
Scarring	Rare	Common	None
Location	Buccal and labial mucosa, lateral tongue, floor of mouth	Palate, oropharynx, lips	All sites
Comments	Resembles viral infections, induced by trauma, hematologic abnormalities	Common in HIV, may be initial manifestation of GI disease	Not caused by herpesvirus infection
Therapy	Topical or systemic corticosteroids, antibiotics, analgesics	Topical, intralesional or systemic corticosteroids, immunosuppressive agents	Topical corticosteroids and analgesics

HIV, Human immunodeficiency virus; *GI,* gastrointestinal.

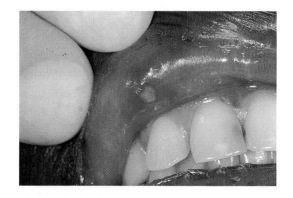

FIG. 9-1   Minor recurrent aphthous stomatitis lesions almost always occur on nonkeratinized mucosa such as the labial vestibule.

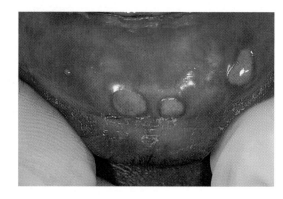

FIG. 9-2   Multiple "canker sores" are common and may cause significant pain.

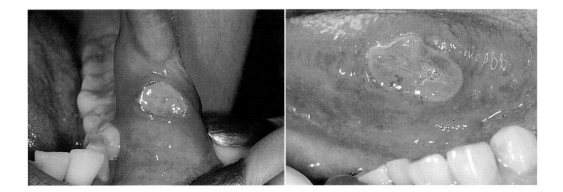

FIG. 9-3   Major aphthous stomatitis lesions are large, deep, and painful and generally persist for up to a month before healing.

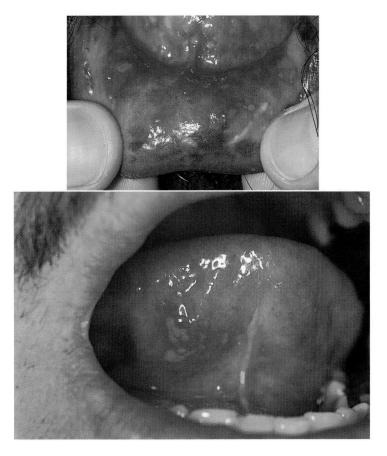

FIG. 9-4   Herpetiform recurrent aphthae are characterized by the presence of multiple oral ulcerations that resemble oral herpes simplex infections. These are a variant of aphthous stomatitis and are not caused by human herpesvirus type 1 infection.

develop ulcerations that are clinically indistinguishable from recurrent aphthous ulcerations. All forms of aphthae are also commonly observed in patients infected with human immunodeficiency virus (HIV) and a number of systemic viral infections such as herpangina and hand-foot-and-mouth disease. Behçet's disease, cyclic neutropenia, complex aphthosis (oral and genital ulcers), syndrome of periodic fever, pharyngitis and aphthous stomatitis, and the MAGIC syndrome (mouth and genital ulcers with inflamed cartilage) display lesions that cannot be clinically differentiated from RAS. Biopsying an ulcer will reveal only nonspecific histologic features; however, it may be useful to exclude other diseases, especially those of viral origin. The great majority of patients with RAS have no underlying abnormalities, and the diagnosis is established by clinical findings and a history of spontaneously healing ulcerations.

All therapies are palliative, and none results in permanent remission. Oral rinses with analgesic or protective properties containing diphenhydramine elixir, dyclonine hydrochloride, Kaopectate, Maalox, and sucralfate, alone or in combination, may suffice in mild cases. Antimicrobial rinses using either chlorhexidine gluconate, tetracycline, or Listerine hasten resolution of ulcerations. Potent topical corticosteroids are the most effective agents in reducing duration and symptoms of RAS. Short courses of systemic corticosteroids are highly effective but should be reserved for those with major aphthae. Colchicine, dapsone, and perhaps pentoxifylline shorten the duration of active ulceration, reduce the frequency of attacks, and can be administered chronically with proper monitoring. Their efficacy, however, has never been confirmed in double-blind studies. Severe cases require immunosuppressive therapy with either thalidomide, azathioprine, or cyclosporine.

BEHÇET'S DISEASE

Behçet's disease is a rare multisystem disorder that can affect any organ system, arises frequently in the third decade of life, and most commonly affects individuals of Mediterranean or Japanese descent. The disease is partly defined by the oral manifestations that are present in all patients. Oral ulcerations are the most consistent finding, and their occurrence is necessary in establishing a diagnosis of Behçet's disease. The international criteria for classification of Behçet's disease have defined the oral lesions as minor, major, and herpetiform aphthous ulcerations, observed by a physi-

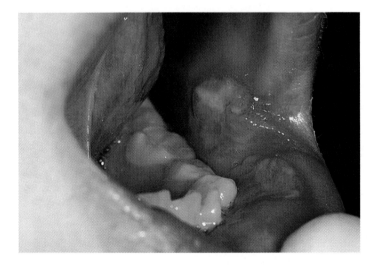

FIG. 9-5 Behçet's disease characterized by painful and recurrent oral ulcerations identical to recurrent aphthous stomatitis.

cian or reliably reported by a patient, that recur at least three times in one 12-month period. Oral aphthae are often the initial manifestation of the disease, and, when they occur in children, the oral lesions commonly precede the onset of systemic involvement by many years. Although the ulcerations in Behçet's disease are often indistinguishable from those of recurrent aphthous stomatitis, several distinctions are generally observed. The oral aphthae in Behçet's, unlike most recurrent aphthous stomatitis lesions, are usually continuously present, recur at the same site, sometimes cause extensive scarring, commonly exceed six in number, have ill-defined erythematous borders, are of varying sizes, and often develop on the soft palate and oropharynx (Fig. 9-5). Complex aphthosis refers to a group of patients who experience continuous oral and genital ulcerations and who sometimes progress to Behçet's disease.

Although the etiology of Behçet's disease is unknown, a strong association with certain haplotypes suggests that genetic factors are important in the development of this disorder. Immunologic abnormalities have been reported, and an infectious etiology in genetically susceptible individuals has also been proposed.

The histology of oral lesions resembles that obtained from skin biopsies. A chronic inflammatory infiltrate at the basal and prickle layers of the mucosa is observed in early lesions, and endothelial proliferation and vasculitis with a perivascular infiltrate subsequently develop.

Topical therapy for the oral lesions consists of the same treatment for recurrent aphthous stomatitis. A large number of immunosuppressive and cytotoxic agents used for those patients with systemic disease produce significant improvement of the oral lesions.

LICHEN PLANUS

Lichen planus is a common mucocutaneous disorder affecting 1% to 2% of the population. Patients with oral lichen planus display cutaneous lesions in approximately 20% of cases, whereas patients with cutaneous lichen planus exhibit oral manifestations in greater than 50% of cases. The disease affects women much more commonly than men, and it occurs most frequently in the fifth to sixth decades of life.

The oral lesions can be classified as one of three types: (1) reticular, characterized by white lines, plaques, and papules; (2) erythematous; and (3) erosive, defined as ulcerations and bullae. Reticular lesions are the most distinctive oral features of this disease, are asymptomatic, and do not require therapy (Figs. 9-6 and 9-7). Erythematous and erosive lesions are a potential cause of sig-

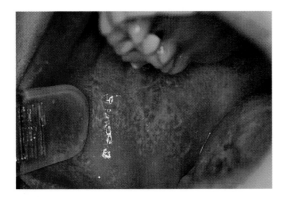

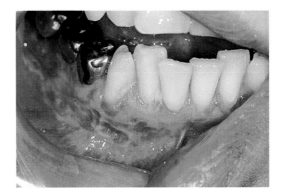

FIG. 9-6   White reticular lines and plaques on the buccal mucosa are the most common manifestation of oral lichen planus.

FIG. 9-7   Reticulated lesions of lichen planus may develop on any oral mucosal surface and are especially common on the gingivae.

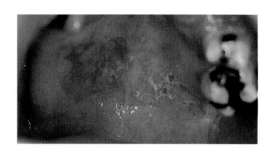

FIG. 9-8   Erythematous lesions of oral lichen planus coexist with white reticulated lesions on the palate.

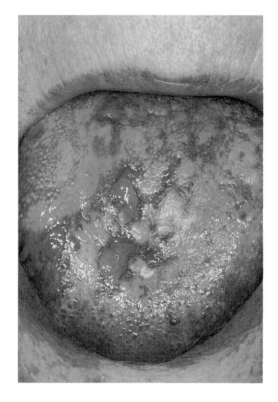

FIG. 9-9   Tongue demonstrating all three types of lesions in oral lichen planus: white reticulated plaques, erythema, and erosions.

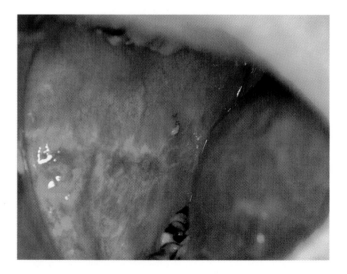

FIG. 9-10   Buccal mucosa revealing characteristic lesions of reticulation, erythema, and early ulceration. Lichen planus is exacerbated by trauma as evidenced by the small blister at the site of trauma.

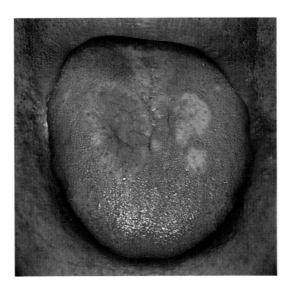

FIG. 9-11   Asymptomatic white-pink plaques on the dorsal tongue are pathognomonic for oral lichen planus.

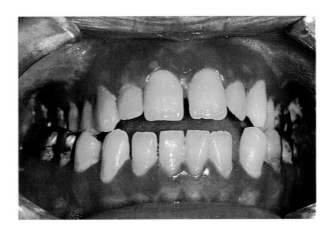

FIG. 9-12   Oral lichen planus may present as a desquamative gingivitis, which often requires immunofluorescence to differentiate the disease from other blistering disorders. In this case, reticulated lesions of the right upper vestibule are present and are highly suggestive of lichen planus.

nificant pain; they are almost always accompanied by reticulated lesions, a helpful feature in formulating a diagnosis (Figs. 9-8 to 9-10). When present, asymptomatic, white-pink plaques on the dorsal surface of the tongue are pathognomonic of oral lichen planus (Fig. 9-11). Postinflammatory hyperpigmentation, a common sequela of cutaneous lichen planus, infrequently occurs in the mouth.

Oral lichen planus may affect any site in the oral cavity but has a predilection for the buccal mucosa and tongue. Patients may present with a desquamative gingivitis without other visible oral lesions (Fig. 9-12). Other mucosal surfaces, including the esophagus, larynx, conjunctiva, and bladder, are infrequently affected; however, the genital mucosa commonly displays features of lichen planus necessitating a careful genital examination.

Lichenoid stomatitis is most likely a heterogenous group of disorders with identical clinical and histologic features. In some patients the oral lesions may result from a hypersensitivity to medications, most commonly nonsteroidal antiinflammatory or antihypertensive agents. In others, resolution of oral lesions may occur after replacement of dental restorations when allergy to these compounds is detected. An oral allergy should be suspected when the disease is localized to the mucosa immediately adjacent to a dental restoration, especially one that is old, worn, and cracked. Lichen planus may be a manifestation of an underlying hepatic abnormality, and liver function tests and a hepatitis profile may be warranted in patients with oral lichen planus. In the majority of cases classified as oral lichen planus, the etiology is unknown, although there is evidence that the disease is caused by an immunologically mediated process.

A definitive diagnosis requires a biopsy, preferably from a reticulated lesion. Histologic features include liquefaction degeneration of the basal cell layer accompanied by a bandlike lymphocytic infiltrate in the submucosa. When the clinical diagnosis is questionable, a biopsy for direct immunofluorescence should be obtained. Although the findings are nonspecific and include fibrin deposition at the mucosal-submucosal junction and absorption of immunoreactants by cytoid bodies, they help exclude other vesiculoerosive diseases.

Considerable controversy exists regarding the premalignant potential of oral lichen planus. Most accept an overall incidence of malignant transformation of 1%, with the majority of carcinomas arising on the tongue from erythematous or erosive lesions. Failure to recognize lichenoid dysplasia as a distinct histologic entity and precursor of oral cancer may account for some of the confusion. All patients with lichen planus should be examined at regular intervals, and use of agents that are known to be oral carcinogenic agents including tobacco and alcohol should be minimized and eliminated if possible.

Potent topical corticosteroids are the most effective and commonly used therapy for oral lichen planus. Intralesional injections of triamcinolone hasten resolution of erosive lesions. Systemic corticosteroids should be reserved for acute exacerbations because their chronic use is limited by their inherent side effects. Topical cyclosporine or tretinoin can augment the effects of topical corticosteroids in refractory cases. Systemic therapy using hydroxychloroquine, etretinate, azathioprine, or cyclosporine may be needed for patients with progressive and erosive disease. Candidiasis frequently complicates therapy and, when identified, should be treated with topical or systemic agents. An optimal oral hygiene program should be instituted because plaque and calculus that accumulate on the teeth exacerbate gingival lichen planus.

CHRONIC ULCERATIVE STOMATITIS WITH STRATIFIED EPITHELIUM-SPECIFIC ANTINUCLEAR ANTIBODY

Chronic ulcerative stomatitis with stratified epithelium-specific antinuclear antibody has all of the clinical and histologic features of oral lichen planus and is defined by a unique immunofluorescence pattern. A perilesional biopsy specimen reveals particulate antinuclear antibody reacting with the lower third of the substrate epithelium only on stratified epithelial substrates, such as the esophagus of a monkey or guinea pig. High titers of circulating antinuclear antibodies can also be detected by indirect immunofluorescent studies. Hydroxychloroquine and topical corticosteroids are the preferred treatments.

PEMPHIGUS

Pemphigus refers to a group of chronic autoimmune diseases that manifest clinically as blisters and erosions of epithelial surfaces of the skin and mucous membranes. In these disorders, circulating autoantibodies are directed against normal epithelial structural proteins that have been identified as cadherins. These pathogenic autoantibodies, when passively transferred in vivo, reproduce the clinical features of pemphigus.

Pemphigus most commonly develops in the fourth to sixth decades of life, although its occurrence in childhood is well recognized. The disease occurs more frequently in Ashkenazic Jews and is associated with the expression of HLA-DR4 and HLA-DR6 haplotypes. Although several clinical variants of the disease have been described, pemphigus vulgaris is the most frequent and severe form.

Oral lesions in pemphigus vulgaris and pemphigus vegetans are common and represent the initial manifestation of these diseases in more than 75% of cases. Pemphigus may be confined to the oral cavity, although in the majority of cases, blisters on the skin appear months after the development of oral lesions. Unfortunately, the lack of recognition of the oral manifestations often results in a substantial delay in diagnosis. Large, painful oral erosions that start as bullae rapidly rupture and result in pain, bleeding, and difficulty in mastication (Fig. 9-13). All of the mucosal surfaces may be involved, but the soft palate is affected in almost all cases followed in frequency by the buccal mucosa, tongue, and gingiva. Hypertrophic vegetative ulcerations on the buccal mucosa (Fig. 9-14) and severe desquamative gingivitis (Fig. 9-15) are commonly observed. A positive Nikolsky's sign, induced by

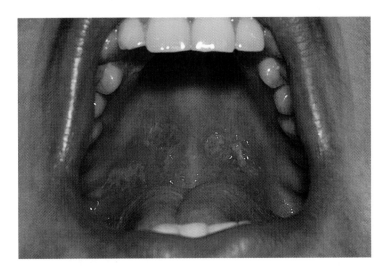

FIG. 9-13   Pemphigus vulgaris most frequently affects the soft palate and is characterized by large and confluent painful ulcerations.

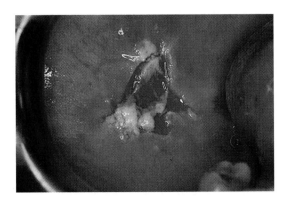

FIG. 9-14   The oral ulcerations on the buccal mucosa in pemphigus are hyperkeratotic and persistent.

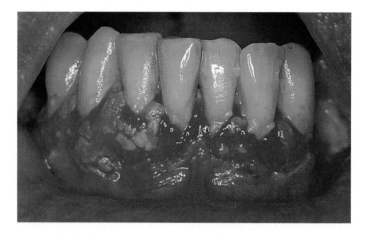

FIG. 9-15   The desquamative gingivitis that results from pemphigus is severe, more so than with any other vesiculoerosive disease.

rubbing the blister or epithelium adjacent to an erosion, causing it to slough, is characteristically seen in pemphigus but usually not with other blistering disorders. Oral manifestations are unusual in pemphigus foliaceus and pemphigus erythematosus.

Histologically, pemphigus is characterized by the formation of vesicles, or bullae, above the basal layer of the epidermis. Acantholytic cells are often seen singly or in clusters in the cavity of the blister accompanied by neutrophils and lymphocytes. Direct immunofluorescence, displaying immunoglobulins of the IgG class bound to the intercellular spaces of the oral mucosa, is a more reliable method of diagnosing pemphigus.

The chronic administration of systemic corticosteroids is the treatment of choice for oral lesions of pemphigus. Patients who do not respond to this treatment or those unable to tolerate corticosteroids require alternative immunosuppressive therapy with azathioprine, cyclosporine, cyclophosphamide, oral and parenteral gold, and plasmapheresis. Beneficial effects have been reported with potent topical corticosteroids as adjuvant therapy. Declining serial indirect immunofluorescent titers and a negative direct immunofluorescent biopsy are both indicative of remission and valuable in monitoring the response to therapy.

PARANEOPLASTIC PEMPHIGUS

Paraneoplastic pemphigus is a recently described syndrome that is characterized by a vesiculobullous eruption with distinct autoantibodies in patients with underlying malignant neoplasms. The oral manifestations are an early presenting feature and result in severe pain. Whereas the cutaneous lesions are variable in appearance, resembling those of pemphigus, bullous pemphigoid, erythema multiforme, and lichen planus, the oral lesions almost always resemble oral pemphigus. The lips are eroded and crusted (Fig. 9-16), and intraorally, large, ragged ulcerations are commonly observed on the lips, gingiva, tongue, and palate (Fig. 9-17). Suprabasilar acantholysis is present histologically when biopsies of skin or oral mucosal blisters are sampled. Direct immunofluorescence demonstrates deposition of IgG and complement in the intercellular spaces of the epidermis as in pemphigus, and immunoreactants may also be found along the basement membrane zone in paraneoplastic pemphigus. Indirect immunofluorescence reveals serum autoantibodies that are highly specific for paraneoplastic pemphigus binding to rodent urinary bladder epithelium (transitional epithelium).

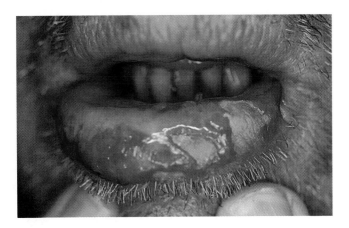

FIG. 9-16 Paraneoplastic pemphigus almost always involves the lips, which become ulcerated and crusted.

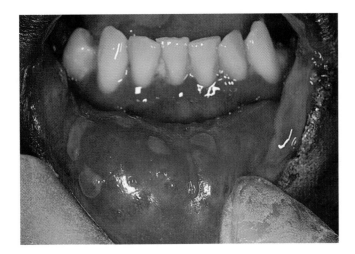

FIG. 9-17 Intraoral features of paraneoplastic pemphigus include diffuse erosions on the lips and labial vestibule.

Underlying associated neoplasms include non-Hodgkin's lymphoma, leukemia, thymoma, spindle cell neoplasms, Waldenström's macroglobulinemia, and Castleman's disease. The prognosis is good in patients with benign tumors that are surgically excised; most patients, however, have malignant neoplasms and die because of their disease or complications of therapy.

PEMPHIGOID

Bullous pemphigoid and cicatricial pemphigoid are autoimmune, blistering mucocutaneous diseases characterized by the separation of the overlying epithelium from its stroma. Both are diseases of the elderly, with the majority of patients older than 65, although they may occur at any age, even in infancy.

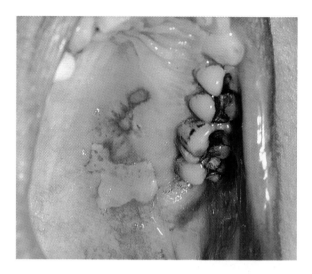

FIG. 9-18 Large erosions, such as these on the palate, develop in approximately one fourth of patients with bullous pemphigoid.

Bullous pemphigoid is a cutaneous disorder clinically characterized by tense bullae and occasionally vesicles, erythematous papules, and urticarial plaques. The disease may be localized, but in most patients it is widespread, with blisters distributed most commonly on the arms, legs, groin, and axillae. The oral cavity is affected in approximately 15% to 25% of cases. Ulcerations of varying sizes typically affect the buccal mucosa, tongue, and palate (Fig. 9-18). Occasionally, intact blisters occur intraorally, but the mouth lesions generally are not a source of significant pain. Unlike pemphigus, the oral lesions accompany and do not predate the onset of cutaneous blister formation. Treatment of the cutaneous lesions with either systemic corticosteroids, immunosuppressive agents, or tetracycline and nicotinamide results in the resolution of oral lesions.

Cicatricial pemphigoid is a chronic disease that predominantly affects the mucous membranes and occasionally the skin. Females are afflicted twice as often as males. The oral cavity and eyes are most frequently involved, although other mucous membranes including the pharynx, larynx, esophagus, nasal mucosa, and genitalia may be affected. Cicatricial pemphigoid has a wide spectrum of disease manifestations, with some patients displaying only oral or ocular involvement and others displaying involvement of multiple sites. The disease often results in scarring, significant debilitation, and suffering.

The most common and characteristic oral finding in cicatricial pemphigoid is a desquamative gingivitis (Figs. 9-19 and 9-20). Reddened and ulcerated gingivae and alveolar mucosa result in bleeding and pain. A distinctive feature that aids in the establishment of the correct diagnosis is the patchy involvement of these structures; diffuse involvement is far less common. Ulcerations and blisters of the palate and tongue may occur, although the gingiva frequently is the only site of involvement.

As the disease develops in the elderly, the patients' gingival findings are often mistakenly attributed to poor oral hygiene. Histopathologic features of a biopsy from a mucosal bulla include a subepithelial blister with an underlying mixed inflammatory infiltrate. A definitive diagnosis requires a positive direct immunofluorescence test from nonulcerated, erythematous tissue revealing deposits of immunoglobulins and complement components on the basilar pole of the basal epithelial cells, most commonly C3 and IgG. Indirect immunofluorescent studies to detect circulating antibasement

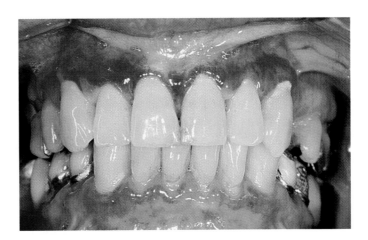

FIG. 9-19   Cicatricial pemphigoid is characterized most frequently by a patchy, desquamative gingivitis. The gingivae are generally not uniformly involved.

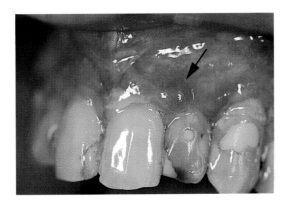

FIG. 9-20   Pemphigoid is a subepidermal blistering disease; therefore intact blisters in the oral cavity, typically on the gingiva, are occasionally found.

membrane antibodies have helped classify this heterogenous disease group; however, they are less consistent than those seen in pemphigus.

When the oral lesions are mild and localized, potent topical and intralesional corticosteroids are all that are needed to control the inflammation. The intermittent administration of systemic corticosteroids is beneficial; however, when chronic therapy is required or when steroids are ineffective or contraindicated, dapsone should be used. Immunosuppressive agents including azathioprine and cyclophosphamide should be reserved for those with progressive disease. Nicotinamide, minocycline, and topical cyclosporine have been reported to be of benefit anecdotally.

ERYTHEMA MULTIFORME, STEVENS-JOHNSON SYNDROME, AND TOXIC EPIDERMAL NECROLYSIS

Erythema multiforme is a group of mucocutaneous disorders with heterogenous clinical manifestations. The "minor" form comprises the majority of cases and is characterized by a self-limiting skin eruption that is often recurrent. Symmetric cutaneous erythematous papules rapidly appear and de-

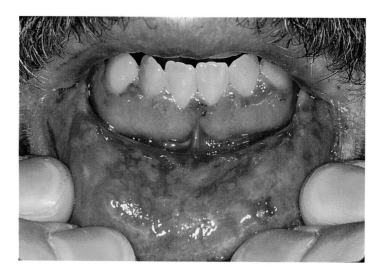

FIG. 9-21   The acute development of erosions covered by a white pseudomembrane is typical of erythema multiforme.

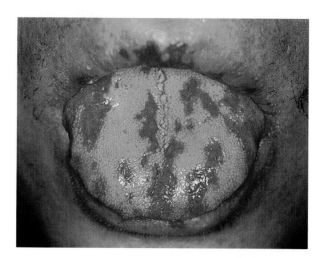

FIG. 9-22   Erythema multiforme with numerous ulcerations of the tongue and lips.

velop a central vesicle or bulla, forming the characteristic target lesion. The incidence of oral lesions varies considerably and ranges from 35% to 65%. Not uncommonly, the disease may be confined to the oral cavity. The clinical oral features include discrete, superficial ulcerations between 1 and 4 mm in diameter covered by a white pseudomembrane and surrounded by erythema (Figs. 9-21 and 9-22). The tongue, buccal and labial mucosa, and lips are most commonly affected, although the ulcerations may be confluent and involve the entire oral mucosa.

The nosology of the "major" form of erythema multiforme remains controversial. A new classification based on the pattern and morphology of skin lesions, as well as on the extent of epidermal detachment, has been accepted and includes Stevens-Johnson syndrome and toxic epidermal necrolysis. The eruption is severe and often accompanied by fever, myalgias, and other constitutional symptoms. Oral involvement is present in almost all cases and accompanies the skin lesions. Severely

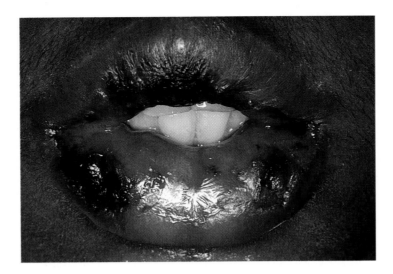

FIG. 9-23   Major erythema multiforme almost always involves the oral mucous membranes and most often results in ulcerations and black eschars of the lips.

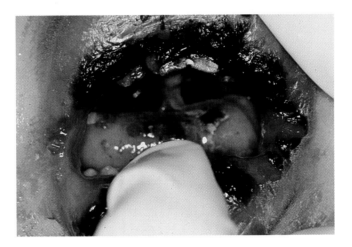

FIG. 9-24   In toxic epidermal necrolysis, the entire oral cavity desquamates and the lips become black and necrotic.

painful and extensive oral bullae, erosions, and mucositis often result in dehydration, decreased nutritional intake, and secondary bacterial infection (Fig. 9-23). Characteristically, the lips are eroded and covered with black hemorrhagic crusts (Fig. 9-24). The extent and severity of oral lesions are similar for the different variants of this disease and do not correlate with the extent of cutaneous epidermal detachment. Ocular and genital mucosal involvement are common.

The cause of erythema multiforme is an immune response to a variety of antigens. In the minor form, recurrent herpes simplex virus infections trigger the disease most frequently. Erythema multiforme major is most often precipitated by infections, notably by *Mycoplasma pneumoniae,* and exposure to medications.

When the disease predominantly affects the oral cavity, systemic corticosteroids are most effective in alleviating symptoms. Levamisole also reduces the severity and frequency of oral erythema multiforme. The treatment of oral lesions in the major form includes maintaining optimal oral hygiene, relieving symptoms by using topical corticosteroids and anesthetics, and minimizing mucosal damage by utilizing a liquid diet.

LUPUS ERYTHEMATOSUS

Lupus erythematosus is an autoimmune disease with a heterogenous spectrum of disease manifestations. A diverse group of subtypes has been defined based on the clinical findings and laboratory abnormalities. A careful assessment of the oral cavity in patients suspected of having lupus is invaluable in obtaining diagnostic information. Discoid lupus erythematosus describes a clinical variant with characteristic skin lesions that either are localized to the skin or are part of a systemic disease process. Distinctive oral lesions are found in up to 30% of patients with discoid lupus and are identified by patches of erythema with radiating white striae and, occasionally, telangiectasias at the periphery (Figs. 9-25 and 9-26). Although any mucosal surface may be involved, the buccal mucosa, vermilion border, gingiva, and labial mucosa are most constantly affected. Infrequently, patients may display oral discoid lesions without evidence of the disease elsewhere. The oral lesions are chronic, and, because they commonly ulcerate or become secondarily infected with *Candida,* they tend to be painful.

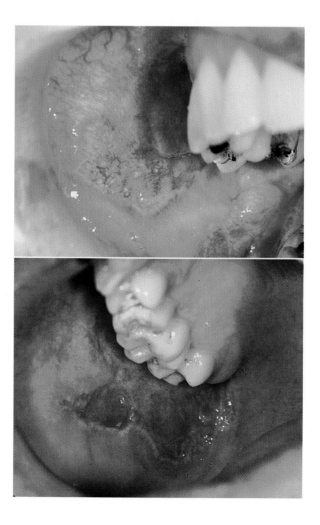

FIG. 9-25 Typical lesions of discoid lupus erythematosus characterized by patches of erythema surrounded by white striae and telangiectases. Lesions develop most frequently on the buccal mucosa.

Oral ulceration is an American College of Rheumatology criterion for the diagnosis of systemic lupus erythematosus. In the majority of instances, the ulcerations are painless and must be detected by a thorough oral examination. Approximately 25% of patients will develop recurrent ulcerations of various sizes, most frequently on the hard palate, centrally and posteriorly. Although the ulcerations are observed most commonly when the systemic disease is active, oral ulcerations are not associated with laboratory changes, nor do they represent a necrotizing vasculitis as some have speculated. Diffuse petechial erythema of the hard palate is the most frequent oral manifestation of systemic lupus erythematosus (Fig. 9-27), and discoid lesions are also commonly detected in the oral cavity. Significantly lowered salivary flow rate is observed and may indicate subclinical involvement of salivary glands.

Similar oral lesions have been documented in other lupus subtypes including subacute cutaneous lupus, neonatal lupus, drug-induced lupus, and mixed connective tissue disease; however, their incidence is unknown.

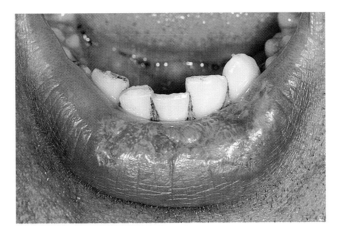

FIG. 9-26   Discoid lupus erythematosus of the lower lip resembles oral lichen planus. Lesions are exacerbated by sunlight.

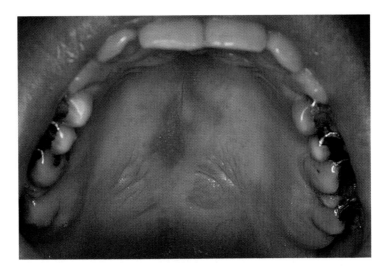

FIG. 9-27   Palatal erythema is the most common oral manifestation of systemic lupus erythematosus.

The histology of the lesions of oral lupus, regardless of the morphology, is an interface reaction similar to that seen in cutaneous lesions of systemic lupus. Direct immunofluorescence from oral lesions corresponds to lesional skin biopsy specimens from patients with systemic involvement and is almost always positive. The lupus band test from nonlesional oral mucosal biopsies is similar to that obtained from skin unexposed to the sun.

Topical corticosteroids hasten the resolution of oral lupus lesions. Intralesional corticosteroids are needed for painful discoid lesions, which generally are refractory to treatment, even with systemic antimalarial agents.

DERMATITIS HERPETIFORMIS

Dermatitis herpetiformis, a disease that most often presents in the second and third decades of life, is characterized by an intensely pruritic cutaneous eruption that is symmetrically distributed on the extensor surfaces. The majority of patients have an associated gluten-sensitive enteropathy, which is usually asymptomatic. Additional associations include an increased risk for gastrointestinal malignancies, a frequent occurrence with other autoimmune diseases, and an increased frequency of HLA-A1, HLA-B8, HLA-DR3, and HLA-Dqw2 haplotypes. The diagnosis is firmly established by detecting granular deposits of IgA and often C3 at the dermoepidermal junction from normal appearing perilesional skin. The oral mucosa is commonly involved, although a careful examination is required to detect abnormalities. Superficial ulcerations precipitated by minimal trauma and diffuse areas of erythema are observed most frequently on the buccal mucosa and tongue (Fig. 9-28). Intact bullae may be noted infrequently. More than half of patients with dermatitis herpetiformis exhibit tooth enamel defects similar to those observed in patients with celiac disease. Even when there are no visible oral lesions, a biopsy from the buccal mucosa for direct immunofluorescence reveals granular IgA deposits. The oral lesions respond to therapy with either dapsone or sulfapyridine or to dietary therapy that avoids gluten.

LINEAR IgA DISEASE

Linear IgA disease is an uncommon disorder that is characterized by a vesiculobullous eruption that occurs in the fifth to sixth decades of life. Some patients display tense blisters resembling those in bullous pemphigoid, and others demonstrate vesicular eruptions similar to dermatitis herpetiformis.

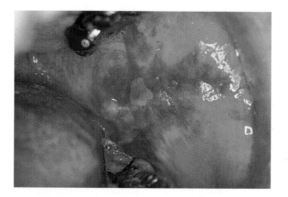

FIG. 9-28   Dermatitis herpetiformis commonly involves the oral cavity, and lesions are characterized by erosions developing in areas subjected to trauma.

The disease has been defined on the basis of immunofluorescent findings consisting of linear deposits of IgA along the dermoepidermal junction. Although a diverse group of diseases, malignancies, infections, and drugs have been associated with linear IgA disease, their significance has not been well established.

Oral manifestations of this disease are common and may be present in almost all cases. Generally, they occur simultaneously with skin lesions, although they may be the initial manifestation of the disease. Nonspecific, painful, large ulcerations occur most commonly on the tongue, palate, and buccal mucosa (Figs. 9-29 and 9-30). A significant number of patients exhibit a diffuse desquamative gingivitis indistinguishable from cicatricial pemphigoid. Direct immunofluorescent studies from perilesional oral biopsies are a reliable method of demonstrating linear IgA deposits. The oral lesions

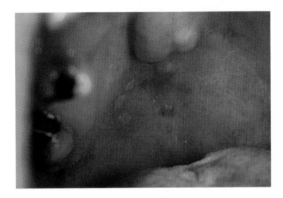

FIG. 9-29   Erosions and vesicles are frequently observed on the palate in linear IgA disease.

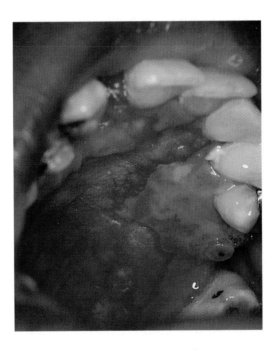

FIG. 9-30   Extensive oral ulcerations are typical in patients with linear IgA disease and may be the sole manifestation of the disease.

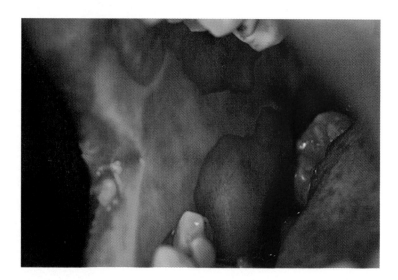

FIG. 9-31   Familial benign pemphigus. Oral serpiginous ulcerations resemble cutaneous lesions.

respond to dapsone or sulfapyridine, which are used to treat cutaneous lesions. Topical corticosteroids hasten resolution of the oral ulcerations and systemic steroids are rarely required.

FAMILIAL BENIGN PEMPHIGUS

Also known as Hailey-Hailey disease, familial benign pemphigus is a rare autosomal dominant condition that begins in the second or third decade of life. The cutaneous eruption originates as vesicles that rupture and become covered with crusts. Often the lesions form moist, vegetative plaques with serpiginous borders. Sites of predilection include the intertriginous folds such as the axillae, groin, inframammary, and perianal areas. Oral mucosal lesions have been well described and consist of ulcerations and painful papules that may appear vegetative and resemble cutaneous lesions (Fig. 9-31). Trauma, which is known to induce skin lesions, also results in oral ulcerations most commonly on the tongue and buccal mucosa. Treatment with topical steroids and antibiotics is beneficial for oral and cutaneous lesions.

EPIDERMOLYSIS BULLOSA

Epidermolysis bullosa (EB) describes a group of more than 20 inherited, phenotypically different disorders that are all characterized by skin fragility and blister formation. Tissue separation, occurring spontaneously or after mechanical trauma, develops at variable depths in the skin depending on the specific type of EB.

EB can be classified into three major types based on light and electron microscopic findings: EB simplex, junctional EB, and dystrophic EB. Oral involvement is common in all forms of EB, and the recognition of the different patterns of involvement in the various forms of this disease may help establish a specific diagnosis. The most severe oral involvement occurs in the recessive dystrophic form, with patients almost always exhibiting oral lesions. Oral tissue fragility and widespread blisters result in ulcerations and scarring characterized by microstomia, complete vestibular obliteration, and ankyloglossia (Fig. 9-32). By comparison, the oral cavity of patients with dominant dystrophic EB is affected with a similar frequency but without scarring. Patients with junctional EB and EB simplex frequently demonstrate ulcerations (90% and 50%, respectively) that heal without scarring (Fig.

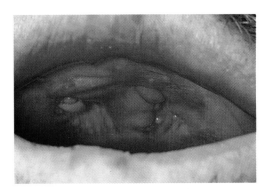

FIG. 9-32   Recessive dystrophic epidermolysis bullosa results in extensive ulcerations, microstomia, and complete vestibular obliteration.

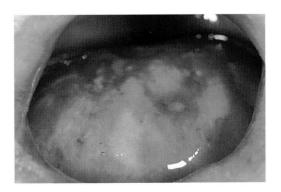

FIG. 9-33   Dominant dystrophic epidermolysis bullosa with extensive and severely painful tongue ulcerations.

9-33). The oral manifestations of the inversa subtype of EB dystrophic recessive are ankyloglossia, loss of tongue papillae, and obliteration of the oral vestibule between the lips and gingiva. Oral milia are present in all major EB categories, most prevalently in the dystrophic forms. Alterations of the teeth are common, with enamel hypoplasia present in all junctional EB patients. Dental caries is greatly increased in dystrophic and junctional EB patients compared with patients with other EB types or unaffected individuals.

The diagnosis and classification of patients with EB are achieved by demonstrating the level of skin cleavage by electron microscopy and immunohistochemical techniques.

All therapies are palliative and preventive, aimed at minimizing physical and chemical trauma to the oral cavity. Maintaining adequate nutrition is accomplished more readily if the teeth are adequately preserved. Early and aggressive dental intervention can ensure optimal dental health and oral function, even in the most severely affected individuals with EB.

EPIDERMOLYSIS BULLOSA ACQUISITA

Epidermolysis bullosa acquisita (EBA) is a rare disorder that is characterized by blistering of the skin and mucous membranes resulting in scarring. The disease is acquired and has been reported in all

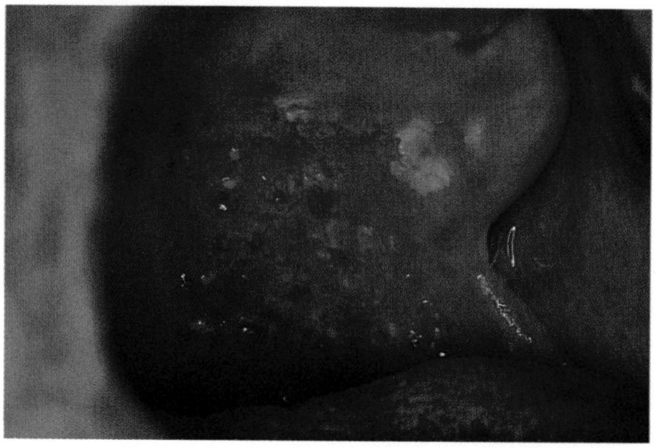

FIG. 9-34   Intact blisters and ulcerations on the palate are a common manifestation of epidermolysis bullosa acquisita.

age groups, although the majority of patients are older than 40 years. Blisters arise most commonly on areas of the skin and mouth subjected to trauma. These include the dorsal surfaces of the hands, elbows, knees, and ankles. A generalized blistering form is also recognized. The oral manifestations, which have been noted but not characterized in detail, include ulcerations and bullae on the buccal mucosa, palate, and tongue (Fig. 9-34). A desquamative gingivitis sometimes is evident, and, in general, the lesions often resemble those of pemphigoid. The disease can also predominantly or exclusively affect the oral cavity with minimal or no skin involvement.

Histologic evaluation reveals a subepidermal blister identical to that obtained from patients with pemphigoid. Immunofluorescent studies of perilesional skin exhibit linear IgG immune deposits at the dermal-epidermal junction in all cases. The most definitive test for establishing this diagnosis is demonstration of autoantibodies from patients' serum reacting against type VII collagen.

Minimizing trauma to the oral cavity by removing sharp dental restorations and limiting oral habits, including cheek and lip biting, results in fewer ulcerations. Immunosuppressive agents are commonly used to control disease activity.

REITER'S SYNDROME

The clinical triad of urethritis, arthritis, and conjunctivitis has classically defined Reiter's syndrome, although a significant number of patients do not present with all the symptoms. The high incidence of HLA-B27 and venereal infections signifies the importance of genetic and environmental factors in Reiter's syndrome. The condition occurs almost exclusively in men, and a possible association with HIV infection has been noted. Psoriasis and pustular psoriasiform lesions, termed *keratoderma blennorrhagicum,* occur most frequently on the soles and palms. Balanitis circinata, characterized by crusted serpiginous papules and vesicles, appears on the genitalia.

The oral mucosal lesions occur in up to one half of all patients with Reiter's syndrome. The initial lesions start as painless papules that coalesce into plaques and eventually develop into superficial ulcerations. A white circinate border often surrounds the ulcerations, which occur commonly on the buccal mucosa, lips, and gingiva. The most frequent oral manifestation of Reiter's syndrome is a sharply demarcated erosion on the hard palate (Fig. 9-35). Lesions on the tongue are clinically identical to geographic tongue. Fortunately, all of these lesions are asymptomatic.

Histologically, the lesions resemble psoriasis with parakeratosis, elongation of the rete ridges, intraepithelial microabscess formation, and polymorphonuclear leukocyte infiltration of the epithe-

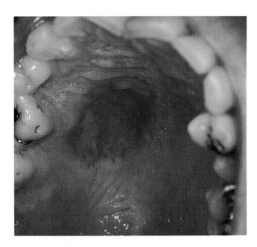

FIG. 9-35   Sharply demarcated ulcers on the hard palate are the most common oral manifestation of Reiter's syndrome.

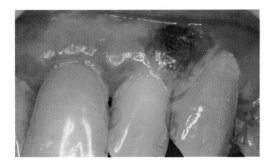

FIG. 9-36   Angina hemorrhagica bullosa. Blood blisters may spontaneously appear on any mucosal surface and are not associated with underlying disease.

lium. Treatment of Reiter's syndrome consists of nonsteroidal antiinflammatory medications for joint symptoms. Immunosuppressive agents are used for severe arthritis and cutaneous disease.

ANGINA BULLOSA HEMORRHAGICA

Angina bullosa hemorrhagica is characterized by the sudden appearance of one or more blood blisters in the oral cavity (Fig. 9-36). Although the lesions develop predominantly at the junction of the hard and soft palate, angina bullosa hemorrhagica may occur on any oral mucosal surface. After minutes or hours, the blisters spontaneously rupture, forming ulcerations that heal without scarring. The blisters are often painful and recurrences are common. The disease is seen most frequently in the elderly, occurs equally in men and women, and develops in the absence of any identifiable systemic disorders. Although the cause is unknown, many cases have been precipitated by the use of steroid inhalers for the treatment of asthma and obstructive airway diseases. Other identifiable causes include trauma from dental procedures and the ingestion of certain foods. No therapy is needed other than reassuring patients of the benign nature of the condition.

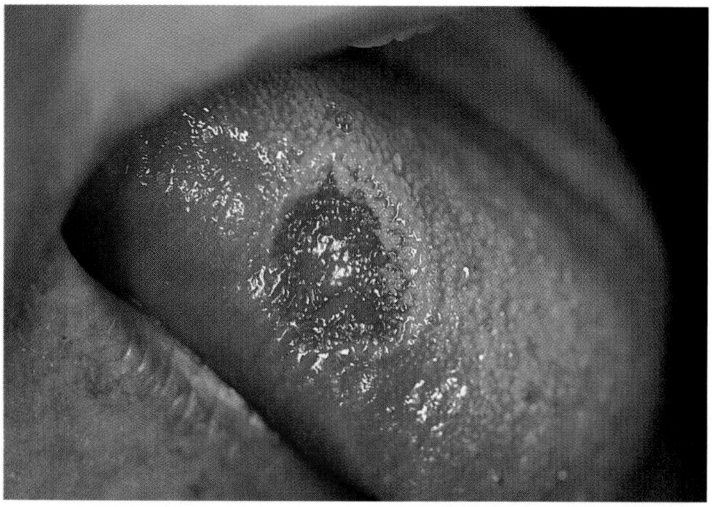

FIG. 9-37   Eosinophilic ulcer of the tongue may persist for months and mimic malignancy.

EOSINOPHILIC ULCER

Eosinophilic ulcer, also known by many names including traumatic granuloma and Riga-Fede disease, is an uncommon condition that represents a benign reactive process. Although the cause remains unknown, antecedent trauma is believed to be an important etiologic factor in approximately 50% of cases. The role of a T-cell–mediated mechanism is also supported by several investigations.

Clinically, the majority of lesions occur on the tongue, buccal mucosa, and lip and present as ulcerations with firm indurated borders (Fig. 9-37). The lesions are often greater than 1.5 cm in diameter and symptomatic in only one third of cases. Nonulcerated submucosal masses and multiple lesions occur infrequently. The disease can present at any age, and its incidence peaks during the fourth to fifth decades of life.

Histologically, a dense cellular infiltrate consisting of lymphocytes, eosinophils, histiocytes, and plasma cells extends from the ulcer base through the submucosa into skeletal muscle. Muscle degeneration, necrosis, and regenerative myocytes are also observed. Immunohistochemical staining of the large mononuclear cells in the infiltrate reveals these to be comprised of a mixture of macrophages, "dendrocytes," and S-100–positive connective tissue cells.

Eosinophilic ulcer may mimic oral malignancies both clinically and histologically. Once these lesions are properly identified, the administration of either topical or systemic steroids may hasten their resolution. Regardless of therapy, spontaneous healing usually takes weeks to months, with recurrences noted in 10% of cases.

ULCERATIVE STOMATITIS RESULTING FROM CHEMOTHERAPY, RADIATION, AND BONE MARROW TRANSPLANTATION

Oral mucositis occurring as a consequence of cytotoxic therapy is a major cause of morbidity in cancer patients. Direct stomatologic effects from antineoplastic agents include reduced mucosal thickening and keratinization, superficial sloughing, intense erythema, and ulcerations. Edema and serration of the lateral borders of the tongue are frequent findings. Pain is intense and often limits the administration of chemotherapy and food intake. The disruption and compromise of oral mucosal barriers can result in the development of infection and hemorrhage. Aggressive chemotherapeutic regimens result in a greater incidence of oral mucositis compared with treatment of solid tumors.

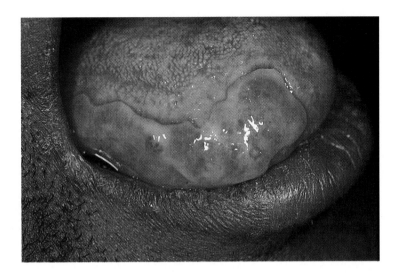

FIG. 9-38   Large painful ulcerations develop in almost all bone marrow transplant recipients and resolve when the absolute neutrophil count rises.

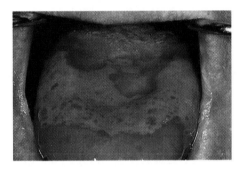

FIG. 9-39   Radiation therapy for head and neck malignancies results in painful ulcerations covered with a fibrinous exudate. (Lynch DP: *Postgrad Med* 75:191, 1984.)

Ulcerative stomatitis complicates bone marrow transplantation in almost all cases. Most lesions occur on nonkeratinized mucosa subjected to trauma including the tongue and buccal and labial mucosa (Fig. 9-38). The oral ulcers usually begin 3 days after marrow infusion and persist until the absolute neutrophil count rises above 750 cells/ml. Pain is commonly severe, necessitating the administration of narcotics for analgesia. The reactivation of herpes simplex virus infections in the oral cavity can be prevented by the prophylactic administration of acyclovir to patients with antibody titers against herpes simplex virus. Candidiasis is the most frequent oral infection in bone marrow transplant recipients and can be prevented by prophylaxis with either topical or systemic antifungal agents. Oral ulcerations may also result from bacterial and fungal infections and systemic diseases such as graft-versus-host (GVH) disease.

Radiation for head and neck cancers can result in mucositis after the first week of therapy and may persist for 2 to 3 weeks after the completion of treatment. Initially the oral mucosa appears reddened and swollen; however, as therapy progresses, painful areas of ulceration covered with a fibrinous exudate develop (Fig. 9-39). Xerostomia, rampant dental caries, taste loss, osteoradionecrosis, oral infections, and trismus are frequent postradiation complications.

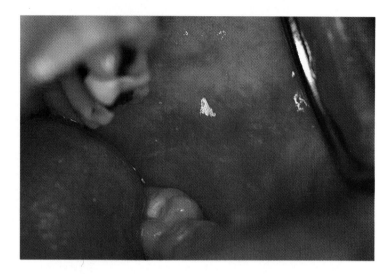

FIG. 9-40   Acute graft-versus-host disease. Oral lesions are common and are characterized by areas of erythema, sometimes resembling lichen planus.

Attempts to minimize or prevent chemotherapy and radiation mucositis have been relatively unsuccessful. Topical steroids may hasten the resolution of ulcerations. Although the presence and extent of oral complications depend on the type of malignancy, age of the patient, and total dosage of chemotherapy, patients who maintain an optimal oral hygiene program tend to experience less severe mucositis. Topical anesthetics and coating agents may provide some benefit.

GRAFT-VERSUS-HOST DISEASE

Graft-versus-host (GVH) disease remains a common cause of morbidity and mortality after allogenic bone marrow transplantation despite the use of HLA-identical donors and the administration of immunosuppressive drugs. The early recognition of oral manifestations can lead to a correct diagnosis, the institution of appropriate therapy, and prolonged survival.

Acute GVH disease occurs in the first 100 days after transplantation, with an incidence ranging from 25% to as high as 78%. Oral manifestations of acute GVH disease are common and are characterized by diffuse erythema, lichenoid changes, xerostomia, inflamed minor salivary gland duct orifices, and sometimes ulcerations (Fig. 9-40). Although all sites may be affected, the disease is most evident on the tongue and labial and buccal mucosa. The oral changes observed are nonspecific and difficult to differentiate from other causes of erythema including pretransplant chemotherapy, conditioning, posttransplantation immunosuppressive drugs and infections. Oral acute GVH disease lesions may precede the onset of systemic disease; however, they usually accompany systemic signs and symptoms. Persistent oral mucositis that occurs beyond 21 days after bone marrow transplantation or lichen planuslike lesions are strongly suggestive of acute GVH disease.

The onset of chronic GVH disease occurs between 100 and 400 days posttransplantation and develops in 25% to 40% of allogenic bone marrow transplant recipients. Oral findings are present in up to 80% of cases, are often included as one of the criteria for establishing a diagnosis, and may be the only manifestation of the disease. Diffuse mucosal erythema, often with distinct telangiectases, is observed most frequently. White reticulated lesions and erosions clinically identical to oral lichen planus are the most characteristic changes and occur in one third of patients (Fig. 9-41). Mucosal atrophy characterized by loss of filiform papillae and gingival stippling are subtle changes that should

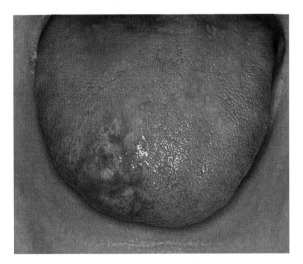

FIG. 9-41   Chronic graft-versus-host disease. Oral lesions are diagnostic and may be the only manifestation of the disease. The lesions are clinically and histologically identical to oral lichen planus.

be searched for. Oral pain and dryness are reported by more than one half of patients with chronic GVH disease.

The histopathologic changes of acute and chronic oral GVH disease are similar and consist of a subepithelial mononuclear infiltrate with basal vacuolar degeneration. Labial salivary gland biopsies revealing infiltrating lymphocytes and ductal epithelial necrosis in combination with an abnormal oral examination are diagnostic of GVH disease.

In addition to systemic therapy for the disease, the oral lesions of GVH disease can be treated by the application of topical corticosteroids and topical cyclosporine. Therapy with psoralens and ultraviolet A light is also beneficial.

SUGGESTED READINGS

Recurrent aphthous stomatitis

Brice SL, Jester JD, Huff JC: Recurrent aphthous stomatitis, *Curr Probl Dermatol* 3:113, 1991.

Field EA, Brookes V, Tyldesley WR: Recurrent aphthous ulceration in children: a review, *Int J Pediatr Dent* 2:1, 1992.

Hayrinen-Immonen R: Immune-activation in recurrent oral ulcers (ROU), *Scand J Dent Res* 100:222, 1992.

Herlofson BB, Barkvoll P: Sodium lauryl sulfate and recurrent aphthous ulcers: a preliminary study, *Acta Odontol Scand* 52:257, 1994.

MacPhail LA et al: Recurrent aphthous ulcers in association with HIV infection: description of ulcer types and analysis of T lymphocyte subsets, *Oral Surg Oral Med Oral Pathol* 71:678, 1991.

Nolan A et al: Recurrent aphthous ulceration and food sensitivity, *J Oral Pathol Med* 20:473, 1991.

Nolan A et al: Recurrent aphthous ulceration: vitamin B1, B2 and B6 status and response to replacement therapy, *J Oral Pathol Med* 20:389, 1991.

Scully C: Are viruses associated with aphthae and oral vesiculo-erosive disorders? *Br J Oral Maxillofac Surg* 31:173, 1993.

Ship JA: Recurrent aphthous stomatitis: an update, *Oral Surg Oral Med Oral Pathol Oral Radiol Endod* 81:141, 1996.

Vincent SD, Lilly GE: Clinical, historic, and therapeutic features of aphthous stomatitis: literature review and open clinical trial employing steroids, *Oral Surg Oral Med Oral Pathol* 74:79, 1992.

Behçet's disease

Frances TC: Recurrent aphthous stomatitis and Behçet's disease: a review, *Oral Surg* 30:476, 1980.

Helm TN et al: Clinical features of Behçet's disease: report of four cases, *Oral Surg Oral Med Oral Pathol* 72:30, 1991.

Jorizzo JL: Behçet's disease: an update based on the International Conference held in Paris, France, June 30-July 1, 1993, *J Eur Acad Dermatol Venereol* 3:215, 1994.

Kim DK, Chang SN, Lee ES: Clinical manifestations of childhood-onset Behçet's disease, *Pediatr Dermatol* 11:95, 1994.

McCalmont TH: Behçet's disease. In Arndt KA et al, editors: *Cutaneous medicine and surgery: an integrated program in dermatology,* Philadelphia, 1996, WB Saunders.

Main DM, Chamberlain MA: Clinical differentiation of oral ulceration in Behçet's disease, *Br J Rheumatol* 31:767, 1992.

Lichen planus

Bagan JV et al: Oral lichen planus and chronic liver disease: a clinical and morphometric study of the oral lesions in relation to transaminase elevation, *Oral Surg Oral Med Oral Pathol* 78:337, 1994.

Barnard NA et al: Oral cancer development in patients with oral lichen planus, *J Oral Pathol Med* 22:421, 1993.

Brown RS et al: A retrospective evaluation of 193 patients with oral lichen planus, *J Oral Pathol Med* 22:69, 1993.

Eisen D: The therapy of oral lichen planus, *Crit Rev Oral Biol Med* 4:141, 1993.

Eisen D: A comprehensive guide to management of oral lichen planus, *Fitzpatrick's J Clin Derm* 3:50, 1995.

Chronic ulcerative stomatitis with stratified epithelium-specific antinuclear antibody

Beutner EH et al: Ten cases of chronic ulcerative stomatitis with stratified epithelium-specific antinuclear antibody, *J Am Acad Dermatol* 24:781, 1991.

Church LF, Schosser RH: Chronic ulcerative stomatitis associated with stratified epithelial specific antinuclear antibodies, *Oral Surg Oral Med Oral Pathol* 73:579, 1992.

Pemphigus

Anhalt GJ: Pemphigus vulgaris and the pemphigus disease spectrum. In Arndt KA et al, editors: *Cutaneous medicine and surgery: an integrated program in dermatology,* Philadelphia, 1996, WB Saunders.

Amagai M, Klaus-Kovtun V, Stanley JR: Autoantibodies against a novel epithelial cadherin in pemphigus vulgaris, a disease of cell adhesion, *Cell* 67:869, 1991.

Bystryn JC, Steinman NM: The adjuvant therapy of pemphigus: an update, *Arch Dermatol* 132:203, 1996.

Chrysomallis F et al: Treatment of oral pemphigus vulgaris, *Int J Dermatol* 33:803, 1994.

Gorsky M, Raviv M, Raviv E: Pemphigus vulgaris in adolescence: a case presentation and review of the literature, *Oral Surg Oral Med Oral Pathol* 77:620, 1994.

Helander SD, Rogers RS III: The sensitivity and specificity of direct immunofluorescence in disorders of mucous membranes, *J Am Acad Dermatol* 30:65, 1994.

Lamey PJ et al: Oral presentation of pemphigus vulgaris and its response to systemic steroid therapy, *Oral Surg Oral Med Oral Pathol* 74:54, 1992.

Ratnam KV, Pang BK: Pemphigus in remission: value of negative direct immunofluorescence in management, *J Am Acad Dermatol* 30:547, 1994.

Paraneoplastic pemphigus

Anhalt GJ et al: Paraneoplastic pemphigus: an autoimmune mucocutaneous disease associated with neoplasia, *N Engl J Med* 323:1729, 1990.

Helm TN et al: Paraneoplastic pemphigus: a distinctive autoimmune vesiculobullous disorder associated with neoplasia, *Oral Surg Oral Med Oral Pathol* 75:209, 1993.

Liu AY et al: Indirect immunofluorescence on rat bladder transitional epithelium: a test with high specificity for paraneoplastic pemphigus, *J Am Acad Dermatol* 28:69, 1993.

Pemphigoid

Ahmed AR, Kurgis BS, Rogers RS III: Cicatricial pemphigoid, *J Am Acad Dermatol* 24:987, 1991.

Capecchi M, Ficarra G, Pagni L: Benign pemphigoid of the mucous membranes: the clinical and histopathological aspects in 20 patients, *Minerva Stomatol* 43:423, 1994.

Mutasim DF, Pelc NJ, Anhalt GJ: Cicatricial pemphigoid, *Dermatol Clin* 11:499, 1993.

Sarret Y et al: Salt-split human skin substrate for the immunofluorescent screening of serum from patients with cicatricial pemphigoid and a new method of immunoprecipitation with IgA antibodies, *J Am Acad Dermatol* 24:952, 1991.

Vincent SD, Lilly GE, Baker KA: Clinical, historic, and the therapeutic features of cicatricial pemphigoid: a literature review and open therapeutic trial with corticosteroids, *Oral Surg Oral Med Oral Pathol* 76:45, 1993.

Erythema multiforme, Stevens-Johnson syndrome, and toxic epidermal necrolysis

Bastuji-Garin S et al: Clinical classification of cases of toxic epidermal necrolysis, Stevens-Johnson syndrome, and erythema multiforme, *Arch Dermatol* 129:92, 1993.

Farthing PM et al: Characteristics of the oral lesions in patients with cutaneous recurrent erythema multiforme, *J Oral Pathol Med* 24:9, 1995.

Lozada-Nur F, Gorsky M, Silverman S: Oral erythema multiforme: clinical observations and treatment of 95 patients, *Oral Surg Oral Med Oral Pathol* 67:36, 1989.

Schofield JK, Tatnall FM, Leigh IM: Recurrent erythema multiforme: clinical features and treatment in a large series of patients, *Br J Dermatol* 128:542, 1993.

Lupus erythematosus

Ben-Aryeh H et al: Whole saliva in systemic lupus erythematosus, *Oral Surg Oral Med Oral Pathol* 75:696, 1993.

Burge SM et al: The lupus band test in oral mucosa, conjunctiva and skin, *Br J Dermatol* 121:743, 1989.

Jonsson R et al: Oral mucosal lesions in systemic lupus erythematosus: a clinical, histopathological and immunopathological study, *J Rheumatol* 11:38, 1984.

Karjalainen TK, Tomich CE: A histopathologic study of oral mucosal lupus erythematosus, *Oral Surg Oral Med Oral Pathol* 67:547, 1989.

Schiodt M, Halberg P, Hertzner B: A clinical study of 32 patients with oral discoid lupus erythematosus, *Int J Oral Surg* 7:85, 1978.

Urman JD et al: Oral mucosal ulceration in systemic lupus erythematosus, *Arthritis Rheum* 21:58, 1978.

Dermatitis herpetiformis

Ahmed AR et al: Major histocompatibility complex susceptibility genes for dermatitis herpetiformis compared with those for gluten-sensitive enteropathy, *J Exp Med* 178:2067, 1993.

Aine L, Maki M, Reunala T: Coeliac-type dental enamel defects in patients with dermatitis herpetiformis, *Acta Derm Venereol* 72:25, 1992.

Fraser NG, Kerr NW, Donald D: Oral lesions in dermatitis herpetiformis, *Br J Dermatol* 89:439, 1973.

Hietanen J, Reunala T: IgA deposits in the oral mucosa of patients with dermatitis herpetiformis and linear IgA disease, *Scand J Dent Res* 92:230, 1984.

Seah PP et al: Immunoglobulins in the skin in dermatitis herpetiformis and coeliac disease, *Lancet* 360:611, 1972.

Linear IgA disease

Chan LS, Regezi JA, Cooper KD: Oral manifestations of linear IgA disease, *J Am Acad Dermatol* 22:362, 1990.

Kelly SE et al: A clinicopathological study of mucosal involvement in linear IgA disease, *Br J Dermatol* 119:161, 1988.

Leonard JN et al: The relationship between linear IgA disease and benign mucous membrane pemphigoid, *Br J Dermatol* 110:307, 1984.

Porter SR, Bain SE, Scully CM: Linear IgA disease manifesting as recalcitrant desquamative gingivitis, *Oral Surg Oral Med Oral Pathol* 74:179, 1992.

Prost C et al: Diagnosis of adult linear IgA dermatosis by immunoelectron microscopy in 16 patients with linear IgA deposits, *J Invest Dermatol* 92:239, 1989.

Familial benign pemphigus

Botvinick I: Familial benign pemphigus with oral mucous membrane lesions, *Cutis* 12:371, 1973.

Burge SM: Hailey-Hailey disease: the clinical features, response to treatment and prognosis, *Br J Dermatol* 126:275, 1992.

Epidermolysis bullosa

Wright JT, Fine JD: Hereditary epidermolysis bullosa, *Semin Dermatol* 13:102, 1994.

Wright JT, Fine JD, Johnson L: Dental caries risk in hereditary epidermolysis bullosa, *Pediatr Dent* 16:427, 1994.

Wright JT et al: Oral involvement of recessive dystrophic epidermolysis bullosa inversa, *Am J Med Genet* 47:1184, 1993.

Wright JT, Fine JD, Johnson L: Hereditary epidermolysis bullosa: oral manifestations and dental management, *Pediatr Dent* 15:242, 1993.

Epidermolysis bullosa acquisita

Chan LS, Chen M, Woodley DT: Epidermolysis bullosa acquisita in the elderly: clinical manifestations, diagnosis, and therapy, *J Geriatr Dermatol* 4:47, 1996.

Gammon WR et al: Epidermolysis bullosa acquisita: a pemphigoid-like disease, *J Am Acad Dermatol* 11:820, 1984.

Reiter's syndrome

Fotiou G, Laskaris G: Reiter's syndrome oral manifestations, *Hell Stomatol Chron* 32:148, 1988.

Hammer JE, Graykowski E: Oral lesions compatible with Reiter's disease: a diagnostic problem, *J Am Dent Assoc* 69:560, 1964.

Kane-Wanger GF: Reiter's syndrome. In Arndt KA et al, editors: *Cutaneous medicine and surgery: an integrated program in dermatology,* Philadelphia, 1996, WB Saunders.

Pindborg JJ, Gorlin RJ, Asboe-Hansen G: Reiter's syndrome, *Oral Surg Oral Med Oral Pathol* 16:551, 1963.

Angina bullosa hemorrhagica

Brigitte DM, van der Waal I: Blood blisters of the oral mucosa (angina bullosa haemorrhagica), *J Am Acad Dermatol* 31:341, 1994.

Stephenson P et al: Angina bullosa haemorrhagica: clinical and laboratory features in 30 patients, *Oral Surg Oral Med Oral Pathol* 63:560, 1987.

Eosinophilic ulcer

El-Mofty SK et al: Eosinophilic ulcer of the oral mucosa: report of 38 new cases with immunohistochemical observations, *Oral Surg Oral Med Oral Pathol* 75:716, 1993.

Elzay RP: Traumatic ulcerative granuloma with stromal eosinophilia, *Oral Surg Oral Med Oral Pathol* 55:497, 1983.

Mezei MM et al: Eosinophilic ulcer of the oral mucosa, *J Am Acad Dermatol* 33:734, 1995.

Regezi JA et al: Oral traumatic granuloma, *Oral Surg Oral Med Oral Pathol* 75:723, 1993.

Ulcerative stomatitis resulting from chemotherapy, radiation, and bone marrow transplantation

Carl W: Oral complications of local and systemic cancer treatment, *Curr Opin Oncol* 7:320, 1995.

Dreizen S: Description and incidence of oral complications, *NCI Monogr* 9:11, 1990.

Wingard JR et al: Oral mucositis after bone marrow transplantation, *Oral Surg Oral Med Oral Pathol* 72:419, 1991.

Woo SB et al: A longitudinal study of oral ulcerative mucositis in bone marrow transplant recipients, *Cancer* 72:1612, 1993.

Verdi CJ: Cancer therapy and oral mucositis: an appraisal of drug prophylaxis, *Drug Saf* 9:185, 1993.

Graft-versus-host disease

Barrett AP, Bilous AM: Oral patterns of acute and chronic graft-v-host disease, *Arch Dermatol* 120:1461, 1984.

Epstein JB, Reece DE: Topical cyclosporine A for treatment of oral chronic graft-versus-host disease, *Bone Marrow Transplant* 13:81, 1994.

Hiroki A et al: Significance of oral examination in chronic graft-versus-host disease, *J Oral Pathol Med* 23:209, 1994.

Hsiao M et al: Oral manifestations of acute graft-versus-host disease following marrow transplantation, *J Dent Res Spec Issue* 67:202, 1988.

Schubert MM, Sullivan KM: Recognition, incidence, and management of oral graft-versus-host disease, *NCI Monogr* 9:135, 1990.

Schubert MM et al: Oral manifestations of chronic graft-v-host disease, *Arch Intern Med* 144:1591, 1984.

CHAPTER 10

Disorders of Pigmentation

Abnormal pigmentation of the oral cavity can result from a variety of exogenous and endogenous etiologic factors (Table 10-1). When the pigmentation is diffuse, a thorough oral examination and medical history are required to identify a specific cause. Focal areas of intraoral pigmentation that cannot be identified with certainty necessitate biopsy to exclude oral melanoma.

EXOGENOUS ORIGIN

Pharmacologic Agents

A large group of systemic medications, notably the antimalarials, minocycline, amiodarone, and clofazimine, may result in a characteristic blue appearance of the oral mucosa, most commonly of the hard palate and gingiva (Fig. 10-1). The chronic administration of high doses of minocycline for acne may result in blue-black pigmentation of the alveolar bone. After 1 year, more than 10% of patients taking 200 mg of minocycline daily develop this abnormality and the incidence increases to 20% after 4 years of therapy. The bone pigmentation is most visible beneath the semitransparent anterior maxillary and mandibular alveolar mucosa, although it is often apparent on the hard palate and the lingual mandibular alveolar bone. If the antibiotic is not discontinued, the pigmentation may be permanent; however, its presence, although unsightly, is not harmful. Azidothymidine and ketoconazole, commonly prescribed for human immunodeficiency virus (HIV)-positive patients, produce darkly pigmented patches on the tongue, buccal mucosa, and palate. In contrast, adrenocorticotropic hormone (ACTH), busulfan, oral contraceptives, and the phenothiazine drugs may cause brown pigmentation of various oral mucous membranes. Generally, drug-induced pigmentation does not seem to correlate with the dose and duration of the medication. Even when the offending drug is withdrawn, the pigmentation may persist for months to years. Fixed drug eruptions (the appearance of a lesion in the same location each time a drug is administered), characterized by darkly pigmented lesions of the tongue, can occur in people who use antibiotics and phenobarbital and in heroin addicts.

Amalgam Tattoos

Amalgam tattoos represent the most common exogenous cause of oral pigmentation. Dental filling materials (amalgam) may be accidentally or inadvertently introduced into soft tissue during surgical and dental procedures, resulting in a permanent tattoo. Almost half of amalgam tattoos are located on the gingiva and alveolar mucosa, and more than 20% occur on the buccal mucosa. Clinically, the lesions are macular, asymptomatic, and vary in size, although the majority are less than 0.4 cm (Figs. 10-2 and 10-3). The lesions are discovered most frequently during the third decade of life and twice as often in women. They appear blue, gray, and, infrequently, black depending on the depth at which the particles lodge. The color of these tattoos helps differentiate them from oral melanoma, nevi, and melanotic macules, which are most often brown. Several lesions are occasionally discovered in a patient. Amalgam pigmentation can usually be recognized clinically and the diagnosis supported by a dental history. Radiographically, amalgam tattoos can be diagnosed by their opaque appearance, but

Table 10-1 Hyperpigmentation of the Oral Mucosa

ORIGIN	COMMENTS
EXOGENOUS	
Foreign materials	Amalgam tattoos; lead; carbon; bark, seeds, and leaves of various plants; tobacco and alcohol; cosmetic gingival tattoos
Pharmacologic agents	Minocycline, azidothymidine, quinidine, antimalarials, clofazimine, ketoconazole, amiodarone, oral contraceptives, phenolphthalein, chlorpromazine, busulfan, doxorubicin
Fixed drug eruption	Antibiotics and heroin
Heavy metal exposure	Bismuth, arsenic, lead, mercury, silver, tin, copper, brass, zinc, cadmium, chromium, manganese
ENDOGENOUS	
Systemic diseases	Addison's disease, Albright's syndrome, Peutz-Jeghers syndrome, neurofibromatosis, hemochromatosis, β-thalassemia, Wilson's disease, acromegaly, hyperpituitarism, hyperthyroidism, most nutritional deficiencies, human immunodeficiency virus, syndrome of cardiac myxomas, spotty pigmentation and endocrine overactivity, soft palate pigmentation associated with pulmonary disease, Laugier-Hunziker syndrome, acanthosis nigricans
Neoplasms	Nevi, oral and labial melanotic macules, malignant melanoma
Reactive processes	Oral melanoacanthoma, postinflammatory hyperpigmentation

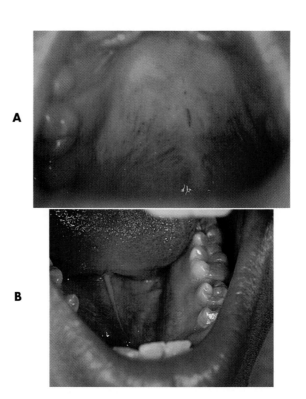

FIG. 10-1   Diffuse blue pigmentation of the hard palate **(A)** and lingual alveolar bone beneath the semitransparent alveolar mucosa **(B)** is an adverse reaction triggered by chronic minocycline therapy.

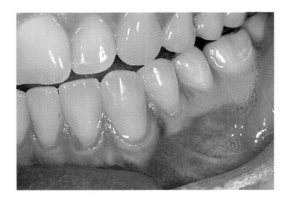

FIG. 10-2   Amalgam tattoos occur most frequently on the gingiva and have a characteristic slate-gray color.

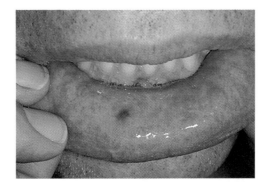

FIG. 10-3   Amalgam tattoo developing after dental filling material was accidentally introduced into the lower lip during a dental procedure.

this feature is noted in fewer than 25% of cases. Energy dispersive x-ray microanalysis is a more sensitive and accurate diagnostic method for detecting amalgam particles. The pattern of amalgam dispersal by routine radiography is also a reliable method of postmortem identification by forensic dentists.

Histologically, amalgam appears as dark granules and irregular solid fragments along collagen bundles and blood vessels. Dark granules are also present intracellularly within macrophages, multi-nucleated giant cells, endothelial cells, and fibroblasts. In approximately one third of patients with amalgam tattoos, the amalgam elicits a surrounding chronic inflammatory infiltrate.

Amalgam tattoos require no treatment unless they cannot be differentiated from other causes of pigmentation. A Q-switched ruby laser may be used as therapy for cosmetic reasons.

Heavy Metal-Induced Pigmentation

Much of the literature regarding heavy metal-induced pigmentation originates from the first half of this century when preparations containing heavy metals were used medicinally. Presently, accidental and occupational exposure to compounds containing these substances occurs infrequently. Bismuth, which had been used as a treatment for syphilis, produces a thin but prominent blue-black line involving the marginal gingiva surrounding the teeth. Pigmentation also commonly develops on the buccal mucosa, lips, and tongue. In patients with optimal oral hygiene, the incidence of pigmenta-

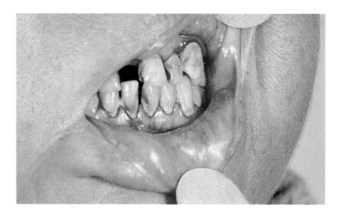

FIG. 10-4 Accidental or occupational exposure to heavy metals may result in blue or gray pigmentation typically affecting the gingiva.

tion is reduced from 75% to less than 10%. When bismuth is discontinued, the hyperpigmentation usually resolves over several months. Lead poisoning results in a lead line (Burton's line) identical to that produced by bismuth (Fig. 10-4). Diffuse pigmentation, metallic taste, and deposition of lead in the primary teeth of children also have been reported. The hyperpigmentation resulting from mercury poisoning, characterized by diffuse grayish discoloration of the alveolar gingiva, probably represents postinflammatory changes and not deposition of salts as with bismuth and lead. Ulcerations, increased salivation, and diffuse loosening of the teeth with periodontal destruction are common with chronic exposure. Arsenic exposure results in widespread inflammation, especially of the gingiva, and oral hyperpigmentation. Argyria (silver pigmentation) produces a permanent, diffuse, bluish-gray pigmentation with a shiny metallic luster of the oral cavity unlike that seen with other metals, most commonly of the hard palate. Silver nitrate applied as a caustic agent to oral ulcerations produces a transient dark black discoloration caused by the deposition of silver. Copper can produce a blue-green line on the gingiva, whereas chrome and cadmium exposure results in a deep orange stain of the teeth and gingiva. Unexplained or unusual pigmentation of the oral cavity, especially when confined to the gingiva, should prompt a search for possible metal exposure.

Miscellaneous Foreign Materials

A diverse group of foreign materials introduced into the oral cavity produce color changes of oral soft tissues. Particles of pencils, various dyes, and ink accidentally introduced into the mucosa; plant materials used by some for oral hygiene aids; and gingival tattoos performed for cosmetic reasons induce pigmentary changes that can usually be diagnosed by a complete history and physical examination. Patients who consume tobacco can develop smoker's melanosis characterized by hyperpigmentation, usually on the mandibular gingiva of the anterior teeth and occasionally on the buccal mucosa and palate. The oral pigmentation abnormalities of alcoholics, recognized by areas of depigmentation surrounded by hyperpigmentation, can serve as a useful screening tool.

ENDOGENOUS ORIGIN

A large group of systemic diseases manifest oral pigmentation. Postinflammatory hyperpigmentation, commonly observed on the skin, also develops in the oral cavity, especially in patients with chronic inflammatory conditions such as oral lichen planus (Fig. 10-5). In hemochromatosis, up to 15% of patients display diffuse bronzing of the oral mucosa secondary to hemosiderin deposition

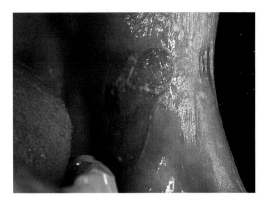

FIG. 10-5   Oral lichen planus and other inflammatory conditions may result in postinflammatory hyperpigmentation, a phenomenon commonly observed on the skin.

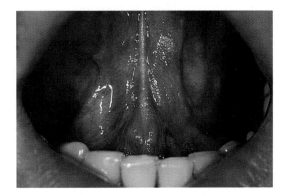

FIG. 10-6   The detection of oral hyperpigmentation may uncover an underlying systemic disorder, in this case, hemochromatosis.

(Fig. 10-6). Endocrine abnormalities including acromegaly and Albright's syndrome result in a reddish brown hyperpigmentation of the oral mucosa. Patients with β-thalassemia commonly display oral brown pigmentation that is diffuse and caused by the metallic deposition from hemoglobin degradation products.

Oral pigmentation may alert the clinician to a systemic illness. Pigmentation on the lateral surfaces of the soft palate resembling melanotic macules is reportedly a marker for chronic pulmonary disease and bronchogenic carcinoma. The complex of life-threatening cardiac myxomas, spotty pigmentation, and endocrine overactivity is a recently recognized syndrome transmitted as an autosomal dominant trait (Carney syndrome). Spotty facial pigmentation and pigmented macules of the lips are present in approximately 50% of cases. Patients with HIV disease frequently display melanotic hyperpigmentation of the oral mucosa characterized by well-circumscribed macules in some patients and diffuse involvement in others. Adrenal insufficiency and pharmacologic agents are responsible for a significant number of cases, but in the majority, the cause is unknown. The oral manifestations of Addison's disease and Peutz-Jeghers syndrome are of great significance and are discussed later in this chapter.

Focal areas of pigmentation in the oral cavity can be caused by a variety of neoplasms and reactive processes that are described in the next section. These necessitate histologic differentiation from oral melanomas because, clinically, they resemble one another.

Melanotic Macules

Intraoral and labial melanotic macules are relatively common lesions that were defined as distinct entities in the 1970s. Clinically, pigmented macules that are shaded blue, black, and, most commonly, brown appear with greatest frequency on the lips followed by the palate, gingiva, and buccal mucosa (Fig. 10-7). Although the majority are solitary, multiple lesions occur especially when located on buccal mucosa (Fig. 10-8). Melanotic macules are usually well circumscribed and average 6 mm in size with the exception of buccal mucosal lesions that tend to be greater than 10 mm. Labial melan-

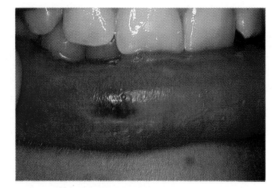

FIG. 10-7   The labial melanotic macule is a distinct lesion that is well circumscribed and darkly pigmented and has no malignant potential.

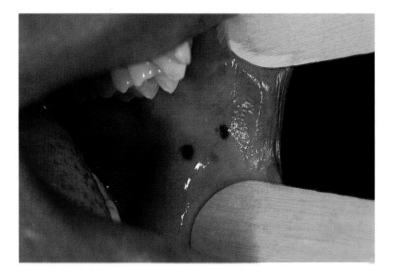

FIG. 10-8   Melanotic macules may develop at any age and are usually multiple when they occur on the buccal mucosa.

otic macules are diagnosed most commonly in the 20- to 30-year age group, whereas intraoral lesions are noted in patients older than 40. All melanotic macules occur more commonly in women than in men and affect all races equally.

Histologically, the lesions are characterized by the presence of melanin in the basal cell layer, lamina propria, or both. In contrast to simple lentigines, melanotic macules do not exhibit elongation of the rete ridges and lack melanocytic activity. In contrast to oral nevi and melanomas, melanotic macules, when studied immunohistochemically, are HMB-45 negative.

Because melanotic macules are completely innocuous and have no malignant potential, semiannual observation for changes in color, size, and shape is acceptable. However, many lesions, especially those occurring intraorally on the palate and gingiva, cannot be clinically differentiated from incipient melanomas and other causes of pigmentation. Such lesions and others that are ulcerated, exophytic, or atypical should be excised.

Oral Nevi

Oral nevi occur infrequently (0.1% of the general population), with fewer than 400 cases reported in the literature. Although they occur at any age and in all races, they are most frequently diagnosed during the third and fourth decades of life. More than 80% of intraoral nevi are less than 1 cm and almost half measure from 0.1 to 0.3 cm. Intraoral nevi are usually well circumscribed, and approximately two thirds are raised in contrast to oral melanotic macules, melanoma, and physiologic pigmentation (Figs. 10-9 and 10-10). Oral nevi usually appear in shades of gray, brown, and blue and

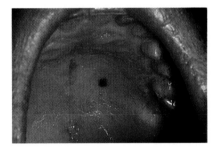

FIG. 10-9   Oral nevi occur most often on the palate and should be excised because they cannot be clinically differentiated from early melanomas.

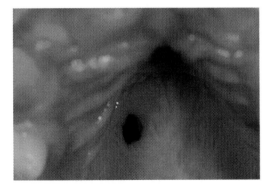

FIG. 10-10   Oral blue nevus, which is the most common type of nevus that develops on the palate.

therefore are most commonly confused with amalgam tattoos. A significant number may be non-pigmented and resemble oral fibromas.

When examined histologically, more than one half of oral nevi are of the intramucosal type and one third are common blue nevi. Compound, junctional, combined, and congenital nevi comprise the remaining cases. Intramucosal nevi occur most commonly on the buccal mucosa, whereas blue nevi are predominantly discovered on the hard palate.

The malignant potential of oral nevi has yet to be determined, and dysplastic nevi have not been described in the oral cavity. Nevertheless, oral nevi and melanomas both occur with greatest frequency on the palate, and nevi may represent the pigmentation that precedes the development of one third of oral melanomas. Furthermore, oral nevi cannot be clinically differentiated from early oral melanomas. The excision of all suspected oral nevi is, therefore, justified.

Oral Melanoacanthoma

Although intraoral melanoacanthomas are rare, their recognition is underscored by their clinical and histologic similarities to oral melanoma. Almost all cases have occurred in blacks with a mean age of 26 years, ranging from 9 to 45 years. Females are more than three times as likely to be affected as males.

Clinically, lesions are typically darkly pigmented, unilateral, and sharply demarcated with a rough, irregular, textured surface. The lesions, which measure 1 to 3 cm and occur most frequently on the buccal mucosa, often have morphologic features of either patches or plaques (Fig. 10-11). Bilateral, diffuse, and nodular involvement are atypical, rare variants.

Histologic examination reveals large, dendritic melanocytes uniformly distributed through all layers of the epithelium. The epithelium is hyperplastic and spongiotic with occasional intraepithelial vesicular formation. Unlike other entities colonized with dendritic melanocytes, including squamous cell carcinomas and acral lentiginous melanomas, melanoacanthomas lack nuclear pleomorphism and mitoses.

Oral melanoacanthomas are believed to be a reactive phenomenon to trauma. This is supported by the location of the majority of lesions in areas subjected to oral trauma and their sudden appearance. Many cases have regressed spontaneously after removal of irritants or performance of a biopsy. In all cases, tissue examination is required to differentiate these lesions from other causes of oral pigmentation.

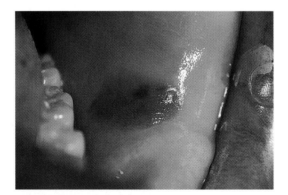

FIG. 10-11   Oral melanoacanthomas occur most frequently in young, black females and are characterized by a well-circumscribed, brown plaque with a rough textured surface.

Peutz-Jeghers Syndrome

Peutz-Jeghers syndrome, a syndrome of mucocutaneous hyperpigmentation and gastrointestinal polyposis, is well recognized and inherited as autosomal dominant with a high degree of penetrance. Although the syndrome appears in infancy, the diagnosis is not established until the third decade of life in part because of the failure to recognize the oral manifestations. Pigmented macules, often confluent and varying in size and shades of brown, appear in almost all cases on the lips and buccal mucosa (Fig. 10-12). Other oral sites may be involved and pigmented oral fibromas have also been described. Cutaneous macular pigmentation of the extremities and face is less frequently observed. The cutaneous lesions fade and often disappear during adulthood; however, the intraoral pigmentation always persists, a feature that aids in establishing a definitive diagnosis. Unfortunately, the intraoral macules have no distinguishing properties that separate them from other systemic diseases that cause oral pigmentation. Furthermore, microscopic examination of an oral lesion is nonspecific and reveals increased melanin in the basal layer without an increased number of melanocytes. Patients with oral and perioral pigmentation require a gastroenterology evaluation to search for concomitant intestinal polyps. Early detection of this syndrome will prevent delay in diagnosing malignant transformation of the hamartomatous polyps, a complication reported to occur in 2% to 3% of cases. Extracolonic malignancies of the breast, testicles, and ovaries are even more prevalent, necessitating continued surveillance.

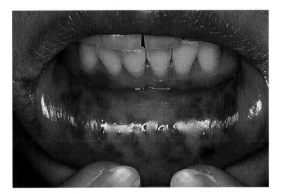

FIG. 10-12   Peutz-Jeghers syndrome demonstrating multiple pigmented macules of the lower lip. The lesions may often be the most prominent manifestation of the disease.

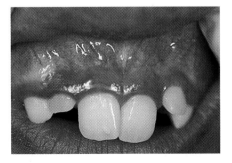

FIG. 10-13   Diffuse bronzing of the gingiva in a white child with Addison's disease.

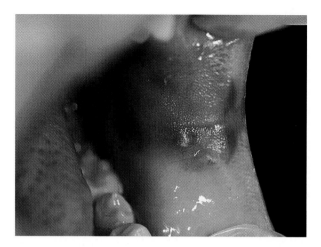

FIG. 10-14 Addison's disease may present with focal or diffuse areas of hyperpigmentation, most frequently in areas subjected to trauma such as the buccal mucosa.

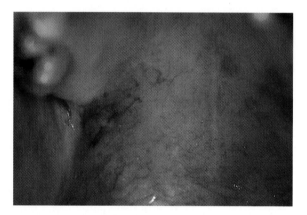

FIG. 10-15 Patients with the Laugier-Hunziker syndrome display single or confluent areas of hyperpigmentation that may simulate a number of systemic diseases. Pigmented longitudinal streaks of the fingernails are almost always present.

Addison's Disease

Adrenocortical insufficiency may be idiopathic or result from a number of infections and tumors affecting the adrenal cortex. The insufficient secretion of glucocorticoids and mineralocorticoids results in increased circulating ACTH, which in turn causes increased hyperpigmentation of the skin and mucous membranes. In one third of cases the pigmentation is the initial sign of the disease and is characterized by a diffuse darkening and bronzing of all of the skin. Oral manifestations include discrete macules and patches of pigmentation or diffuse involvement of the oral structures (Figs. 10-13 and 10-14). Areas subjected to trauma including the buccal mucosa, tongue, and gingiva are preferentially affected. Skin pigmentation usually returns to normal with replacement therapy of corticosteroids; however, the oral pigmentation commonly persists. Histologic examination is generally not required and is of minimal value because it resembles other causes of increased melanin in the basal layer. Systemic symptoms that accompany the oral hyperpigmentation include fatigue, gastrointestinal distur-bances, hypotension, and electrolyte abnormalities.

Laugier-Hunziker Syndrome

The importance of Laugier-Hunziker syndrome, a rarely reported syndrome, is that the oral findings simulate those recognized in a number of systemic diseases. Multiple pigmented macules, either sin-gular or confluent, in shades of brown and black, occurring exclusively in whites, arise most fre-quently on the lips, buccal mucosa, palate, and gingiva (Fig. 10-15). Patients often simultaneously develop darkly pigmented, longitudinal streaks on the fingernails and, less frequently, the toenails. Occasionally, brown pigmentation develops on the neck and genitalia.

Histologically, oral lesions reveal an accumulation of melanin in the cells of the basal layer and an increase in the number of melanophages in the papillary dermis. Electron microscopic studies demonstrate mature melanosomes in the basal layer of keratinocytes.

This benign condition should be differentiated from other causes of oral pigmentation including Addison's disease and Peutz-Jeghers syndrome by the lack of systemic findings. The oral lesions persist and require no therapy because they have no malignant potential.

SUGGESTED READINGS

Pigmentation abnormalities

Birek C, Main JH: Two cases of oral pigmentation as-sociated with quinidine therapy, *Oral Surg Oral Med Oral Pathol* 66:59, 1988.

Birt B, From L, Main LP: The diagnosis of melanotic and other pigmented lesions of the lips and oral mu-cosa (dark spots in the mouth), *J Otolaryngol* 7:203, 1978.

Cook CA, Lund BA, Carney JA: Mucocutaneous pig-mented spots and oral myxomas: the oral manifes-tations of the complex of myxomas, spotty pigmen-tation, and endocrine overactivity, *Oral Surg Oral Med Oral Pathol* 63:175, 1987.

Eisen D: Minocycline-induced oral hyperpigmenta-tion, *Lancet* 349:400, 1997.

Eisen D, Voorhees JJ: Oral melanoma and other pig-mented lesions of the oral cavity, *J Am Acad Der-matol* 24:527, 1991.

Ficarra G et al: Oral melanotic macules in patients in-fected with human immunodeficiency virus, *Oral Surg Oral Med Oral Pathol* 70:748, 1990.

Granstein RD, Sober AJ: Drug- and heavy metal-in-duced hyperpigmentation (review), *J Am Acad Der-matol* 5:1, 1981.

Merchant HW, Hayes LE, Ellison LT: Soft palate pig-mentation in lung disease, including cancer, *Oral Surg Oral Med Oral Pathol* 41:726, 1976.

Natali C et al: Oral mucosa pigment changes in heavy drinkers and smokers, *J Natl Med Assoc* 83:434, 1991.

Amalgam tattoos

Ashinoff R, Tanenbaum D: Treatment of an amalgam tattoo with the Q-switched ruby laser, *Cutis* 54:269, 1994.

Buchner A, Hansen LS: Amalgam pigmentation (amalgam tattoo) of the oral cavity: a clinicopatho-logical study of 268 cases, *Oral Surg Oral Med Oral Pathol* 49:139, 1980.

Daley TD, Gibson D: Practical applications of energy dispersive x-ray microanalysis in diagnostic oral pathology, *Oral Surg Oral Med Oral Pathol* 69:339, 1990.

Owens BM, Johnson WW, Schuman NJ: Oral amalgam pigmentations (tattoos): a retrospective study, *Quintessence Int* 23:805, 1992.

Slabbert H, Ackermann GC, Altini M: Amalgam tattoo as a means for person identification, *J Forensic Odontostomatol* 9:17, 1991.

Heavy metal-induced pigmentation

Dummett CO: Oral tissue changes (IV), *Quintessence Int* 11:67, 1980.

Dummett CO: Pertinent considerations in oral pig-mentations, *Br Dent J* 158:9, 1985.

Powell JP, Cummings CW: Melanoma and the differ-ential diagnosis of oral pigmented lesions, *Laryn-goscope* 88:1252, 1978.

Melanotic macules

Buchner A, Hansen LS: Melanotic macule of the oral mucosa: a clinicopathological study of 105 cases, *Oral Surg Oral Med Oral Pathol* 48:244, 1979.

Ho KKL et al: Labial melanotic macule: a clinical, histopathologic, and ultrastructural study, *J Am Acad Dermatol* 28:33, 1993.

Kaugars GE et al: Oral melanotic macules, *Oral Surg Oral Med Oral Pathol* 76:59, 1993.

Weathers DR et al: The labial melanotic macule, *Oral Surg Oral Med Oral Pathol* 42:196, 1976.

Oral nevi

Buchner A, Hansen LS: Pigmented nevi of the oral mucosa: a clinicopathological study of 36 new cases and review of 155 cases from the literature. Part II. Analysis of 191 cases, *Oral Surg Oral Med Oral Pathol* 63:676, 1987.

Buchner A et al: Melanocytic nevi of the oral mucosa: a clinicopathologic study of 130 cases from northern California, *J Oral Pathol Med* 19:197, 1990.

Grossman JR, Miller A: Intraoral junctional nevus: review of the literature and report of a case, *J Oral Surg* 33:275, 1975.

King O, Blankenship F, King W: Frequency of pigmented nevi in the oral cavity, *Oral Surg Oral Med Oral Pathol* 23:82, 1967.

Oral melanoacanthoma

Goode RK et al: Oral melanoacanthoma: review of the literature and report of ten cases, *Oral Surg Oral Med Oral Pathol* 56:622, 1983.

Tomich CE, Zunt SL: Melanoacanthosis (melanoacanthoma of the oral mucosa), *J Dermatol Surg Oncol* 16:231, 1990.

Wright JM: Intraoral melanoacanthoma: a reactive melanocytic hyperplasia, *J Periodontol* 59:53, 1988.

Zemtsov A, Bergfeld WF: Oral melanoacanthoma with prominent spongiotic intraepithelial vesicles, *J Cutan Pathol* 16:365, 1989.

Peutz-Jeghers syndome

Burdick D, Prior JT: Peutz-Jeghers syndrome: a clinicopathologic study of a large family with a 27-year follow-up, *Cancer* 50:2139, 1982.

Flageole H et al: Progression toward malignancy of hamartomas in a patient with Peutz-Jeghers syndrome: case report and literature review, *Can J Surg* 37:231, 1994.

Shapiro L, Zegarelli DJ: The solitary labial lentigo: a clinicopathologic study of twenty cases, *Oral Surg Oral Med Oral Pathol* 31:87, 1971.

Addison's disease

Kong MF, Jeffcoate W: Eighty-six cases of Addison's disease [see comments], *Clin Endocrinol* 41:757, 1994.

Nomura K, Demura H, Saruta T: Addison's disease in Japan: characteristics and changes revealed in a nationwide survey, *Intern Med* 33:602, 1994.

Schurer N, Zumdick M, Goerz G: Hyperpigmentation in primary adrenal cortex insufficiency: Addison disease, *Hautarzt* 44:300, 1993.

Laugier-Hunziker syndrome

Koch SE, Leboit PE, Odom RB: Laugier-Hunziker syndrome, *J Am Acad Dermatol* 16:431, 1987.

Veraldi S et al: Laugier-Hunziker syndrome: a clinical, histopathologic and ultrastructural study of four cases and review of the literature, *J Am Acad Dermatol* 25:632, 1991.

CHAPTER 11

Genodermatoses

COWDEN SYNDROME

Cowden syndrome, or multiple hamartoma syndrome, is an autosomal dominant genodermatosis that is characterized by multiple benign and malignant neoplasms of ectodermal, endodermal, and mesodermal origin. The oral lesions of this disorder generally precede the onset of malignancies and, because they are consistent and diagnostic in their appearance, their recognition is of paramount importance.

The oral manifestation most commonly encountered is papillomatosis, which is present in approximately 90% of cases. Smooth-surfaced and flesh-colored or white papules measuring 1 to 4 mm in diameter occur primarily on the gingiva, tongue, lips, and palate (Fig. 11-1). The lesions often coalesce, giving rise to the "cobblestone" appearance. The papillomas are asymptomatic and remain unchanged once present. Although the age of onset of oral lesions has not been well documented, the lesions most likely develop during childhood and are usually noted by the second or third decade of life. Histologic features of oral papillomas are nonspecific and consist of elongation of the rete ridges with overlying epithelial hyperplasia and acanthosis. The following are a number of other consistently reported oral manifestations of Cowden syndrome.

Routinely present	Inconsistently present
Papillomas	High-arched palate
Fissured tongue	Hypoplasia of soft palate
Caries	Malformed maxilla or mandible
Periodontal disease	Macroglossia

Cutaneous verrucous papules on the face, specifically periorbitally, periorally, and preauricularly, clinically resemble warts but microscopically are tricholemmomas. These are pathognomonic for the disease and are present in the majority of patients by the third to fourth decade of life. Acral papules on the hands, hyperkeratotic pits of the palms and soles, sclerotic fibromas, and a diverse group of benign and malignant cutaneous neoplasms are also frequently encountered.

Another feature of this syndrome is the development of gastrointestinal polyps in as many as 50% of patients, with malignant degeneration occurring infrequently. Progressive macrocephaly with mild to moderate delay in psychomotor development is present in one third of patients and has recently been emphasized as a marker for this disease.

Abnormalities of the thyroid are the most common extramucocutaneous manifestation of Cowden syndrome. More than one half of patients develop goiter and adenomas, whereas far fewer develop thyroid carcinoma. Fibrocystic disease of the breast is especially prevalent, and up to one third of women with Cowden syndrome develop breast cancer. Thus the presence of benign oral and cutaneous papillomas should prompt a thorough investigation to detect occult internal malignancies.

FIG. 11-1   Papillomatosis of the gingiva characterized by coalescing, minute, mucosal-colored papules is characteristic of Cowden syndrome.

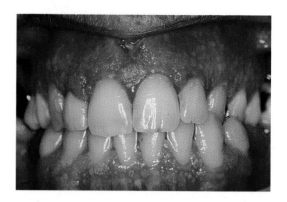

Table 11-1   Oral Manifestations of Dyskeratosis Congenita

MANIFESTATIONS	COMMENTS
Leukoplakia	Most consistent feature; tongue and buccal mucosa; premalignant
Lichenoid eruption	Clinically resembles erosive lichen planus; ages 5-15 years old, precedes onset of leukoplakia
Periodontitis	Severe destruction of alveolar bone, gingival inflammation and recession; resembles juvenile periodontitis
Dental abnormalities	Caries and premature tooth loss, enamel defects, hyperpigmentation of teeth, short-blunted root formation, taurodontism
Oral cancer	Squamous cell carcinomas can develop within leukoplakia as early as the teenage years

DYSKERATOSIS CONGENITA

Dyskeratosis congenita, also known as the Zinsser-Cole-Engman syndrome, is a well-recognized, multisystem disorder strongly associated with hematologic complications and malignancies. Although the disease is genetically transmitted heterogeneously, the majority of cases occur in males and the recent linkage to Xq28 supports an X-linked mode of inheritance. Distinct cutaneous features appear during childhood. These include a striking grayish-brown reticulated hyperpigmentation interspersed with hypopigmentation and accompanied by telangiectatic erythema and atrophy. The face, neck, and upper trunk are initially involved, but the pigmentation generally progresses with age to involve other cutaneous sites. Dystrophic or absent fingernails and toenails are a prominent feature of the syndrome, which is usually evident by the age of 10 years.

A large number of oral findings have been reported in patients with dyskeratosis congenita (Table 11-1). Oral leukoplakia is a constant feature of this disease and occurs on any mucosal surface, most frequently on the tongue and buccal mucosa (Fig. 11-2). The lesions are apparent by the second decade of life and are preceded by a spontaneously healing vesicular and ulcerative oral eruption during the teenage years. Histologically, the white plaques are characterized by slight thickening of the epithelium with atypia of keratinocytic nuclei, hyperkeratosis, and parakeratosis.

Early recognition of oral leukoplakia may lead to early detection of internal malignancies. The oral leukoplakic patches have a high propensity to undergo malignant change usually by the third to fourth decades of life. Oral squamous cell carcinomas appear most frequently on the tongue, often

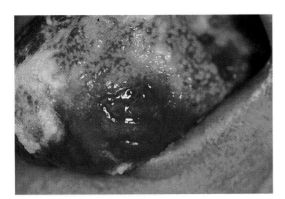

FIG. 11-2   Leukoplakia in dyskeratosis congenita is generally not uniform in its appearance and has a high propensity to undergo malignant change as in this patient with squamous cell carcinoma of the left anterior portion of the tongue.

with fatal results; therefore patients should be subjected to continual and careful oral surveillance. Cytokeratin profiles of oral biopsy specimens reveal an unusually immature state of tissue differentiation and may indicate early malignant degeneration.

Severe alveolar bone loss and gingival inflammation, especially affecting the tissues surrounding the incisors and first molars and resembling juvenile periodontitis, are other common oral manifestations of dyskeratosis congenita. Decayed teeth and tooth abnormalities including hypomineralized teeth, taurodontism, short blunted roots, thin enamel, and brown hyperpigmented teeth have also been reported in patients with this syndrome.

Hematologic abnormalities and their complications are common and are the most frequent cause of death. Aplastic anemia usually occurs in one half of all patients and develops during the second decade of life. Skeletal abnormalities and delayed mental development affect approximately one fourth of patients. In addition to oral cancer, malignancies may develop at other sites, especially in the gastrointestinal tract.

Dyskeratosis congenita and Fanconi's anemia share many clinical features, often making it difficult to distinguish one from the other. In addition to differences in hematologic abnormalities, leukoplakia and tooth abnormalities are routinely present in dyskeratosis congenita and are almost never observed in Fanconi's anemia. The diagnosis of dyskeratosis congenita is also supported by the presence of oral leukoplakia in heterozygous relatives.

DARIER'S DISEASE

Darier's disease, also known as Darier-White disease or keratosis follicularis, is an autosomal dominantly inherited cutaneous disease with prominent oral features and neuropsychiatric problems. The skin lesions usually develop in the first two decades of life, although some patients may not display clinical features of the disease until they are elderly. The cutaneous lesions are characterized by warty brown papules and plaques, which are often aggravated by exposure to sunlight. They almost always appear in a seborrheic dermatitis distribution including the chest, shoulders, back, forehead, scalp, and behind the ears. Additionally, flexural involvement, particularly axillae, groin, and inframammary folds, is common. Palmar pits and keratotic papules are evident in most patients, as are small warty papules on the dorsal surfaces of the hands. Pathognomonic nail changes consist of red and white linear bands extending from the base of the nail across the lunula to the free margin terminating in V-shaped notches or splits. The dystrophic nails are often fragile and painful and involve fingernails more than toenails. The cutaneous eruption often itches and causes body malodor. Patients are also at an increased risk for widespread herpes simplex infections and bacterial skin infections.

The oral manifestations of Darier's disease may be subtle but, when recognized, are present in approximately 50% of cases. White papules of varying size occur either individually in small groups

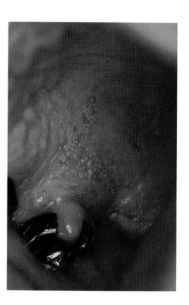

FIG. 11-3   Minute white papules occur typically on the palate in patients with Darier's disease.

or coalesce into plaques (Fig. 11-3). A rough, sandy, granular texture is noted on palpation, especially when extensive cobblestoning is present. The soft and hard palates are most frequently involved, followed by the gingiva, buccal mucosa, and tongue. The oral lesions are totally asymptomatic, with most patients unaware of their presence. The extent of oral involvement generally parallels the severity of the skin eruption. Although the eruption of oral lesions usually follows those of the skin, their presence may help confirm the diagnosis.

Oral salivary gland involvement in Darier's disease occurs in approximately one third of patients. When questioned, patients complain of recurrent parotid and, less commonly, submandibular gland swelling without clinical evidence of xerostomia. Sialograms may reveal strictures in the terminal duct indicative of obstructive sialadenitis.

The histology of an oral white papule from patients with Darier's disease reveals prominent hyperkeratosis and acanthosis with varying degrees of suprabasal clefting, corps ronds, and grains, particularly in the superficial epithelium. These features are identical to those obtained from cutaneous lesions.

The molecular abnormality in this disorder of keratinization is unknown but may be caused by a mutation in a structural protein resulting in a change in the stability of the adhesion molecules. The gene for Darier's disease has recently been shown to map to chromosome 21q23-124.1.

Topical and systemic agents are beneficial in treating cutaneous lesions but have little effect on oral lesions. Because the oral papules are asymptomatic and are not premalignant, they do not require treatment.

PACHYONYCHIA CONGENITA

Pachyonychia congenita is a rare hereditary disorder of keratinization with distinct cutaneous and oral mucous membrane features. The disease is transmitted autosomal dominantly, with a predilection for Jews and persons of Slavic descent.

Unique nail changes are present in all cases at birth or shortly thereafter and are characterized by yellow-brown discoloration, thickening, and dystrophy. The distal portions of the nails increase in thickness, resulting in a subungual mass that pushes the nail plate upward and elevates it distally. The nails are frequently shed as a result of chronic paronychial infections but continue to regrow abnormally.

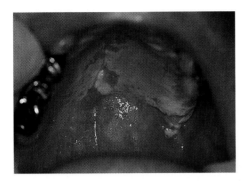

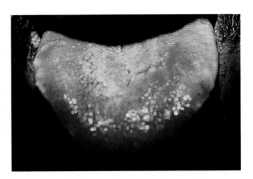

FIG. 11-4   Leukoplakia in patients with pachyonychia congenita may be diffuse in the oral cavity but is not premalignant and requires no treatment.

FIG. 11-5   Leukoplakia of the tongue in pachyonychia congenita is distinctive and characterized by an opaque white thickening with scalloped edges of the lateral surfaces.

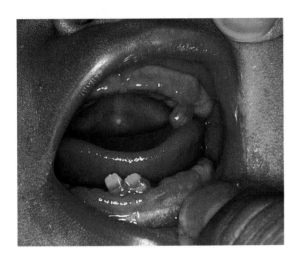

FIG. 11-6   Natal teeth may be the first oral manifestation of pachyonychia congenita, although this anomaly occurs infrequently as an isolated finding. This infant also displays an incidental lymphangioma on the maxillary ridge.

Skin lesions are characterized by symmetric and prominent hyperkeratosis of the palms and soles that produce a keratoderma and are often accompanied by hyperhidrosis and bullae. Sites of pressure are especially vulnerable, developing painful fissuring and bleeding. Verrucous plaques and papules resembling keratosis pilaris occur on the elbows, knees, legs, and buttocks.

A consistent feature of pachyonychia congenita is the presence of oral white plaques that manifest at birth. The lesions may be either focal, appearing most commonly on the tongue, lips, and buccal mucosa, or confluent and cover the entire oral mucosa (Fig. 11-4). Tongue abnormalities are the most recognizable manifestations and are characterized by an opaque white thickening with scalloped edges of the lateral surfaces (Fig. 11-5). Histologic evaluation of the white plaques reveals marked hyperkeratosis and acanthosis with intracellular vacuolization and edema in the superficial epithelial layers. Although the oral lesions are totally innocuous and have no malignant potential, they are frequently infected with *Candida albicans.* Stomatitis and angular cheilitis are less common manifestations of pachyonychia congenita.

The presence of congenital teeth (natal teeth) and neonatal teeth that erupt shortly after birth may be the earliest manifestation of pachyonychia congenita (Fig. 11-6). Natal teeth are often loose because of a structural abnormality and should be extracted to prevent aspiration. In contrast, neonatal teeth are usually well formed and spontaneously exfoliate after several years. Other dental abnormalities, including twinning of the incisor teeth and rampant caries, are occasional associated findings of pachyonychia congenita.

Pachyonychia congenita has been classified into a number of distinct subtypes. In the most prevalent form of the syndrome, also called Jadassohn-Lewandowsky syndrome, oral white plaques are a prominent feature, whereas patients with the rarer Jackson-Lawler syndrome lack oral mucosal involvement but commonly display natal and neonatal teeth. Various keratin mutations in epidermal structures have recently been shown to correlate with the specific abnormalities observed in each form of pachyonychia congenita.

MULTIPLE ENDOCRINE NEOPLASIA TYPE 2B

Multiple endocrine neoplasia (MEN) type 2B is a rare and serious disorder that, when recognized early by the characteristic oral manifestations, can result in the prompt detection and treatment of multiple cancers. Although the syndrome is transmitted autosomal dominantly with complete penetrance and variable phenotypical expressivity, more than one half of cases arise as sporadic mutations.

Medullary thyroid carcinoma develops in almost all patients with this condition and is the most common cause of death. Lymph node metastases at time of surgery are evident in over one half the cases because the cancer tends to be bilateral, multicentric, aggressive, and less amenable to surgical cure. Elevated levels of calcitonin produced by the tumors, in conjunction with computed tomography (CT) scans, may indicate the extent of the disease, although most clinicians advocate prophylactic thyroidectomy as soon as the syndrome is established. As thyroid carcinomas develop at a median age of 15 and as early as the first year of life, early recognition of MEN 2B with prophylactic thyroidectomy is of paramount importance.

Approximately 50% of patients with MEN develop a second type of malignancy, the pheochromocytoma. These arise typically during the second or third decade of life and are often preceded by diffuse or nodular adrenal medullary hyperplasia. The diagnosis can be confirmed by 24-hour urine collection assaying for increased vanillylmandelic acid and catecholamines and by demonstrating adrenal masses with various imaging techniques. In undiagnosed cases, cardiovascular crisis during surgical procedures can result in morbidity and death.

The most distinctive feature of MEN 2B is multiple oral neuromas, which are present in all cases. The benign, asymptomatic lesions may develop at birth or during the first several years of life. Clinically, pink nodules, occurring either singly or more commonly in groups, are found on the mucosal surfaces of the lips, anterior dorsal tongue, anterior buccal mucosa, and less frequently on the palate, gingivae, ventral tongue, and covering the entire dorsal tongue (Fig. 11-7). The lesions on the lips appear lumpy and protrude as a result of the multiple lesions that arise on their mucosal surfaces.

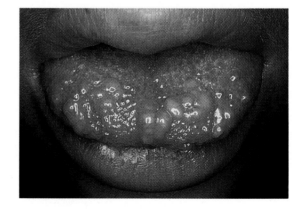

FIG. 11-7 The most distinctive finding in patients with multiple endocrine neoplasia type 2B is the presence of oral neuromas, which typically arise on the anterior tongue.

The neuromas are firm, with the consistency of rubber, when palpated. Whereas the lip and tongue lesions are generally sessile, the buccal mucosal lesions are pedunculated. Histologically, they are identical to plexiform neuromas, consisting of an encapsulated collection of myelinated and un-myelinated nerve fibers. Neuromas are also commonly present on the conjunctiva and eyelids. Other oral manifestations of lesser significance but consistently noted include a high arched palate and dental abnormalities including caries and widely spaced teeth.

Gastrointestinal symptoms occur in 90% of patients as a result of ganglioneuromatosis affecting the entire alimentary canal. Chronic constipation from birth is an early manifestation, and megacolon often complicates the condition. A classic marfanoid habitus, including musculoskeletal abnormalities, is displayed by virtually all adults with MEN 2B.

The gene for MEN 2B has been localized to the region of chromosome 10, which contains the RET proto-oncogene. Genetic testing is not yet available as it is for other forms of MEN. All patients and their first-degree relatives should be screened for the characteristic mucocutaneous manifestations because early identification has been shown to greatly increase the chance of survival.

WHITE SPONGE NEVUS

White sponge nevus is a rare autosomal dominant disorder of squamous epithelial differentiation with characteristic clinical and histologic features. Clinically, white, thickened, and folded spongy plaques occur most frequently in a bilateral distribution on the buccal mucosa. The tongue, labial mucosa, alveolar ridges, and floor of the mouth are also commonly involved, and occasionally all oral surfaces may be affected (Fig. 11-8). The plaques may intermittently peel away, but they invariably recur. The condition is present at birth or shortly thereafter; however, infrequently the clinical manifestations are first noted during the adult years. The lesions are asymptomatic and remain unchanged throughout the patient's life except during pregnancy, at which time the plaques may become more pronounced. Oral microflora may also play a role in stimulating the lesions as evidenced by the clinical improvement of white sponge nevus with tetracycline. Malignant transformation has been reported in only a single case.

The oral cavity is always involved, and in approximately 15% to 30% of cases the mucous membranes of the nose, esophagus, vagina, anus, or penis may also be affected.

Histologic and clinical findings are characteristic enough to differentiate white sponge nevus from other causes of congenital leukokeratosis including pachyonychia congenita. Irregular hyperkeratosis, acanthosis, extensive vacuolization of the suprabasal keratinocytes, and compact aggregates of keratin intermediate filaments in the upper spinous layers are noted microscopically. Mutations in both keratin 4 and keratin 13 have recently been demonstrated in patients with white sponge

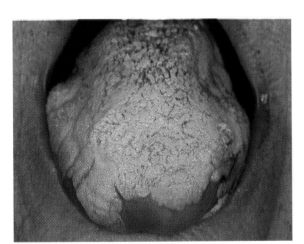

FIG. 11-8   Thick, folded, white spongy plaques may cover all oral mucosal surfaces in white sponge nevus, but the lesions are totally innocuous.

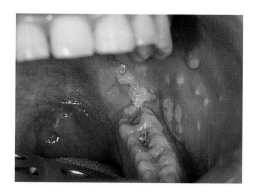

FIG. 11-9 Patients with focal dermal hypoplasia frequently demonstrate warty-type growths in the oral cavity.

nevus. Because the white plaques are restricted to mucosal epithelia and the suprabasal cell histopathology parallels the tissue-specific expression of keratins 4 and 13 in the differentiating cell layers, the mutations in these keratins are responsible for the white sponge nevus phenotype.

FOCAL DERMAL HYPOPLASIA

Also known as Goltz syndrome, focal dermal hypoplasia is an X-linked recessive disorder associated with multiple severe mesenchymal defects. Developmental skin lesions present at birth are diverse in appearance and include skin atrophy in linear symmetric streaks with telangiectasia, yellow-red nodules representing herniation of subcutaneous adipose tissue, alopecia and hair defects, hyperpigmentation, and hypopigmentation. Multiple skeletal abnormalities are frequently displayed, especially syndactyly and polydactyly. Ophthalmologic defects such as strabismus and anophthalmia are strongly associated with focal dermal hypoplasia.

The oral mucous membranes are affected in at least one half of cases and are characterized by papillomas, clinically indistinguishable from oral warts. The lesions most often occur in groups and are found on the lips, gingivae, tongue, palate, and buccal mucosa (Fig. 11-9). Lesions of the gingivae are often accompanied by erythema and may cause bleeding and periodontal defects. When the lesions are excised for diagnostic, cosmetic, or functional purposes, they occasionally recur. Microscopically, the lesions resemble fibromas. Additionally, the palatal mucosa may exhibit a striated character identical to the linear streaking of the hypoplastic skin.

Notching and clefting of the alveolar ridges are commonly encountered. Tooth abnormalities are also predictably found in patients with focal dermal hypoplasia and include anodontia, enamel defects, and morphologic defects in size and shape of the dentition. Malocclusion, precocious dental caries, delayed eruption, and hyperdontia are less frequently noted. All affected individuals should have regular oral and dental evaluations.

INCONTINENTIA PIGMENTI

Also known as the Bloch-Sulzberger syndrome, incontinentia pigmenti is an X-linked dominant disorder that is usually lethal in males. The disease is characterized by a cutaneous eruption that starts either at birth or shortly thereafter and progresses through stages with vesicles, verrucous plaques, hyperpigmentation, and hypopigmentation. Although each clinical stage may appear sequentially, variable morphologic lesions may occur concurrently or randomly. Extracutaneous manifestations include hair and nail defects in one half of cases, ocular defects in approximately one third of cases, and central nervous system disorders and skeletal abnormalities in 10% to 15% of cases. Incontinentia pigmenti may also be associated with an increased frequency of childhood malignant neoplasms.

The cutaneous signs of incontinentia pigmenti in adults are often subtle or nonexistent. Thus early detection of female carriers or establishment of a diagnosis of incontinentia pigmenti in adults

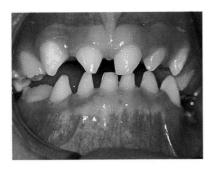

FIG. 11-10   Incontinentia pigmenti frequently affects both sets of dentitions and is characterized by hypodontia and conical-shaped teeth.

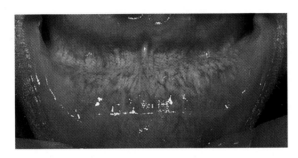

FIG. 11-11   The presence of yellow plaques on the labial mucosa, identical in appearance to cutaneous lesions, is diagnostic of pseudoxanthoma elasticum.

without an accurate neonatal history can be difficult. The presence of extracutaneous manifestations is often required to support the clinical diagnosis. Oral cavity abnormalities characterized by dental defects occur in more than 80% of patients and are the most significant and constant diagnostic extracutaneous features. In contrast to the skin eruptions, dental abnormalities, which affect both the deciduous and permanent dentition, persist. Dental defects (Fig. 11-10) include hypodontia usually of the lateral incisors, conical shaped crowns most commonly affecting the upper anterior teeth and resembling ectodermal dysplasia, malformed crowns with accessory cusps, and delayed eruption.

The gene for incontinentia pigmenti has been precisely localized on the long arm of the X chromosome. Prenatal diagnosis is possible by deoxyribonucleic acid (DNA) marker analysis.

PSEUDOXANTHOMA ELASTICUM

Pseudoxanthoma elasticum is an inherited disease usually transmitted in an autosomal recessive pattern. Elastic fibers of the skin, retinae, and cardiovascular system become progressively calcified, resulting in pathologic changes in each of these organ systems. Distinctive yellow-orange papules and plaques become confluent on the skin, giving it a cobblestone or orange peel appearance. The lesions are characteristically localized to the flexural sites including the neck, antecubital and popliteal fossae, axillae, and groin. Ocular manifestations include angioid streaks, which are present in almost all cases. Hypertension, myocardial infarction, and stroke are cardiovascular complications, whereas gastrointestinal hemorrhage is a result of vascular involvement.

Oral manifestations are evident in approximately 5% of patients with pseudoxanthoma elasticum. The lesions may be subtle and easily overlooked, often mistaken for Fordyce's spots; the true incidence of oral involvement is probably much higher than reported. The inner aspect of the lip, especially the lower and the buccal mucosa are favored sites of involvement. The oral lesions appear identical to those present on the skin and are also distinctly yellow (Fig. 11-11). Mucosal involvement may occur in the absence of skin lesions but, when accompanied by systemic findings, permits the diagnosis of pseudoxanthoma elasticum. Microscopically, oral lesions reveal fragmented and calcified elastic fibers in the middle dermis. Special elastic stains (e.g., von Kossa's stain) can be used to demonstrate thick, twisted collagen fibrils and confirm the diagnosis. Genetic counseling is crucial for all patients.

ORAL-FACIAL-DIGITAL SYNDROMES

A large and diverse group of conditions sharing many abnormal clinical characteristics is collectively known as the oral-facial-digital syndromes. At least nine distinct clinical types have been identified; however, a larger number of syndromes with phenotypic similarity has not yet been precisely classified.

Prominent findings consist of digital malformations including clinodactyly, brachydactyly, and polydactyly. Facial deformities are frequently encountered and are characterized by an upper cleft lip, ocular hypertelorism, and micrognathia. The oral manifestations are varied in appearance but are pronounced in each of the subtypes of oral-facial-digital syndromes identified. A constant and distinctive abnormality is the presence of multiple hyperplastic frenula extending from the gingivae to the labial mucosa (Fig. 11-12). Tongue clefts are also present in all types of the oral-facial-digital syndromes. Lingual and gingival nodules (Fig. 11-13), microscopically identified as hamartomas, a high-arched or cleft palate, and tooth abnormalities including missing teeth, small teeth, supernumerary teeth, and malpositioned teeth are less consistently observed and may occur in only some of the subtypes. A variety of cutaneous and miscellaneous abnormalities are also frequently present depending on the specific syndrome. Recommended diagnostic tests include a skeletal survey, CT scans, ophthalmologic evaluation, and dental examination.

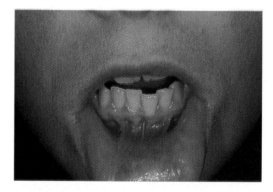

FIG. 11-12 Multiple hyperplastic frenula attaching the lower labial mucosa to the gingiva is a characteristic finding in the oral-facial-digital syndromes.

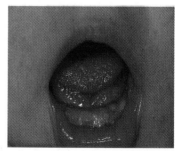

FIG. 11-13 The child of the patient in Fig. 11-12 exhibiting tongue and gingival nodules, representing mucosal hamartomas in the oral-facial-digital syndromes.

XERODERMA PIGMENTOSUM

Xeroderma pigmentosum is an autosomal recessive dermatologic disease that is characterized by a profound sensitivity to ultraviolet light because of a defect in the DNA repair mechanism resulting in severe actinic damage and skin cancers. Skin abnormalities are noted early in life and consist of diffuse freckling limited to the sun-exposed areas. With age, telangiectases, angiomas, depigmentation, atrophy, ulcerations, and eventually squamous cell carcinomas, basal cell carcinomas, and melanomas develop. Skin cancers usually develop by the time the patient is 8 years old. Ocular abnormalities are as common and are characterized by photophobia, severe keratitis, ulcerations, and cancers of the ocular tissues. A variety of neurologic defects are frequently encountered.

The oral cavity is a common site of involvement in patients with xeroderma pigmentosum. Children and teenagers have a significantly increased risk for the development of squamous cell carcinomas. The majority form on the anterior one third of the tongue and probably result from the effects of ultraviolet radiation. Oral cancers are also increased in frequency on the palate and gingiva. Actinic damage in the oral cavity may manifest as lingual telangiectases, ulcerations, and leukoplakia. Lip abnormalities and cancers are identical in appearance to the intraoral changes but are often more pronounced. Periodic oral cavity examinations should be performed in all patients and persistent ulcerations and neoplasms subjected to biopsy. Ultraviolet-cured dental resin restorations should not be used in these patients. Oral carcinogenic agents including alcohol and tobacco should also be avoided. The life span of patients with xeroderma pigmentosum is greatly diminished as a result of malignancies.

FAMILIAL DYSAUTONOMIA

Familial dysautonomia, also known as Riley-Day syndrome, is an autosomal recessive disorder that occurs almost exclusively in Ashkenazic Jews. Early in life, neurologic defects become evident and are characterized by difficulty in swallowing, aspiration, profuse sweating, absent lacrimation resulting in corneal ulcerations, vomiting, fainting spells, and emotional instability. Postural hypotension and paroxysmal hypertension develop later in life. Frequent bouts of aspiration result in recurrent pneumonia, which is often fatal. An asymmetric facial appearance with a transverse elongated mouth and facial drooping is apparent.

The diagnosis is determined by the clinical signs and symptoms because no specific laboratory test or enzyme defect has been demonstrated. A useful diagnostic and pathognomonic feature is the absence or severe decrease in the number of fungiform and circumvallate tongue papillae. Because taste buds are normally located at the base of these papillae, there is decreased sensitivity to sweet and bitter tastes and infrequent intake of food. Patients with Riley-Day syndrome have also been consistently shown to have a marked reduction in dental caries, which may result from reduced sugar intake or change in the salivary composition and content caused by chronic autonomic denervation. Additional oral features include self-inflicted oral injuries and mutilation, which occur in approximately one third of patients (Fig. 11-14). Tongue, lip, and cheek biting, as well as bruxism (tooth

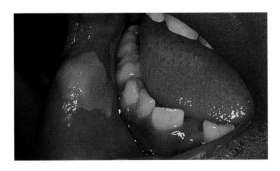

FIG. 11-14   Self-inflicted oral injuries and mutilation are common features in children with familial dysautonomia.

grinding), oral lacerations, and self-extraction of teeth are the most common injuries observed. Elimination of sharp edges of teeth and restorations is helpful. Severe chronic gingivitis is also common and is most likely the result of neglected oral hygiene.

Recently, the familial dysautonomia gene was mapped to chromosome 9q31-33, permitting reliable prenatal diagnosis.

LIPOID PROTEINOSIS

Lipoid proteinosis, an autosomal recessive condition, is also known as hyalinosis cutis et mucosae or Urbach-Wiethe disease. The disorder is characterized by unique deposits of hyaline material in the connective tissue of the skin and mouth, as well as in every organ, especially the brain. The disease is usually diagnosed shortly after birth because affected infants are unable to cry and they exhibit a hoarse voice as a result of laryngeal involvement. Skin lesions arise early and appear as waxy yellow papules accompanied with diffuse thickening, particularly in the flexural surfaces. Skin fragility results in ulcerations that heal leaving linear, depressed scars, particularly on the face. A pathognomonic feature is the accumulation of papules on the edges of the eyelids that resemble a string of beads. Scalp involvement often leads to alopecia. Neurologic complications are present in the majority of patients and are attributed to a distinctively shaped intracranial calcification in the hippocampus or temporal lobes.

The mouth is perhaps the most common and severely affected location in patients with lipoid proteinosis. Characteristic pinkish-yellow papules and plaques develop in childhood and increase in severity with age. All of the oral surfaces may be involved, but the lesions are most common on the lower lip where they impart a pebbly and cobblestone appearance (Fig. 11-15). The tongue surface develops ulcerations with subsequent loss of papillae. As the disease progresses, the tongue eventually becomes thickened, enlarged, and bound to the floor of the mouth, thus inhibiting protrusion. Buccal mucosa involvement is characterized by recurrent and painful parotitis attributed to blockage of Stensen's duct by the hyaline infiltrates. Palpation of the oral mucosal reveals a rigid consistency resembling hard rubber. Microscopic examination of oral lesions reveals characteristic deposits of amorphous eosinophilic material in the dermis that stain intensely with periodic acid-Schiff stain.

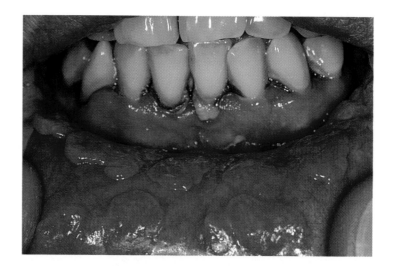

FIG. 11-15   Pink papules and plaques imparting a pebbly surface to the mucosa develop most frequently on the lower lip in patients with lipoid proteinosis.

A number of dental abnormalities are known to commonly occur and may be the only identifiable signs of heterozygous carriers. These include congenital absence of teeth and severe enamel hypoplasia, especially involving the maxillary lateral incisors, cuspids, and premolars. Therapy is palliative and directed toward alleviating the complications of the disease.

CONGENITAL ERYTHROPOIETIC PORPHYRIA

Also known as Günther's disease and first described in 1911, congenital erythropoietic porphyria is an autosomal recessive disease of heme biosynthesis. The defective activity of uroporphyrinogen III synthase results in the accumulation of the isomer I series of porphyrins in erythroid cells. The abnormal porphyrins are deposited in various tissues, bones, and teeth. Although most patients manifest symptoms in the neonatal period, adult onset cases have been reported.

Mutilating skin lesions characterized by blisters, atrophy, pigmentation, and hirsutism are caused by the marked cutaneous photosensitivity. Chronic hemolytic anemia with splenomegaly is frequently present.

Erythrodontia (red-stained teeth) of both the primary and permanent dentitions is a distinctive feature of the disease and may be its first manifestation (Fig. 11-16). The discoloration of the incisors is uniformly dark brown, whereas the canines and molars exhibit the characteristic reddish hue. The teeth are best examined under ultraviolet light using a Wood's light; a reddish-pink fluorescence is seen. The permanent teeth are less intensely discolored than the primary teeth. Dental discoloration is caused by the preferential deposition of porphyrins in the dentin and, to a lesser extent, in the enamel. Cosmetic restorative dental procedures can significantly improve the appearance of the teeth. Atrophic scars on the sun-exposed portions of the lips and localized advanced periodontitis are additional oral features commonly found in patients with Günther's disease.

HEREDITARY BENIGN INTRAEPITHELIAL DYSKERATOSIS

Hereditary benign intraepithelial dyskeratosis is an autosomal dominant disorder that affects both the oral cavity and eyes. The majority of reported patients have been from a triracial population in North Carolina; however, cases have appeared elsewhere and the disease is probably underreported and underrecognized.

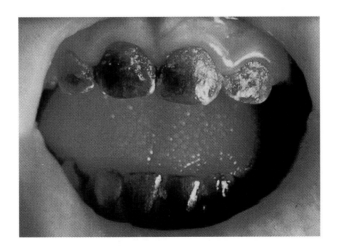

FIG. 11-16   Red-stained teeth are a distinctive feature of congenital erythropoietic porphyria.

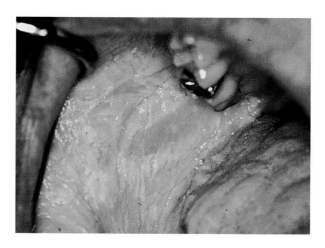

FIG. 11-17   Soft, white, spongy plaques on the buccal mucosa develop in infancy in patients with hereditary benign intraepithelial dyskeratosis.

Oral manifestations appear in infancy and are characterized by white, thickened plaques that are spongy and soft to palpation (Fig. 11-17). The lesions are asymptomatic and adult patients may be unaware of their presence. Any oral site may be involved, but the buccal and labial mucosa are favored locations. Clinically, they appear identical to the white plaques found in the white sponge nevus syndrome. Microscopically, oral lesions reveal dyskeratosis, acanthosis, parakeratosis, and a variable degree of subepithelial inflammation. Ultrastructurally, numerous vesicular bodies in immature dyskeratotic cells, densely packed tonofilaments filling the cytoplasm of mature dyskeratotic cells, and desmosomes in mature dyskeratotic cells have been demonstrated. The syndrome is recognized by the presence of ocular lesions accompanying the oral lesions. Foamy, gelatinous, bilateral limbal conjunctival plaques and chronic relapsing courses of ocular irritation and photophobia are the typical ocular manifestations.

The white plaques have no malignant potential. Both the ocular and oral lesions are resistant to medical and surgical treatments.

PAPILLON-LEFÈVRE SYNDROME

Papillon-Lefèvre syndrome is a disorder that is inherited in an autosomal dominant fashion and manifests during childhood. Clinically, patients develop thickening of the stratum corneum of the skin on the palms and soles. Discrete, thickened, red, scaly plaques that often extend onto the dorsal surfaces of the fingers and toes occur in these areas. Pain, fissuring, and cracking are accompanied by fetid hyperhidrosis. Calcification of the falx cerebri and of other parts of the brain is also associated with the syndrome.

Concurrent with the onset of skin lesions, children with Papillon-Lefèvre syndrome develop precocious periodontal disease characterized by marked inflammation and swelling of the gingivae (Fig. 11-18). Severe destruction of the alveolar bone accompanied by hemorrhage and pain results in the exfoliation of all of the deciduous teeth. The gingivae revert to normal until the permanent teeth erupt, at which time the process of inflammation and destruction is repeated and persists throughout the teenage years. The activities of the skin and oral lesions parallel each other and have been shown to be seasonal. The occurrence of *Actinobacillus actinomycetemcomitans* in affected children and extended family members suggests that this organism may be important in the pathogenesis of the periodontal disease process.

A number of studies have documented the efficacy of systemic retinoids, especially etretinate and acitretin, in treating both the skin and mouth lesions. With early and prolonged administration, patients may be able to maintain their permanent teeth even after therapy is discontinued. These com-

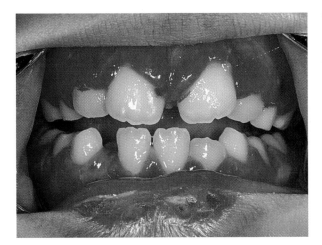

FIG. 11-18   The exfoliation of teeth in patients with Papillon-Lefèvre syndrome is preceded by an episode of severe inflammation and swelling of the gingiva.

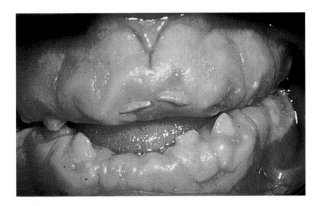

FIG. 11-19   The gingivae are firm, smooth, and minimally inflamed, often obscuring all of the teeth in gingival fibromatosis.

pounds have significant adverse events and require careful monitoring. Additionally, beneficial results can sometimes be achieved with aggressive oral hygiene measures using topical and systemic antimicrobial agents.

GINGIVAL FIBROMATOSIS

In the majority of patients with gingival fibromatosis, the disease is inherited primarily in an autosomal dominant pattern and less commonly in an autosomal recessive mode. The disorder is characterized by progressive enlargement of the gingivae, which begins in childhood and persists indefinitely. The gingival papillae are initially involved, and, with age, the attached gingival tissues become affected. The entire gingivae of the maxilla and mandible may be involved, or the disease may be localized to portions of each. The gingivae of both the buccal and lingual surfaces are usually firm to palpation, smooth, minimally inflamed, and partially or completely obscure the teeth (Fig. 11-19). Histopathologic findings from the gingival lesions include thickening of the epithelium and hyperplasia of interlacing collagen bundles, forming an avascular mass. Ultrastructurally, fibroblasts exhibiting rough-surfaced endoplasmic reticulum, cells with vesicular nuclei resembling mast cells,

Table 11-2   Syndromes Associated with Gingival Fibromatosis

SYNDROME	MANIFESTATIONS
Zimmermann-Labland syndrome	Dysplasia of terminal phalanges and nails, hepatosplenomegaly, facial dysmorphism
Ramon syndrome	Cherubism, mental retardation, epilepsy, arthritis
Cross syndrome	Hypopigmentation, oligophrenia, athetosis
Rutherford syndrome	Corneal dystrophy, delayed tooth eruption
Murray syndrome	Multiple hyaline dermal tumors, recurrent infections
Miscellaneous associations	Sensorineural hearing loss, hypertrichosis, Klippel-Trénaunay-Weber syndrome, epilepsy, mental retardation

and mostly types I and III collagens can be demonstrated. Although these nonspecific findings are helpful, the diagnosis is based on the clinical presentation.

Several well-defined genetic syndromes with gingival fibromatosis as a prominent feature have been documented, necessitating a systemic evaluation of all children with gingival enlargement. The most commonly associated abnormalities include hypertrichosis and epilepsy (Table 11-2).

Surgical resection of the enlarged tissue by laser or scalpel is the preferred treatment, although recurrences are common.

ECTODERMAL DYSPLASIAS

The ectodermal dysplasias are a diverse group of genetic disorders that share abnormalities related to a developmental defect in ectodermally derived structures. More than 100 conditions are classified under this heading with variable clinical features and modes of inheritance. After hair and skin, the teeth are affected most frequently in this group of syndromes.

The triad of hypohidrosis, hypotrichosis, and hypodontia constitute the major manifestations of the well-recognized X-linked recessive variant. Dental anomalies are a prominent feature and consist of partial or complete anodontia. The teeth present are usually hypoplastic and peg or conical shaped, especially the anterior teeth (Fig. 11-20). When the skin and hair defects are noted and the condition is suspected, tooth abnormalities may be demonstrated by radiographs before the teeth erupt. Delayed eruption, microdontia, enamel defects, and supernumerary teeth are frequent additional developmental defects found in other types of ectodermal dysplasias. Leukoplakia involving various oral surfaces may be noted in the hidrotic form of ectodermal dysplasia.

The early construction of partial or compete dental prostheses or the use of endosseous dental implants that are routinely used for elderly patients greatly improves the appearance of children with missing and malformed teeth.

HEREDITARY MUCOEPITHELIAL DYSPLASIA

Hereditary mucoepithelial dysplasia is an autosomal dominant condition that affects multiple organ systems, but the oral mucosal changes are the most characteristic and diagnostic. The defect in this syndrome is presumably caused by a reduction in the number of desmosomes and gap junction formation, resulting in epithelial dyshesion and dyskeratosis. Clinically, the eyes, skin, lungs, and mucosae are affected. The skin lesions consist of rough keratotic papules, psoriasiform plaques, and chronic diffuse alopecia. Ophthalmologic findings include conjunctival erythema and keratitis, nys-

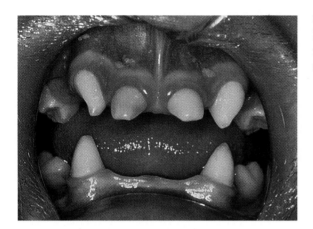

FIG. 11-20   Partial or complete anodontia is a prominent finding in patients with ectodermal dysplasia. The teeth present are usually peg shaped.

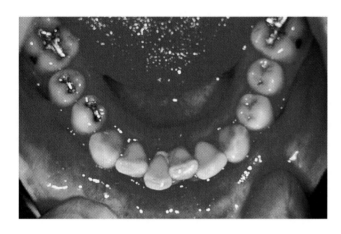

FIG. 11-21   Hereditary mucoepithelial dysplasia characteristically involves the oral mucosa and features fiery red, asymptomatic mucosal surfaces.

tagmus, corneal vascularization, photophobia, and early cataract formation. Recurrent respiratory tract infections and extensive fibrocystic lung disease are serious complications of the disease.

The oral mucosal surfaces, predominantly the palate, gingiva, and tongue, are characteristically fiery red and totally asymptomatic (Fig. 11-21). These changes develop during infancy and persist throughout life. Similar abnormalities may be noted on other mucosal surfaces of the nose, vagina, cervix, urethra, and bladder. Exfoliative cytology from a reddened oral mucosal lesion demonstrating numerous dyskeratotic cells and cytoplasmic vacuolization can be used to confirm the clinical diagnosis. Electron microscopy reveals the defective reduction in desmosomes and intracellular bundles of fibers. Despite these microscopic abnormalities of the mucosae, malignant transformation has not been reported.

ENCEPHALOTRIGEMINAL ANGIOMATOSIS

Encephalotrigeminal angiomatosis, or Sturge-Weber syndrome, is a rare developmental vascular anomaly characterized by involvement of the central nervous system and mucocutaneous structures of the face. The cutaneous lesions of encephalotrigeminal angiomatosis are referred to as nevus flammeus, or port-wine stain, and exhibit a unilateral distribution involving one or more branches of the trigeminal nerve. The extent and location of these lesions determine the risk for developing Sturge-Weber syndrome. The syndrome occurs only if the first branch of the trigeminal nerve is involved. Patients with Sturge-Weber syndrome also develop leptomeningeal angiomas and characteristic

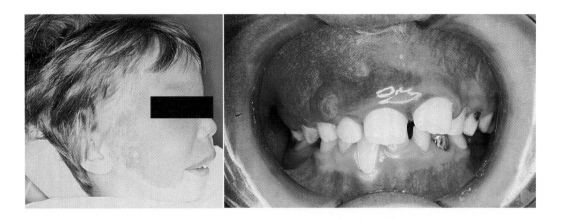

FIG. 11-22   Sturge-Weber syndrome with oral involvement. The increased vascularity results in erythema of the ipsilateral mucosa and accelerated eruption of teeth.

"tram-line" meningeal calcifications, with associated neurologic disorders including seizures and mental retardation. Ipsilateral involvement of the eye is also common, resulting in retinal dysfunction and glaucoma.

Intraorally, the mucosa exhibits analogous vascular changes in approximately one third of cases when the second or third division of the trigeminal nerve is involved. The affected oral mucosal surfaces are redder than the normal mucosa, and the degree of vascular hyperplasia varies from mild to severe. The lips, buccal mucosa, and maxillary gingivae are most frequently affected and, like the skin lesions, remain unilateral. Gingival hyperplasia and macroglossia are less commonly observed. The increased vascularity is usually associated with accelerated eruption of the ipsilateral permanent teeth (Fig. 11-22). Intraoral vascular malformations may result in increased bleeding after dental procedures and extractions.

The treatment of encephalotrigeminal angiomatosis is variable, depending on the severity of the disorder and the extent of involvement. Laser therapy of facial lesions is effective for cosmetic purposes; however, meningeal angiomas must frequently be removed surgically. Care must be taken whenever affected areas are incised because of the propensity for profound hemorrhage.

HEREDITARY HEMORRHAGIC TELANGIECTASIA

Hereditary hemorrhagic telangiectasia, also known as Osler-Rendu-Weber disease, is an autosomal dominant condition that is characterized by a triad of telangiectases of the skin and mucous membranes, repeated hemorrhages, and a genetic occurrence. Epistaxis is a frequent initial manifestation during childhood, but the disorder may not be recognized until the adult years. The oral cavity is almost always affected, with telangiectases appearing most frequently on the lips and anterior tongue (Fig. 11-23) and less often on the buccal mucosa and palate. When subjected to trauma during eating and brushing, these bright red lesions often bleed profusely. The recognition of oral lesions can help establish a definitive diagnosis, especially in patients who lack a positive family history. Microscopically, oral telangiectases reveal dilated, thin-walled vessels, which are constituted predominantly of small venules.

Pulmonary arteriovenous malformations are significantly increased in patients with hereditary hemorrhagic telangiectasia and may be life-threatening if undetected. Vascular lesions may also result in severe gastrointestinal and central nervous system bleeding. Iron deficiency anemia may ensue from chronic blood loss, and vascular malformations may cause complications of the liver and spleen. Treatment is symptomatic and aimed at preventing hemorrhage.

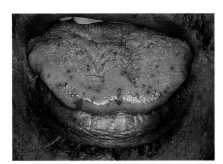

FIG. 11-23 A constant oral feature in hereditary hemorrhagic telangiectasia is the presence of telangiectases on the anterior tongue.

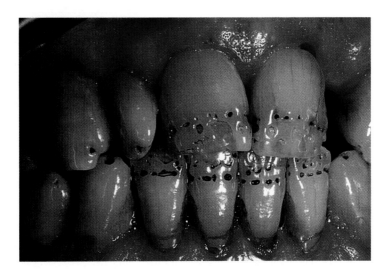

FIG. 11-24 Enamel pitting can be demonstrated in all patients with tuberous sclerosis who are older than 11 years and in the majority of younger patients.

TUBEROUS SCLEROSIS

Tuberous sclerosis is an autosomal dominant disorder of cellular differentiation and proliferation in which a variety of lesions arise in the skin, nervous system, heart, kidney, and other organs. The most frequently recognized clinical features constitute a triad of adenoma sebaceum, epilepsy, and mental retardation. The initial manifestations are usually apparent in the first several years of life and are caused by central nervous system abnormalities including seizures, retardation, and hamartomatous proliferations of neural tissues. A diverse group of visceral defects may be noted including phakomas of the retina, rhabdomyomas of the heart, cysts of the lungs and bones, and benign neoplasms in the kidneys, liver, and gastrointestinal tract. The initial cutaneous manifestations are hypomelanotic macules in the shape of an ash leaf. These occur in the majority of patients and have unique clinical and microscopic features. Pathognomonic angiofibromas on the face appear late in childhood, and another characteristic cutaneous lesion, the shagreen patch, characterized by a flesh-colored plaque resembling the skin of an orange, develops after puberty. The diagnosis of tuberous sclerosis is based on a constellation of clinical findings because there are no markers or blood tests to confirm the diagnosis. The detection of oral abnormalities may greatly contribute to the early recognition of this syndrome.

The presence of dental enamel pitting is a useful marker in screening patients suspected of having tuberous sclerosis (Fig. 11-24). In children younger than 11 years old, pits in the teeth can be demonstrated in approximately 75% of cases, whereas in older children the occurrence is universally present. Usually, several pits of various sizes less than 1 mm in diameter may be noted on the labial sur-

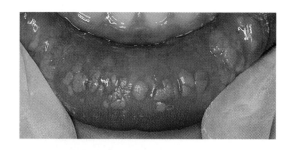

FIG. 11-25   Pink fleshy fibromas develop typically during late childhood in patients with tuberous sclerosis.

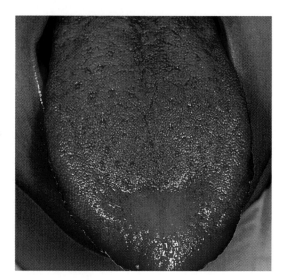

FIG. 11-26   A distinctive and diagnostic feature of the Beckwith-Wiedemann syndrome is the presence of an enlarged, protruding tongue that often becomes ulcerated as a result of trauma.

faces of the teeth, and the number increases with age. The use of red-staining dental plaque disclosing solution aids in identifying the pits.

Approximately one half of all patients with tuberous sclerosis will exhibit oral fibromatosis. Pink or white fibromas occur during late childhood, most frequently on the anterior gingiva, but may also appear on the tongue, lips, buccal mucosa, and palate (Fig. 11-25). Involvement of the gingiva may be diffuse and resemble drug-induced gingival enlargement. Potential carriers of tuberous sclerosis may also exhibit oral fibromas and should be screened for their presence. Recent studies suggest the disease is genetically heterogeneous with at least two gene loci on chromosomes 9 and 16.

BECKWITH-WIEDEMANN SYNDROME

Beckwith-Wiedemann syndrome is a multisystem disorder associated with an increased risk of childhood malignancies. Although the majority of cases appear to be sporadic, the etiology is considered genetic with autosomal dominant inheritance with reduced penetrance. A distinctive and diagnostic feature of the Beckwith-Wiedemann syndrome is the presence of an enlarged and protruding tongue (Fig. 11-26). This abnormality is present at birth and occurs in nearly all patients with the syndrome. The macroglossia is uniform in nature and improves with age as the tongue accommodates to a larger space. Complications of macroglossia are frequently encountered and include malpositioning and malocclusion of the anterior teeth resulting in an open bite, difficulties in speech, and unsightly appearance. Rarely, serious respiratory obstruction may be caused by the enlarged tongue, and anterior partial tongue resections can be performed to correct the defect.

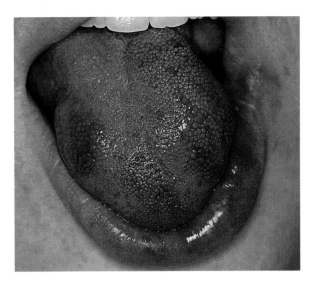

FIG. 11-27   Multiple hemangiomas of the oral cavity are frequently detected and may bleed severely after trauma in the blue rubber bleb nevus syndrome.

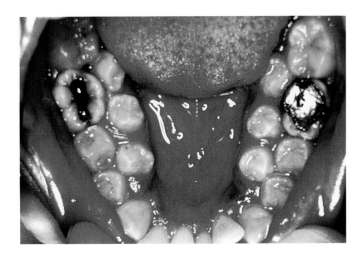

FIG. 11-28   Bone-impacted or, as in this patient, erupted supernumerary teeth are a frequent finding in patients with Gardner's syndrome.

Symptomatic hypoglycemia occurs in approximately one half of cases and may result in permanent brain damage if undetected. Fortunately, it regresses spontaneously by 4 months of age. Abdominal wall defects and newborn infants who are large for gestational age are the major clinical features present in the majority of patients. Minor manifestations include ear pits and creases, facial nevus flammeus, and visceromegaly. Benign hamartomas and malignant neoplasms have been detected with greater frequency in children with Beckwith-Wiedemann syndrome. The majority have been located intraabdominally.

The presentation of macroglossia in a newborn should prompt an investigation to exclude the

Table 11-3   Oral Manifestations of Genodermatosis

DISEASE	ORAL FINDINGS	COMMENTS
Acatalasemia	Recurrent painful ulcers of the dental alveoli; gangrene and destruction of alveolar bone with loss of teeth	Autosomal recessive; catalase enzyme defect; predominantly in the Far East
Angiokeratoma corporis diffusum universale	Punctate angiokeratomas in most patients found on the inner lower lip and sometimes on the buccal mucosa	Fabry's disease; X-linked recessive; error of glycosphingolipid metabolism
Ataxia-telangiectasia	Numerous telangiectasias may be found on the palate and less often on the buccal mucosa, tongue, and lower lip	Autosomal recessive; ocular and cutaneous telangiectasias, cerebellar ataxia, choreoathetosis and pulmonary infections
Blue rubber bleb nevus syndrome	50% to 60% display one or more cavernous hemangiomas in the mouth; severe bleeding with oral trauma (see Fig. 11-27)	Autosomal dominant; multiple hemangiomas of the skin and gastrointestinal tract, often with iron deficiency anemia
Böök's syndrome	Hypodontia of bicuspids (premolars) and sometimes third molars	Autosomal dominant; hyperhidrosis and premature whitening of hair
Chondroectodermal dysplasia	Multiple fibrous bands attaching the gingiva to the inner lip resulting in the obliteration of the mucolabial fold; missing, conical shaped, natal, and malformed teeth	Ellis-van Creveld syndrome; autosomal recessive; polydactyly and chrondrodysplasia of bones, hair, and nails
Chronic granulomatous disease	Oral ulcerations, severe gingivitis, and granulomatous mucositis; female carriers may display oral lupuslike lesions	X-linked recessive; recurrent severe bacterial and fungal infections
Cleidocranial dysplasia	High-arched palate, delay in eruption of teeth and malformed teeth; increase in gingivitis and periodontitis	Autosomal dominant; hypoplasia or absence of clavicles and skull defects
Ehlers-Danlos syndrome	Type VIII: childhood severe periodontal disease with loss of permanent teeth is characteristic; in other types, oral bruising and bleeding and dental anomalies	Type VIII: autosomal dominant; pretibial hyperpigmented atrophic scars but no visceral involvement and only mild joint changes
Familial holoprosencephaly	Single central incisor in affected individuals is characteristic and also present in carriers	Malformation of forebrain and midface: microphthalmia, hypopituitarism, hypotelorism
Gardner's syndrome	Multiple supernumerary teeth is diagnostic; osteomas of mandible early in life; fibromas of buccal mucosa and tongue (see Fig. 11-28)	Autosomal dominant; intestinal polyposis with malignant transformation, bony abnormalities, soft tissue tumors
Maffucci's syndrome	10% develop oral hemangiomas, most frequently of the tongue	May not be genetic; multiple enchondromas, hemangiomas, and increased risk of malignant chondrosarcomas
Marfan's syndrome	Narrow and high-arched palate; tooth abnormalities in size, shape, and spacing; occasionally cleft palate and bifid uvula	Autosomal dominant; abnormalities in eyes, skeletal system, and cardiovascular system
Tricho-dento-osseous syndrome	Small pitted teeth prone to severe caries resulting in decay, discoloration, and gingival abscesses; taurodont molars	Autosomal dominant; congenital kinky hair, amelogenesis imperfecta and brittle nails
Wiskott-Aldrich syndrome	Spontaneous gingival bleeding, purpura and petechiae and ulcerations	X-linked recessive; thrombocytopenic purpura, severe eczema, recurrent infections, lymphoreticular malignancies

Beckwith-Wiedemann syndrome. Early recognition of this disorder may avoid the neonatal complications of apnea, cyanosis, seizures, and respiratory distress.

MISCELLANEOUS SYNDROMES

A number of uncommon genodermatoses may display oral manifestations (Figs. 11-27 and 11-28). These are summarized in Table 11-3.

SUGGESTED READINGS

Cowden syndrome

Fielding CG: Multiple hamartoma syndrome (Cowden's disease): a case report, *Compend Contin Educ Dent* 14:234, 1993.

Hanssen AMN, Fryns JP: Cowden syndrome, *J Med Genet* 32:117, 1995.

Porter S et al: Multiple hamartoma syndrome presenting with oral lesions, *Oral Surg Oral Med Oral Pathol Oral Radiol Endod* 82:295, 1996.

Starink TM: Cowden's disease: analysis of fourteen new cases, *J Am Acad Dermatol* 11:1127, 1984.

Starink TM et al: The Cowden syndrome: a clinical and genetic study in 21 patients, *Clin Genet* 29:222, 1986.

Takenoshita Y et al: Oral and facial lesions in Cowden's disease: report of two cases and a review of the literature, *J Oral Maxillofac Surg* 51:682, 1993.

Dyskeratosis congenita

Anil S et al: Oral squamous cell carcinoma in a case of dyskeratosis congenita, *Ann Dent* 53:15, 1994.

Drachtman RA, Alter BA: Dyskeratosis congenita, *Dermatol Clin* 13:33, 1995.

Ogden GR et al: Cytokeratin profiles in dyskeratosis congenita: an immunocytochemical investigation of lingual hyperkeratosis, *J Oral Pathol Med* 21:353, 1992.

Yavuzyilmaz E et al: Oral-dental findings in dyskeratosis congenita, *J Oral Pathol Med* 21:280, 1992.

Darier's disease

Burge S: Darier's disease: the clinical features and pathogenesis, *Clin Exp Dermatol* 19:193, 1994.

Burge SM, Wilkinson JD: Darier-White disease: a review of the clinical features in 163 patients, *J Am Acad Dermatol* 27:40, 1992.

Ferris T, Lamey PJ, Rennie JS: Darier's disease: oral features and genetic aspects, *Br Dent J* 168:71, 1990.

Macleod RI: The incidence and distribution of oral lesions in patients with Darier's disease, *Br Dent J* 171:133, 1991.

Pachyonychia congenita

Dahl PR, Daoud MS, Daniel Su WP: Jadassohn-Lewandowski syndrome (pachyonychia congenita), *Semin Dermatol* 14:129, 1995.

Daniel Su WP et al: Pachyonychia congenita: a clinical study of 12 cases and review of the literature, *Pediatr Dermatol* 7:33, 1990.

Feinstein A, Friedman J, Schewach-Millet M: Pachyonychia congenita, *J Am Acad Dermatol* 19:705, 1988.

Hersh S: Pachyonychia congenita: manifestations for the otolaryngologist, *Arch Otolaryngol Head Neck Surg* 116:732, 1990.

McLean WHI et al: Keratin 16 and keratin 17 mutations cause pachyonychia congenita, *Nat Genet* 9:273, 1995.

Multiple endocrine neoplasia type 2B

DeLellis RA: Biology of disease: multiple endocrine neoplasia syndromes revisited: clinical, morphologic, and molecular features, *Lab Invest* 72:494, 1995.

Donis-Keller H: The RET proto-oncogene and cancer, *J Intern Med* 238:319, 1995.

Holloway KB, Flowers FP: Multiple endocrine neoplasia 2B (MEN2B)/MEN3, *Dermatol Clin* 13:99, 1995.

Kahn MA, Cote GJ, Gagel GF: RET protooncogene mutational analysis in multiple endocrine neoplasia syndrome type 2B, *Oral Surg Oral Med Oral Pathol Oral Radiol Endod* 82:288, 1996.

O'Riordain DS et al: Multiple endocrine neoplasia 2B: more than an endocrine disorder, *Surgery* 118:936, 1995.

White sponge nevus

Downham TF, Plezia RA: Oral squamous-cell carcinoma within a white sponge nevus, *J Dermatol Surg Oncol* 4:470, 1978.

Jorgenson RJ, Levin LS: White sponge nevus, *Arch Dermatol* 117:73, 1981.

Richard G et al: Keratin 13 point mutation underlies the hereditary mucosal epithelia disorder white sponge nevus, *Nat Genet* 11:453, 1995.

Rugg EL et al: A mutation in the mucosal keratin K4 is associated with oral white sponge nevus, *Nat Genet* 11:450, 1995.

Focal dermal hypoplasia

Goltz RW et al: Focal dermal hypoplasia syndrome: a review of the literature and report of two cases, *Arch Dermatol* 101:1, 1970.

Greer RO, Reissner MW: Focal dermal hypoplasia: current concepts and differential diagnosis, *J Periodontol* 6:330, 1989.

Sule RR, Dhumawat DJ, Gharpuray MB: Focal dermal hypoplasia, *Cutis* 53:309, 1994.

Incontinentia pigmenti

Cohen PR: Incontinentia pigmenti: clinicopathologic characteristics and differential diagnosis, *Cutis* 54:161, 1994.

Dutheil P et al: Incontinentia pigmenti: late sequelae and genotypic diagnosis: a three-generation study of four patients, *Pediatr Dermatol* 12:107, 1995.

Landy SJ, Donnai D: Incontinentia pigmenti (Bloch-Sulzberger syndrome), *J Med Genet* 30:53, 1993.

Milam PE, Griffin TJ, Shapiro RD: A dentofacial deformity associated with incontinentia pigmenti: report of a case, *Oral Surg Oral Med Oral Pathol* 70:420, 1990.

Pseudoxanthoma elasticum

Goette DK, Carpenter WM: The mucocutaneous marker of pseudoxanthoma elasticum, *Oral Surg* 51:68, 1981.

Katagiri K et al: Heterogeneity of clinical features of pseudoxanthoma elasticum, *J Dermatol* 18:211, 1991.

Lebowohl M et al: Classification of pseudoxanthoma elasticum: report of a consensus conference, *J Am Acad Dermatol* 30:103, 1994.

Oral-facial-digital syndromes

Gorlin RJ, Psaume J: Orodigitofacial dysostosis—a new syndrome: a study of 22 cases, *J Pediatr* 61:520, 1962.

Toriello HV: Heterogeneity and variability in the oral-facial-digital syndromes, *Am J Med Genet* 4:149, 1988.

Toriello HV: Oral-facial-digital syndromes, 1992, *Clin Dysmorph* 2:95, 1993.

Xeroderma pigmentosum

Kraemer KH, Lee MM, Scotto J: Early onset of skin and oral cavity neoplasms in xeroderma pigmentosum, *Lancet* 1:56, 1982.

Kraemer KH, Lee MM, Scotto J: DNA repair protects against cutaneous and internal neoplasia: evidence from xeroderma pigmentosum, *Carcinogenesis* 5:511, 1984.

Patton LL, Valdez IH: Xeroderma pigmentosum: review and report of a case, *Oral Surg Oral Med Oral Pathol* 71:297, 1991.

Familial dysautonomia

Mass E, Gadoth N: Oro-dental self mutilation in familial dysautonomia, *J Oral Pathol Med* 23:273, 1994.

Mass E et al: Dental and oral findings in patients with familial dysautonomia, *Oral Surg Oral Med Oral Pathol* 74:305, 1992.

Lipoid proteinosis

Chaudhary SJ, Dayal PK: Hyalinosis cutis et mucosae, *Oral Surg Oral Med Oral Pathol Oral Radiol Endod* 80:168, 1995.

Israel H: Gingival lesions in lipoid proteinosis, *J Periodontol* 63:561, 1992.

Konstantin K et al: Lipoid proteinosis, *J Am Acad Dermatol* 27:293, 1992.

Simpson HE: Oral manifestations in lipoid proteinosis, *Oral Surg Oral Med Oral Pathol* 33:528, 1972.

Congenital erythropoietic porphyria

Cabrerizo-Merino CC et al: Stomatological manifestations of Günther's disease, *J Pedod* 14:113, 1990.

Fayle SA, Pollard MA: Congenital erythropoietic porphyria-oral manifestations and dental treatment in childhood: a case report, *Quintessence Int* 25:551, 1994.

Hereditary benign intraepithelial dyskeratosis

McLean IW et al: Hereditary benign intraepithelial dyskeratosis: a report of two cases from Texas, *Ophthalmology* 88:164, 1981.

Sadeghi EM, Witkop CJ: Ultrastructural study of hereditary benign intraepithelial dyskeratosis, *Oral Surg Oral Med Oral Pathol* 44:567, 1977.

Witkop CJ et al: Hereditary benign intraepithelial dyskeratosis: oral manifestations and hereditary transmission, *Arch Pathol* 70:696, 1960.

Papillon-Lefèvre syndrome

Blanchet-Bardon C et al: Acitretin in the treatment of severe disorders of keratinization: results of an open study, *J Am Acad Dermatol* 24:982, 1991.

Hattab FN et al: Papillon-Lefèvre syndrome: a review of the literature and report of 4 cases, *J Periodontol* 66:413, 1995.

Ishikawa I, Umeda M, Laosrisin N: Clinical, bacteriological, and immunological examinations and the treatment process of two Papillon-Lefèvre syndrome patients, *J Periodontol* 65:364, 1994.

Stabholz A, Taichman NS, Soskolne WA: Occurrence of *Actinobacillus actinomycetemcomitans* and anti-leukotoxin antibodies in some members of an extended family affected by Papillon-Lefèvre syndrome, *J Periodontol* 66:653, 1995.

Gingival fibromatosis

Bakaeen G, Scully C: Hereditary gingival fibromatosis in a family with the Zimmerman-Laband syndrome, *J Oral Pathol Med* 20:457, 1991.

Bozzo L et al: Hereditary gingival fibromatosis: report of an extensive four-generation pedigree, *Oral Surg Oral Med Oral Pathol* 78:452, 1994.

Takagi M et al: Heterogeneity in the hereditary gingival fibromatoses, *Cancer* 68:2202, 1991.

Witkop CJ: Heterogeneity in the gingival fibromatoses, *Birth Defects* 7:215, 1971.

Ectodermal dysplasias

Gorlin R, Cohen M, Levin S: *Syndromes of the head and neck,* New York-Oxford, 1990, Oxford University Press.

Guckes AD et al: Using endosseous dental implants for patients with ectodermal dysplasia, *J Am Dent Assoc* 122:59, 1991.

Levin LS: Dental and oral abnormalities in selected ectodermal dysplasia syndromes, *Birth Defects* 24:205, 1988.

Hereditary mucoepithelial dysplasia

Rogers M, Kourt G, Cameron A: Hereditary mucoepithelial dysplasia, *Pediatr Dermatol* 11:133, 1994.

Scheman AJ et al: Hereditary mucoepithelial dysplasia, *J Am Acad Dermatol* 21:351, 1989.

Witkop CJ et al: Clinical, histologic, cytologic and ultrastructural characteristics of the oral lesions from hereditary mucoepithelial dysplasia, *Oral Surg Oral Med Oral Pathol* 46:645, 1978.

Encephalotrigeminal angiomatosis

Sujansky E, Conradi S: Outcome of Sturge-Weber syndrome in 52 adults, *Am J Med Genet* 57:35, 1995.

Tallman B et al: Location of port-wine stains and the likelihood of ophthalmic and/or central nervous system complications, *Pediatrics* 87:323, 1991.

Hereditary hemorrhagic telangiectasia

Austin GB, Quart AM, Novak B: Hereditary hemorrhagic telangiectasia with oral manifestations, *Oral Surg Oral Med Oral Pathol* 51:245, 1981.

Ference BA et al: Life-threatening pulmonary hemorrhage with pulmonary arteriovenous malformations and hereditary hemorrhagic telangiectasia, *Chest* 106:1387, 1994.

Flint SR, Keith O, Scully C: Hereditary hemorrhagic telangiectasia: family study and review, *Oral Surg Oral Med Oral Pathol* 66:440, 1988.

Wescott WB, Correll RW: Hemorrhage associated with telangiectasia, *J Am Dent Assoc* 104:60, 1982.

Tuberous sclerosis

Lygidakis NA, Lindenbaum RH: Oral fibromatosis in tuberous sclerosis, *Oral Surg Oral Med Oral Pathol* 68:725, 1989.

Maclker SB, Shoulars HW, Burker EJ: Tuberous sclerosis with gingival lesions, *Oral Surg Oral Med Oral Pathol* 34:619, 1972.

Mlynarczyk G: Enamel pitting: a common symptom of tuberous sclerosis, *Oral Surg Oral Med Oral Pathol* 71:63, 1991.

Roach ES, Delgado MR: Tuberous sclerosis, *Dermatol Clin* 13:151, 1995.

Scully C, Herts R: Orofacial manifestations in tuberous sclerosis, *Oral Surg* 44:707, 1977.

Tillman HH, De Caro F: Tuberous sclerosis, *Oral Surg Oral Med Oral Pathol* 71:301, 1991.

Beckwith-Wiedemann syndrome

Cohen PR, Kurzrock R: Miscellaneous genodermatoses: Beckwith-Wiedemann syndrome, Birt-Hogg-Dube syndrome, familial atypical multiple mole melanoma syndrome, hereditary tylosis, incontinentia pigmenti, and supernumerary nipples, *Dermatol Clin* 13:211, 1995.

Weng EY, Mortier GR, Graham JM: Beckwith-Wiedemann syndrome: an update and review for the primary pediatrician, *Clin Pediatr* 34:317, 1995.

Oral Manifestations of Systemic Diseases

GASTROINTESTINAL DISEASES
Crohn's Disease

Crohn's disease is characterized by chronic transmural inflammation of the gastrointestinal tract affecting any part from the anus to the mouth. The disease occurs most commonly in adolescents and young adults and twice as often in males as in females.

The oral manifestations are diverse and develop in approximately 10% of patients. However, when oral lesions of Crohn's disease are identified, they represent the initial manifestation of the disease in approximately one third of cases. In these patients, gastrointestinal symptoms are usually not evident and a complete evaluation is needed to demonstrate involvement elsewhere. In the majority of instances the oral lesions of Crohn's disease accompany systemic disease, and the severity of the oral lesions parallels the intestinal activity. Patients with oral Crohn's disease also have a higher incidence of extraintestinal manifestations such as cutaneous, ophthalmologic, or joint involvement. Microscopically, the oral lesions are similar to those seen in active intestinal lesions and are characterized by noncaseating granulomas. More frequently, the oral lesions will reveal less specific findings including focal collection of lymphocytes, lymphoid follicles, and perivascular mononuclear cell infiltrates.

Diffuse swelling of the upper and lower lips associated with mild discomfort is the most constant oral feature of Crohn's disease. Intraoral swelling of the buccal mucosa and tongue may also occur. These traits are clinically and microscopically identical to those of the Melkersson-Rosenthal syndrome. Thus a complete gastrointestinal evaluation is needed in patients with granulomatous cheilitis, even in the absence of systemic symptoms. Furthermore, because these labial and intraoral changes may precede the onset of gastrointestinal involvement by years, especially in children, long-term surveillance is required.

Mucosal nodularity resulting in cobblestoning is a more specific but less frequent oral manifestation of Crohn's disease (Figs. 12-1 and 12-2). The lesions consist of pink or mucosal-colored papules coalescing into firm plaques and occur most often on the inner aspect of the lower lip, buccal mucosa, and palate. These may result in discomfort when eating or speaking.

Aphthouslike ulcerations, which are often linear with hyperplastic borders, may be more prevalent in patients with Crohn's disease and have been reported to occur in 10% of patients with active colonic disease (Fig. 12-3). The ulcers may be mild and asymptomatic or extensive and painful, but they are indistinguishable from recurrent aphthous stomatitis. Mucosal tags appearing on the labial and buccal mucosa and resembling oral fibromas are another reported oral feature of Crohn's disease. These are usually discovered during a routine search for extraintestinal manifestations of the disease.

Patients with active Crohn's disease have a greater frequency of dental infections and decay, which may be caused by the aberrant regulation of the immune response that is considered to play an important role in the pathogenesis of the disease.

Oral Crohn's disease may require no therapy and undergo spontaneous remission. More frequently, the lesions result in significant discomfort and respond to the systemic medications admin-

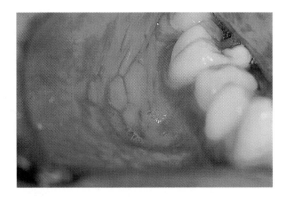

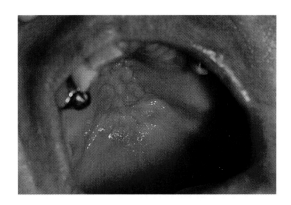

FIG. 12-1   Mucosal nodularity, consisting of coalescing pink papules, develops most often in the buccal mucosa in patients with Crohn's disease.

FIG. 12-2   The recognition of cobblestoning in patients with Crohn's disease may result in a diagnosis before systemic symptoms develop.

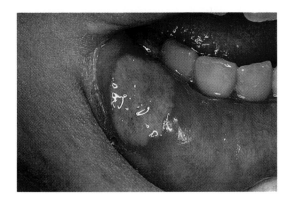

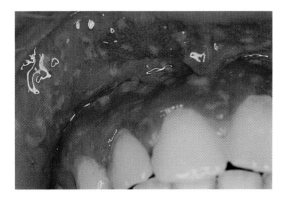

FIG. 12-3   Large and painful aphthouslike ulcerations are commonly observed in patients with active Crohn's disease.

FIG. 12-4   Pyostomatitis vegetans is a highly specific marker for inflammatory bowel disease and is characterized by pustules and erosions that predominantly affect the labial mucosa and gingivae.

istered for the intestinal disease including corticosteroids and sulfasalazine. Topical and intralesional corticosteroids are also effective in treating the oral ulcerations.

Ulcerative Colitis and Pyostomatitis Vegetans

Pyostomatitis vegetans is an oral ulcerative condition that is considered to be a highly specific marker for inflammatory bowel disease. Although the majority of cases are associated with ulcerative colitis, the oral disease may also infrequently occur in association with Crohn's disease, sclerosing cholangitis, or other liver diseases.

The oral disorder is characterized by the appearance of pustules, erosions, and vegetative plaques that predominantly affect the labial and buccal mucosa and the attached gingivae (Fig. 12-4). Minute miliary abscesses and pustules of fairly uniform size develop on an erythematous base and eventually rupture, leading to erosions and ulcerations. These form the pathognomonic "snail track" appearance and occasionally are accompanied by vegetative plaques and fissuring of the buccal mucosa (Fig. 12-5). The oral lesions may be prominent but produce few symptoms.

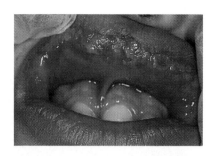

FIG. 12-5   Minute miliary abscesses and pustules of fairly uniform size develop on an erythematous base in a pathognomonic "snail track" pattern in pyostomatitis vegetans.

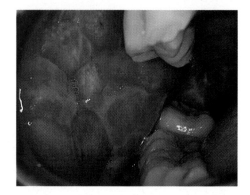

FIG. 12-6   Patients with hepatitis C have an increased incidence of oral lichen planus, usually of the erosive type.

The development of pyostomatitis vegetans usually follows the onset of inflammatory bowel disease. However, in well-documented cases, the oral lesions precede the onset of intestinal disease. When a diagnosis of pyostomatitis vegetans is confirmed, a thorough gastrointestinal evaluation is warranted despite a lack of constitutional symptoms.

The histopathology of oral lesions is characteristic and reveals hyperkeratosis and acanthosis, a dense cellular infiltrate throughout the lamina propria and epithelium comprised of neutrophils, eosinophils, and miliary abscesses, intraepithelially or subepithelially. Results of direct immunofluorescence are typically negative, differentiating pyostomatitis vegetans from pemphigus and pemphigoid. The demonstration of peripheral blood eosinophilia, present in 90% of cases, can help confirm the diagnosis.

The severity of the oral disease parallels the activity of the gastrointestinal disease. In general, pyostomatitis vegetans is refractory to therapy. Usually, the oral lesions regress when the colitis is controlled with various systemic medications, diet, or surgery. Topical and systemic corticosteroids may be effective when the oral lesions are persistent.

Hepatitis and Other Liver Diseases

The simultaneous occurrence of lichen planus (see Chapter 9) and liver disease has been observed by many investigators. Although primary biliary cirrhosis and cryptogenic liver cirrhosis have infrequently been linked with lichen planus, the association of lichen planus with hepatitis appears to be substantial. Specifically, numerous reports have demonstrated a relationship of oral lichen planus with chronic active hepatitis C. The oral lesions are almost always of the erosive type and, in many instances, lead to the discovery of the liver disease (Fig. 12-6). In a prospective trial examining 187 patients with oral lichen planus, more than 20% exhibited elevated liver transaminases and the cause in the majority of patients was chronic active hepatitis C. Similarly, in patients who are known to be infected with the hepatitis C virus, oral erosive lichenoid lesions are detected more frequently than expected. Even when hepatitis is treated with interferon, the oral lesions do not always regress. Histopathologic findings of both lichen planus and hepatitis C are characterized by a T-lymphocytic infiltrate with keratinocyte

Table 12-1   Uncommon Oral Manifestations of Dermatologic Diseases

DISEASE	ORAL FINDINGS
Acute febrile neutrophilic dermatosis (Sweet's syndrome)	Red patches on the buccal mucosa and lesions resembling oral aphthae
Cronkhite-Canada syndrome	Buccal mucosal melanotic hyperpigmentation
Cutaneous T-cell lymphoma	Ulcerations, plaques, and tumors on the gingiva, palate, and tongue; involvement occurs late in the disease (see Chapter 5)
Henoch-Schönlein purpura	Petechiae, most often on palate
Kawasaki disease	Lips are characteristically inflamed, cracked, fissured, and hemorrhagic; oropharynx is bright red; tongue papillae are enlarged and inflamed (strawberry tongue)
Lichen nitidus	Minute and diffuse flat white papules; white plaques on tongue and palate
Lichen sclerosus et atrophicus	White hypopigmented and atrophic plaques most common on inner lips and buccal mucosa
Malignant atrophic papulosis	Atrophic red lesions with telangiectases on buccal mucosa
Multicentric reticulohistiocytosis	Lips, buccal mucosa, and tongue frequently exhibit erythematous, infiltrated papules, and nodules
Pityriasis rubra pilaris	Lesions on tongue identical to geographic tongue
Porokeratosis	Oral lesions may occur in the Mibelli and porokeratosis palmaris et plantaris disseminata types
Sarcoidosis	Superficial or deep-seated red submucosal nodules on buccal mucosa, lips, soft palate, tongue, and gingiva usually in association with lung involvement
Vitiligo	Hypopigmentation of lips, tongue, or other sites
Xanthoma disseminatum	Multiple yellow or orange nodules in various oral locations, most often on the lips and hard palate

and hepatocyte damage, respectively. Therefore it has been postulated that the association of these diseases may be caused by an immune reaction induced by the hepatitis C virus.

It is reasonable to perform liver function tests and measure hepatitis C antibodies in all patents with oral lichen planus, especially those with advanced or erosive disease. A definitive relationship of these disorders, however, has yet to be established.

Primary biliary cirrhosis in the majority of instances results in xerostomia. Less frequent oral manifestations include the appearance of rampant caries, green staining of teeth and mucosa, enamel hypoplasia, and gingival xanthomatosis.

CUTANEOUS DISEASES

A number of disorders with prominent cutaneous manifestations may uncommonly exhibit oral features (Table 12-1). Other skin diseases with pronounced oral findings are discussed in this chapter and in other chapters of this text.

Psoriasis

Psoriasis is a chronic, inflammatory scaling disease of the skin that affects approximately 1% of the population. It can appear at any age but develops most frequently during the third decade of life. The

FIG. 12-7 Intraoral psoriasis is uncommon and characterized by red and white plaques that develop in patients with widespread cutaneous involvement.

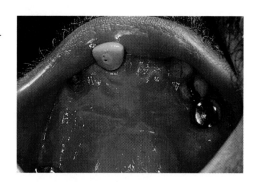

morphology, distribution, and patterns of the skin lesions vary considerably from patient to patient as does the severity of the disease. Generally, psoriatic plaques are well demarcated, erythematous, and covered with silvery scales. The lesions may appear anywhere on the body and are usually symmetrically distributed. Involvement of the nails is also commonly observed.

Oral manifestations have been described but are relatively uncommon. A variety of morphologic lesions have been described, but none are specific and almost all are discovered during routine oral examinations. White, circinate, or serpiginous mucosal patches and plaques on an erythematous base with silvery scales appear clinically and microscopically identical to the skin lesions (Fig. 12-7). These may occur on any oral mucosal surface; but the tongue, buccal mucosa, and palate are favored sites. The lesions are painless but may cause bleeding when subjected to trauma. Oral involvement occurs more commonly in patients with widespread cutaneous psoriasis. The lips are more frequently involved than the oral mucous membranes, and the scaling plaques are often extensions of perioral lesions.

A well-recognized association between psoriasis and geographic tongue has been confirmed by several investigators (see Chapter 4). Whereas the latter condition occurs in only 1% to 2% of the general population, in patients with psoriasis, its incidence approximates 10%. An even greater percentage of psoriatic patients with the severe pustular variety display geographic tongue.

Ectopic geographic tongue lesions, defined as plaques resembling geographic tongue but occurring on mucosal surfaces other than the dorsal tongue, are also significantly increased in patients with psoriasis. These probably represent the same lesions described previously as red, scaly plaques occurring in various oral sites. Both geographic tongue and ectopic geographic tongue are microscopically identical to the cutaneous lesions of psoriasis, supporting the close association of these disorders.

Pityriasis Rosea

Pityriasis rosea is a common dermatosis of unknown etiology that begins with a primary "herald patch" and is followed by a secondary, generalized symmetric eruption. The skin lesions most commonly involve the trunk and follow the natural lines of cleavage. Characteristic morphologic features of pityriasis rosea usually allow for easy diagnosis. Atypical cases may be confused with a large number of dermatologic conditions.

Oral manifestations of pityriasis rosea are probably more common than have been reported, as the oral cavity is rarely examined in patients suspected of having the disorder. When searched for carefully, multiple, erythematous patches, which sometimes are covered with a grayish or white film or accompanied by punctate hemorrhages, are discovered (Fig. 12-8). They are usually irregularly shaped and appear during the most severe phase of the disease. The lesions occur almost exclusively on the buccal mucosa and are more frequent in children than adults. The presence of these oral patches may help establish the diagnosis in atypical cases. The microscopic features from an oral biopsy are nonspecific and include a mixed inflammatory infiltrate in the epithelium and lamina propria with an overlying thickened squamous epithelium.

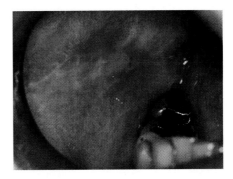

FIG. 12-8   Oral manifestations of pityriasis rosea are more common than reported and consist of erythematous patches on the buccal mucosa, often with punctate hemorrhages.

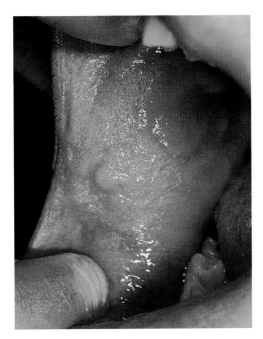

FIG. 12-9   Acanthosis nigricans of the anterior buccal mucosa demonstrating velvety, mucosal-colored, papillomatous growths.

The oral lesions of pityriasis rosea are asymptomatic and do not require therapy. Spontaneous resolution of both the cutaneous and oral eruption occurs after approximately 6 weeks.

Acanthosis Nigricans

Acanthosis nigricans is a cutaneous eruption characterized by the symmetric distribution of hyperpigmented velvety plaques. The most common sites of involvement are the nape and sides of the neck and axillae, although the groin, antecubital and popliteal surfaces, and umbilical areas are also commonly affected. There are eight types of acanthosis nigricans, but of special interest are the forms of the disease associated with internal malignancies and a variety of syndromes, mostly endocrine disorders. Oral manifestations of acanthosis nigricans are common in these forms and may be present in up to 40% of cases.

Characteristic lesions develop most frequently on the tongue and lips and may be the earliest or sole manifestation of the disease. The lips are initially velvety but thicken and enlarge as they become covered by papillomatous growths. These changes are most prominent at the angles of the lips. The palate and buccal mucosa may reveal similar changes (Fig. 12-9). The filiform papillae of the tongue become hypertrophic, resulting in a rough-textured dorsal surface. The gingivae, especially the interdental papillae, may be severely involved and grossly enlarged. Unlike the skin lesions, oral lesions are usually nonpigmented.

Microscopic features that support the diagnosis include marked acanthosis with papillary projections comprised of parakeratotic and hyperplastic epithelium.

The diagnosis of acanthosis nigricans should prompt an investigation for an underlying malignancy. Malignancies, most commonly gastric adenocarcinomas, simultaneously appear with the mucocutaneous eruption or precede its onset in approximately 80% of cases. Uterine, liver, colon, rectal, ovarian, and other malignancies can also be associated with acanthosis nigricans. Thus the recognition of the oral manifestations, which are most pronounced in the malignant form of acanthosis nigricans, can result in the early detection of an often fatal malignancy. Underlying endocrine abnormalities associated with acanthosis nigricans usually result in less prominent oral manifestations. Serious disorders of insulin resistance and compensatory insulin secretion can be harmful if the mucocutaneous features are undetected. The benign forms of acanthosis nigricans are only occasionally accompanied by oral lesions.

Treatment should be directed at the underlying problem. For example, if the malignancy is adequately treated in the early stages, the skin and oral lesions will usually resolve or improve. Unfortunately, these aggressive tumors are usually advanced at the time of diagnosis and are rapidly fatal. Correction of endocrine abnormalities may also lead to the improvement of the eruptions.

HEMATOLOGIC DISEASES
Disorders of Red Blood Cells

The characteristic oral manifestations of a diverse group of disorders with abnormal reduction or increase in red blood cells may be important indicators in the diagnosis of these conditions.

Iron deficiency anemia. Iron deficiency anemia is the most common form of anemia, affecting a significant portion of the population. Disruptions in iron hemostasis are commonly observed during menstruation, pregnancy, and gastrointestinal bleeding. The absence of iron stores in the bone marrow remains the most definitive test for differentiating iron deficiency from other microcytic anemias. Oral features common to all types of anemia include pallor of the mucous membranes. Atrophy of the filiform and fungiform papillae are the initial oral findings, which begin at the tip and lateral margins of the tongue; but as the disease progresses, the entire dorsal surface of the tongue may become reddened, atrophic, and smooth (Fig. 12-10). Patients often complain of a burning and stinging sensation of the tongue before the development of visible changes. Alterations from exfoliated squamous epithelial cells of the tongue revealing microcytosis and changes similar to those from the peripheral blood may be diagnostic. The Plummer-Vinson syndrome is a distinctive entity characterized by iron deficiency anemia accompanied by the oral manifestations previously described in association with esophageal strictures and erosions. The condition occurs most frequently in women who are in their fifth decade of life, and its recognition is important because untreated patients have a significant risk of developing oral carcinomas. Patients respond effectively to well-tolerated oral iron preparations.

Pernicious anemia. Pernicious anemia and other causes of cobalamin (vitamin B_{12}) deficiency are most commonly observed in the elderly, vegetarians, human immunodeficiency virus-infected patients, those with gastrointestinal diseases, and patients with autoimmunity or a family history of pernicious anemia. Assays for cobalamin or its metabolite, methylmalonate, can be used as screening tests for cobalamin deficiency. Burning and excruciating pain of the tongue are constant features of pernicious anemia and often the first indication of the disease. Segments of the tongue or the entire dorsal surface appears inflamed and beefy red. Atrophy of the filiform and fungiform papillae eventually results in an atrophic, smooth, red, glistening tongue (Fig. 12-11). Taste alterations are common, and occasionally aphthae develop on the dorsal surface. Although the glossitis is most characteristic,

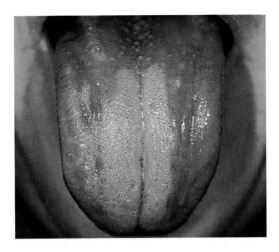

FIG. 12-10   Atrophy of the filiform and fungiform papillae on the lateral dorsal surface of the tongue is an early manifestation of iron deficiency anemia.

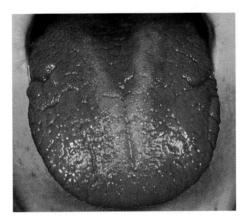

FIG. 12-11   Pernicious anemia almost always results in atrophy of the tongue papillae, which causes the tongue to become smooth, red, and glistening.

an overlooked and underrecognized feature of pernicious anemia is the presence of nonspecific, erythematous patches on the buccal and labial mucosa. Persistent stomatitis of unexplained origin necessitates an evaluation for cobalamin deficiency. Epithelial cells obtained from saliva or buccal mucosal scrapings from patients with pernicious anemia reveal cells with increased nuclear diameter, which may be a diagnostic aid. The oral lesions resolve with replacement therapy.

    Thalassemias. Thalassemias are a group of chronic anemias that result from an inherited abnormality of globin synthesis. In the severe form (thalassemia major), oral manifestations are characterized by protrusion of the anterior upper teeth, resulting in a distinctive prominence of the maxilla. Intraoral pallor and tongue atrophy may also be present.

    Hemolytic disease of the newborn. Isoimmunization is the most common cause of hemolytic disease of the newborn. The availability of anti-D immunoglobulin prophylaxis has dramatically decreased the incidence of the disease resulting from Rh sensitization; however, cases still occur, resulting in perinatal morbidity.

FIG. 12-12   Characteristic purple lips in polycythemia vera.

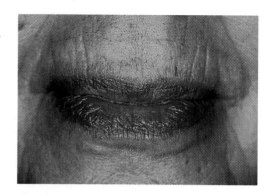

The teeth may exhibit varying shades of brown or blue because of the deposition of bilirubin in enamel. Various degrees of enamel hypoplasia may also develop. Fortunately, only the primary teeth are affected. Intrauterine intravascular transfusion for the treatment of congenital hemolytic anemia resulting from maternal-fetal blood incompatibility has significantly reduced the complications of the disease.

Polycythemia vera. Patients with polycythemia vera, a common myeloproliferative disease characterized by an increased production of red blood cells, typically display a deep purple color of the lips and the mucous membranes (Fig. 12-12). The lips, gingiva, and tongue are most consistently affected. Enlarged gingivae, which often bleed spontaneously, oral petechiae, and hematomas may all occur infrequently. The color of the oral cavity structures reverts to normal as the disease is treated.

Disorders of Platelets

Thrombocytopenia. A diverse group of disorders affect platelets, the cells that form a vascular plug after an initial injury and provide a surface that promotes blood coagulation. Drug-induced platelet dysfunction is the most frequent type of acquired platelet disorder, although chronic renal failure and liver cirrhosis commonly cause prolonged bleeding times. Drug-induced thrombocytopenia is also the primary cause of increased platelet destruction. Idiopathic thrombocytopenic purpura is a common disorder and is a result of rapid platelet destruction caused by circulating antiplatelet antibodies. The acute form typically occurs in children, is commonly associated with a viral infection, and is self-limiting. The chronic form, affecting adults more commonly than children, is characterized by potentially serious exacerbations that often necessitate the use of systemic corticosteroids or splenectomy to prevent hemorrhages. Decreased platelet production resulting from infiltrative bone marrow diseases and nutritional diseases, as well as increased platelet sequestration resulting from splenomegaly, can also cause thrombocytopenia.

Disorders of platelets, regardless of the cause, can manifest clinically as purpura and bleeding of the mucous membranes. The rich vascular structures of the oral cavity are frequently a source of concern and may be an early warning of an underlying platelet abnormality. Bleeding gingiva, often severe and spontaneous, is the most frequent oral manifestation, although petechiae and ecchymoses are also common, especially on the palate. Characteristic reddish-black hemorrhagic bullae in the oral cavity indicate a profound reduction in the platelet count (Fig. 12-13). Oral surgical procedures may be complicated by hemorrhage and should be delayed until the underlying condition is corrected.

Disorders of White Blood Cells

Neutropenia. Although the causes of an abnormal reduction in the number of white blood cells are extremely diverse, the oral manifestations of neutropenia are fairly constant. Oral features include ulcerations and stomatitis, which result from the inability of tissues to respond to trauma or in-

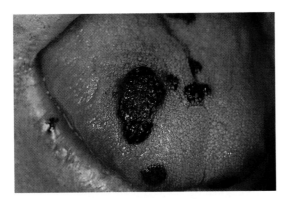

FIG. 12-13   Red-black hemorrhagic bullae are pathognomonic of thrombocytopenia.

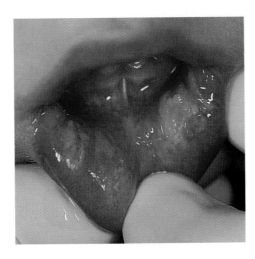

FIG. 12-14   Cyclic neutropenia should be suspected in any patient, especially an infant or child who develops recurrent aphthouslike ulcerations at 3-week intervals.

fection. The severity of oral mucositis generally correlates with the degree of neutrophil reduction. For example, severe oral ulcerations and stomatitis, which develop in almost all recipients of bone marrow transplants, resolve when the absolute neutrophil count recovers to above 500 cells/ml. Furthermore, the changes occur predominantly on the nonkeratinized mucosa, which are not protected from trauma by a cornified layer and are vulnerable to breakdown. Profound neutropenia accompanied by severe oral ulcerations and diffuse stomatitis can be seen in a number of congenital entities including Kostmann's syndrome, reticular dysgenesis, and immune deficiency disorders of B or T lymphocytes. Additionally, a large group of inherited metabolic diseases and phenotypic abnormalities may result in various degrees of neutropenia and hence oral manifestations.

Cyclic neutropenia. Cyclic neutropenia is characterized by regularly recurrent episodes of profound neutropenia, which have a periodicity of approximately 3 weeks (range is 14 to 36 days). The interval tends to remain constant in each patient. The cyclic oscillation in monocytes and reticulocytes is reciprocal to that of the neutrophils, whereas platelet count oscillation parallels the neutrophil cycle. Most patients develop the disease in infancy or childhood; a significant number of patients acquire it as adults and in association with a clonal proliferation of large granular lymphocytes. Approximately one third of patients display an autosomal dominant pattern of inheritance.

The most consistent clinical manifestation of cyclic neutropenia is oral ulcerations that are identical to recurrent aphthous stomatitis (Fig. 12-14). These well-demarcated, superficial ulcerations occur most frequently on the nonkeratinized mucosa and are often accompanied by a severe gingivitis that bleeds readily. As the neutrophil count returns to normal, the ulcerations spontaneously heal and the gingivae revert to their normal healthy appearance. During periods of neutropenia, patients often develop fever, malaise, and cervical lymphadenopathy, important features that may aid in diagnosis.

The diagnosis can be established by demonstrating two cycles of neutropenia (absolute neutrophil counts of less than 1500 per mm^3 for whites and 1000 per mm^3 for blacks). Hemoglobin, lymphocyte, and platelet counts are normal. Cyclic neutropenia is caused by an abnormality in the regulation of early hematopoietic precursor cells. This is supported by bone marrow examination during periods of neutropenia showing maturation arrest in the myeloid cell development at the myelocyte stage.

Peritonitis, segmental bowel necrosis, and septicemia are uncommon complications of cyclic neutropenia. Secondary bacterial infections during episodes of neutropenia necessitate the use of appropriate antibiotics. Recombinant human granulocyte colony-stimulating factor (G-CSF) is now routinely used for a variety of causes associated with neutropenia including cyclic neutropenia. This agent significantly shortens but does not eliminate the period of oscillations and raises the nadir of neutrophil counts. When G-CSF is administered long term to children and adults with this disorder, both the risk of infections and the oral ulcerations are practically eliminated.

Leukemia. Leukemia is a malignancy characterized by the disseminated proliferation of immature white blood cells of the bone marrow accumulating in various tissues of the body. The leukemias are classified according to the type of abnormal proliferating cells and further subdivided into acute and chronic forms, depending on the onset and course of the disease. Oral features are found in all types but are most prominent and prevalent in the acute form of the disease and in the monocytic type. They are a frequent initial manifestation of the disease, and the recognition of specific and characteristic oral changes can result in early therapeutic intervention. Oral complications can result from direct infiltration of the oral structures by malignant cells, the myelosuppressive nature of the disease, or the direct and indirect effects of cytotoxic agents used in treatment.

At presentation the oral mucosa may be noted to be strikingly pale as a result of anemia. Punctate petechiae, ecchymosis, and hemorrhage occur spontaneously and frequently and are often the first manifestations patients notice. These changes most frequently affect the palate, lips, and tongue and reflect underlying thrombocytopenia. When unexplained gingival bleeding and oral petechiae are observed, especially in children, an evaluation for leukemia should be promptly instituted.

Gingival hyperplasia occurs as a result of direct leukemic infiltration of the gingivae. The gums become edematous, pink, fibrotic, and firm and may completely cover the teeth (Fig. 12-15). This oral manifestation of leukemia occurs uncommonly but is the most characteristic and is observed most frequently in the monocytic form. The institution of an optimal oral hygiene regimen may greatly diminish the gingival enlargement.

Painful and deep oral ulcerations covered with a fibrinous pseudomembrane occur in areas subjected to trauma such as the hard palate, buccal mucosa, and tongue. These may be caused by direct oral leukemic proliferation, a diminished granulocyte count, or from cytotoxic and immunosuppressive properties of the antileukemic agents.

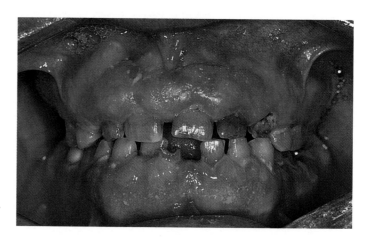

FIG. 12-15 Gingival hyperplasia is the result of leukemic infiltration of the gums and occurs most frequently in the monocytic form of the disease.

Patients with leukemia often experience dental pain and, in the advanced stages, destruction of the periodontal structures and alveolar bone result in loosening of the teeth. Oral bacterial, fungal, and viral infections are significantly increased in frequency, necessitating a high index of suspicion in patients with leukemia exhibiting oral ulcerations. The detection of oral candidiasis by direct culture methods from mucosal smears may prevent significant morbidity as a result of *Candida* septicemia. Leukemic infiltrates involving the salivary glands may result in xerostomia. Neurologic complications of the oral cavity affecting motor and sensory functions may occur because of central and peripheral nervous system involvement. The long-term side effects of chemotherapy in children with leukemia include hypodontia and enamel hypoplasia.

The oral complications of leukemia resolve as the disease is treated with myelosuppressive and immunosuppressive drugs. The maintenance of meticulous oral hygiene cannot be overemphasized. Topical anesthetics and antiseptics may alleviate the pain associated with the oral ulcerations.

Multiple myeloma. Multiple myeloma is a malignancy of plasma cells that synthesize and secrete immunoglobulins. Multiple myeloma comprises nearly one half of all primary bone malignancies, with nearly 15,000 cases reported annually in the United States.

The disease occurs in adults, most frequently in the seventh decade of life, with approximately two thirds of cases arising in men. The disease is more frequent in African-Americans. A serum monoclonal immunoglobulin or urinary monoclonal light-chain protein can be demonstrated by electrophoresis in virtually all patients. The amounts of serum immunoglobulins correlate with tumor load.

The initial presenting symptom of multiple myeloma is often bone pain resulting from bone resorption that is caused by increased osteoclastic activity. Patients frequently display pathologic fractures and hypercalcemia, as well as fever and malaise secondary to bone marrow obliteration by tumor cells. The radiographic findings in multiple myeloma are characteristic, with the presence of multiple, well-circumscribed, "punched-out" radiolucencies, especially of the skull. Up to one third of cases involves the jaws, particularly the mandible. Oral manifestations of multiple myeloma are uncommon and represent secondary changes caused by bone marrow infiltration. These include gingival bleeding and petechiae from platelet deficiencies and nonspecific erythema and ulcerations from neutrophil dysfunction. Jaw involvement results in oral pain and tooth mobility. As 15% to 25% of multiple myeloma cases are associated with amyloidosis, oral manifestations including tongue nodules and tongue enlargement are commonly observed. Solitary soft-tissue plasmacytomas that represent an extramedullary form of myeloma can occasionally arise in the oral cavity. These involve the hard palate and gingiva most frequently and are characterized by dome-shaped masses that may ulcerate (Fig. 12-16).

High-dose chemotherapy and radiotherapy with allogenic or autologous bone marrow transplantation have significantly improved survival in recent years.

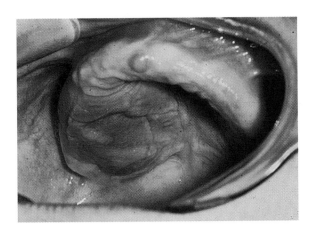

FIG. 12-16   Oral plasmacytomas may develop in multiple myeloma or occur as an isolated finding and arise most frequently on the palate as ulcerated masses.

Langerhans Cell Histiocytosis

Previously referred to as histiocytosis X, Langerhans cell histiocytosis encompasses a diverse spectrum of clinical disorders characterized by proliferation of Langerhans cells.

These cells are derived from bone marrow, function as the major antigen-presenting cell of the skin, display a characteristic immunophenotype, and contain distinctive Birbeck granules.

Three forms of the disease that display oral features are recognized. In general, the gingiva is the most frequent site of involvement in all three types, and the mouth may be the first or only manifestation of the disease.

Letterer-Siwe disease typically occurs in infants and rarely in adults and is characterized by an acute and fulminant course with disseminated visceral involvement, often resulting in death. Skin lesions are almost always evident and consist of papules, plaques, vesicles, and nodules that are often hemorrhagic. The lesions occur in a seborrheic dermatitis pattern. Oral manifestations include large and irregular ulcerations, ecchymoses, advanced gingivitis and periodontitis, and premature tooth loss. These changes often accompany systemic involvement.

Hand-Schüller-Christian disease develops in children and results in diabetes insipidus, proptosis, and lytic bone lesions, although the complete triad occurs in fewer than 25% of affected patients. Skin lesions arise in only one half of affected patients. The oral features may be the initial manifestation of the disorder and are characterized by irregular and persistent ulcerations, most frequently of the palate (Fig. 12-17); severe inflammation and destruction of the gingiva; and ulcerated nodules. These changes may be accompanied by delayed wound healing after tooth extraction, difficulty in mastication, and foul breath.

Eosinophilic granuloma occurs in young adults and is the most common form of Langerhans cell histiocytosis. Monostotic or polyostotic bone lesions may develop in any organ but have a predilection for flat bones. The radiographic appearance is characterized by a well-defined radiolucent destructive process. When the disease involves the jaws, the posterior aspect of the mandible is most commonly affected, resulting in displaced teeth and pathologic fractures. Accompanying these changes is a destructive and painful gingivitis, often with oral ulcerations on the gingiva, palate, and floor of the mouth.

Histologic findings are similar for all oral lesions of Langerhans cell histiocytosis. The infiltrate may be comprised almost entirely of Langerhans cells or be admixed with eosinophils, lymphocytes, and macrophages. Long-standing lesions may exhibit xanthomatous changes with vacuolated cells and giant cells. Langerhans cells can be definitively identified by immunohistochemical studies, as they strongly express S-100 protein in the cytoplasm and HLA-DR.

The disseminated forms of the disease may respond with variable success to cytotoxic drugs administered in conjunction with corticosteroids or radiation. Localized bone lesions in the jaws may

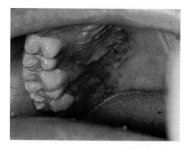

FIG. 12-17   Large and irregular ulcerations of the palate are the most constant oral manifestation of Langerhans cell histiocytosis.

be treated with curettage, excision, or radiation, although recurrences are common, as is spontaneous resolution.

NUTRITIONAL DISORDERS

The mouth is a sensitive indicator of nutritional status because of the assorted hard and soft tissues of the oral cavity and the specific nutritional needs of each. Frequently, oral manifestations of nutritional disorders reflect the initial sign of a deficiency. The severity of oral involvement is generally not proportional to the nutritional shortage, nor are there oral clinical characteristics specific to any one nutritional disorder. Rather, the oral features are variable in their appearance and a careful physical examination, history, laboratory studies, and a high degree of suspicion are required to diagnose specific disorders.

Riboflavin Deficiency

Deficiency of riboflavin, or vitamin B_2, manifests in the oral cavity as tongue alterations. The fungiform papillae enlarge and project over the filiform papillae, which atrophy. Progressive disease may result in smooth atrophic patches and a magenta-colored dorsal surface. Burning and pain are generally mild compared with other vitamin deficiency disorders that cause tongue abnormalities. Angular cheilitis is a frequent manifestation of riboflavin deficiency and is characterized by erythema, maceration, and soggy, white debris at the angles of the mouth (Fig. 12-18). The lesions are most often bilateral and cause discomfort. Deep, moist, and crusted fissures at the corners of the mouth occur in the acute stages and predispose to secondary infection with bacteria and yeast. Cheilitis of the lips represented by swelling, erythema, and denudation of the labial mucosa often accompany these changes.

Niacin Deficiency

The oral manifestations of pellagra are as striking as the better known cutaneous features that are pathognomonic of niacin deficiency. The severe pain associated with erythema, atrophy, and ulcera-

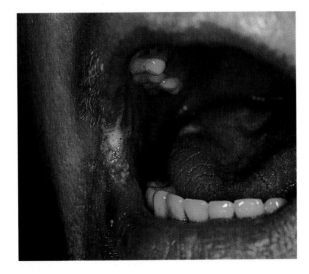

FIG. 12-18   Riboflavin deficiency is characterized by erythema, maceration, and soggy white debris at the angles of the mouth.

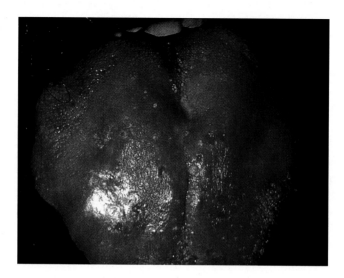

FIG. 12-19   Niacin deficiency results in a severely painful tongue that is beefy red and atrophic, often with ulcerations.

tions of the tongue may be the initial presentation of the deficiency. At first the tongue papillae become reddened and enlarged; however, as the disease progresses, they atrophy, resulting in a smooth, beefy-red surface (Fig. 12-19). Intraoral erythema and ulcerations commonly affect all of the mucous membranes, causing difficulty with food and fluid intake. A severe gingivitis characterized by ulcerated interdental papillae and reddened, necrotic gingivae is commonly observed. Desquamation of the lips and angular cheilitis accompany these changes. Bacteria and fungi frequently infect the compromised oral mucosa. These oral manifestations accompany the systemic abnormalities including diarrhea, dementia, and a marked photosensitivity, most prominently involving the neck and hands.

Folic Acid Deficiency

Folic acid deficiency is observed in patients treated with folic acid inhibitors such as methotrexate or those with various gastrointestinal diseases. Oral epithelial cells are dependent on folic acid for proper maturation; therefore folic acid deficiency results in prominent mucous membrane changes. The changes are nonspecific and consist of atrophy of the tongue papillae, ulcerations predominantly on the dorsal and ventral tongue surfaces, and angular cheilitis. Pain and burning of the tongue are pronounced, and occasionally a diffuse stomatitis with widespread ulcerations occurs.

Pyridoxine Deficiency

Pyridoxine, or vitamin B_6, deficiency results in oral changes characterized by angular cheilitis and a diffuse glossitis. The lesions are painful and the tongue often assumes a purplish and atrophied appearance. The fungiform papillae may remain unchanged or enlarge, appearing prominent on the denuded dorsal tongue surface.

Vitamin C Deficiency

Scurvy, or vitamin C deficiency, develops predominantly in individuals who do not consume fruits and vegetables. More than 50% of patients with scurvy develop a hemorrhagic gingivitis. The interdental papillae are the initial sites of involvement and become reddened and edematous. Tiny hemorrhages appear on the tips of the papillae. The disease proceeds to the marginal and attached gingiva with the development of erythema, desquamation, and ulcerations. Scorbutic gingivitis is painful and causes profuse bleeding as a result of impaired collagen formation and defects in capillary walls

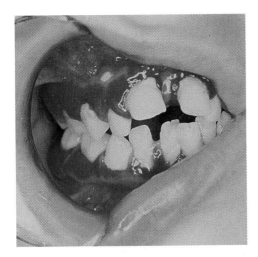

FIG. 12-20 Hemorrhagic gingivitis in untreated scurvy may result in periodontal destruction and alveolar bone degeneration.

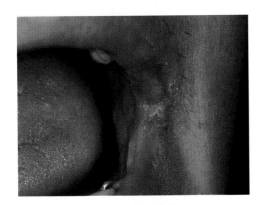

FIG. 12-21 Zinc deficiency in acrodermatitis enteropathica commonly results in ulcerative angular cheilitis.

attributed to vitamin C deficiency. The hemorrhagic gingivae may be fiery red in the acute stages (Fig. 12-20) but become dark blue with time. Aphthouslike ulcerations and hemorrhages of the oral mucous membranes other than the gingivae may also occur. If the gingivae are left untreated, periodontal destruction and alveolar bone degeneration may result in premature loss of teeth. In adults with low plasma ascorbic acid levels, oral mucosal changes include petechiae, lichenoid lesions, and most frequently, leukoplakia.

Vitamin K Deficiency

Hypoprothrombinemia secondary to vitamin K deficiency may cause bleeding to occur anywhere in the body, including the oral cavity. As with other disorders that result in bleeding, the gingivae are the most frequent oral site of involvement. Gingival bleeding is often spontaneous, and profuse bleeding may be triggered by trauma during mastication and oral hygiene. Oral ecchymosis on the palate and buccal mucosa may also be commonly observed.

Zinc Deficiency

Acrodermatitis enteropathica is an autosomal recessive disorder that results from an inability to absorb sufficient amounts of zinc from the diet. The disease manifests shortly after birth and is characterized by an acral and periorificial dermatitis, alopecia, and diarrhea. The symmetric skin eruption initially consists of a vesiculobullous dermatitis, but as the disease progresses, the lesions become thickened and crusted, resembling psoriasis.

Angular cheilitis, often with ulcerations, is almost always present and is an early manifestation of the disease (Fig. 12-21). Nonspecific superficial oral ulcerations frequently develop on the tongue and buccal mucosa as do reddened oral mucosal patches. Secondary infection with candidiasis is an aggravating factor of the skin and oral mucous membrane lesions. Patients with poorly controlled gastrointestinal diseases such as Crohn's disease may also develop zinc deficiency with similar clinical features.

Miscellaneous Vitamin Deficiencies

Thiamine. The oral manifestations of thiamine (vitamin B_1) deficiency are characterized by a vesicular eruption on the buccal mucosa, the floor of the mouth, and, occasionally, the palate. The vesicles ulcerate shortly after they form and are exquisitely painful.

Biotin. Biotin deficiency is most frequently reported in individuals consuming large quantities of raw eggs and results in diverse oral changes. These include dry and crusted lips, patchy atrophy of the tongue papillae resembling geographic tongue, and diffusely reddened oral mucous membranes.

Pantothenic acid, vitamin A, and vitamin D. Glossitis and angular cheilitis can be caused by a deficiency in pantothenic acid. The oral manifestations of vitamin A deprivation, characterized by xerostomia and burning of the mucous membranes, are the result of squamous metaplasia of the minor and major salivary glands. With chronic deprivation, the oral cavity becomes dry and atrophic. Enamel hypoplasia is evident if the deficiency occurs during tooth development. Rickets, resulting from vitamin D deficiency during childhood, causes pronounced changes in the permanent dentition characterized by enamel pitting and hypoplasia.

CONNECTIVE TISSUE DISORDERS

A number of connective tissue diseases display oral manifestations that may aid in establishing a diagnosis (Table 12-2). For example, linear scleroderma causes characteristic oral changes as well as cutaneous changes (Fig. 12-22).

Sjögren's Syndrome

Sjögren's syndrome is an autoimmune disease that affects as many as 3% of women older than 55 years. Apart from dryness of the eyes and mucous membranes, which are the most common clinical findings, systemic involvement frequently results in significant morbidity. This includes myositis, central and peripheral nervous system involvement, interstitial lung disease, hypergammaglobulinemic purpura, renal tubular acidosis, and vasculitis. In addition, lymphoma and Waldenström's macroglobulinemia may develop. Serologic studies in patients with Sjögren's syndrome reveal the presence of anti-Ro (SS-A) and anti-La (SS-B) antibodies in approximately 50% of patients. These autoantibodies are considered pathogenic and are associated with more severe glandular and extraglandular involvement. Although activated epithelial cells and their interaction with T lymphocytes may play a role in the pathogenesis of Sjögren's syndrome, a viral etiology has also been implicated.

Symptoms associated with keratoconjunctivitis sicca (dry eyes) include photophobia, burning, itching, and an inability to produce tears. An abnormal Schirmer's test is the most sensitive method of determining ocular involvement in patients with Sjögren's syndrome.

The oral manifestations of Sjögren's syndrome are not specific to the disease entity because they occur in other conditions in which salivary function is diminished. Xerostomia results in pronounced symptoms including oral dryness, burning mucous membranes (especially of the tongue), and difficulty in swallowing and speaking. The decrease in saliva predisposes patients to oral candidiasis and angular cheilitis and leads to atrophy and erythema of the tongue and buccal mucosa. As discussed in Chapter 14, xerostomia may lead to the development of dental caries, which are atypically located, occurring on the root surfaces adjacent to the gingiva rather than on the occlusal and interproximal surfaces of teeth (Fig. 12-23). An increased incidence of dental caries on the roots of

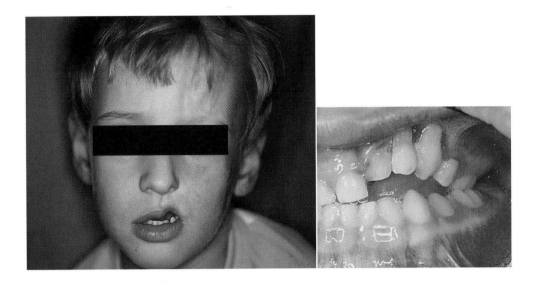

FIG. 12-22   Patients with linear scleroderma of the face often have intraoral involvement consisting of delayed eruption of the ipsilateral maxillary teeth.

Table 12-2   Oral Manifestations of Connective Tissue Diseases

DISEASE	ORAL FINDINGS
Dermatomyositis	Ulcers and erythema of the tongue and palate; telangiectatic erythema of the gingivae and hard palate resembling lupus erythematosus
Systemic sclerosis	Telangiectasia in more than 50% of patients; decreased mouth opening with interincisal distance less than 40 mm; salivary hypofunction; induration of tongue and tongue frenulum resulting in dysarthria; gingival recession as a result of fibrous strictures and increased periodontal disease; about 20% display characteristic extreme widening of the periodontal ligament radiographically
Linear scleroderma	*En coupe de sabre* occurs in children and results in hemiatrophy of the facial structures; atrophy of the lip, palate, and tongue are common; delayed unilateral eruption of teeth (see Fig. 12-23)
Mixed connective tissue	Xerostomia in more than 50% of patients; trigeminal neuropathy with disturbed disease sensory function; infrequent oral ulcerations and telangiectasia

teeth correlates directly with a prolonged oral sugar clearance time in patients. A labial salivary gland biopsy revealing focal lymphocytic sialadenitis is a simple, sensitive, and relatively specific method for determining salivary gland involvement in the diagnosis of Sjögren's syndrome; however, parotid sialography is a more specific and sensitive test. Quantitative salivary gland scintigraphy is also invaluable for the reliable detection of parenchymatous malfunction at an early stage of Sjögren's syndrome. Levels of leukocytes in oral washing from patients with Sjögren's syndrome are elevated, and their reduction can be monitored to assess treatment efficacy.

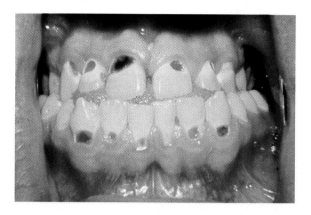

FIG. 12-23 Atypically located dental caries near the gingival margin occurs in patients with severe xerostomia caused by Sjögren's syndrome.

The damage of the salivary gland parenchyma is progressive and irreversible. In the early stages, symptomatic treatment of xerostomia includes stimulating salivary secretion with physiologic sialogogues or pharmacologic agents such as pilocarpine. In the advanced stages when saliva cannot be simulated, saliva substitutes may be tried, although many patients do not find them satisfactory. Mucin-containing lozenges, polymer-based saliva substitutes, and xanthan gum-based saliva substitutes all possess different viscoelastic properties, which may determine why benefits are observed in some patients but not in others. Therefore patients should be encouraged to test a number of different saliva substitutes despite the relative ineffectiveness in many individuals. Rampant caries can be prevented by optimal oral hygiene, frequent applications of topical fluoride, and avoidance of sweets between meals. Oral candidiasis is a frequent complication in patients with xerostomia, especially in edentulous patients, and predisposing factors such as poor oral hygiene and ill-fitting dentures should be corrected.

MULTISYSTEM DISEASES
Melkersson-Rosenthal Syndrome

Melkersson-Rosenthal is classically defined by the triad of recurrent orofacial swelling, relapsing facial paralysis, and fissured tongue. The complete triad, however, occurs in only 10% to 20% of patients. Cheilitis granulomatosa, described by Miescher, consists of swelling of one or both lips and is considered to be an oligosymptomatic form of the Melkersson-Rosenthal syndrome. These conditions develop most frequently during the second and third decades of life but can occur at any age.

Lip swelling is the most consistent feature of the disease and is the initial manifestation in approximately 50% of patients. The labial swelling develops unexpectedly, is usually unilateral and asymmetric, and affects the upper lip more often than the lower lip. As the lips enlarge, erythema, scaling, and fissuring may develop. The swelling spontaneously resolves, but recurrent and prolonged episodes are common. Although the episodes are painless, the lips may remain firmly pronounced unless treatment is initiated.

Intraoral swelling may either accompany the labial swelling or may occur as an isolated finding. The gingiva is enlarged in one fourth of affected patients. The buccal mucosa, palate, and tongue are also commonly involved (Fig. 12-24). The intraoral swelling is often associated with erythema, ulceration, and pain.

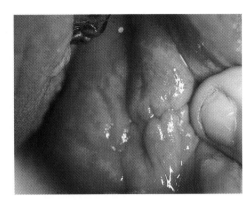

FIG. 12-24   Intraoral swelling of the buccal mucosa is typically observed in the Melkersson-Rosenthal syndrome.

Fissured tongue or lingual plicata is found in approximately two thirds of patients and may be asymptomatic or accompanied by burning, swelling, and taste alterations. This anomaly is commonly found in the general population and is not a specific marker of the syndrome.

Unilateral and episodic facial paralysis develops in approximately one third of patients and is often the first manifestation of the disease. The onset of paralysis is usually preceded by premonitory neural signs. As with labial swelling, the facial palsy is recurrent with prolonged episodes developing as the disease progresses.

Microscopically, small, noncaseating granulomas accompanied by edema, lymphangiectasia, and a perivascular lymphocytic infiltrate are classically observed in oral lesions. Unfortunately, in 50% to 60% of patients with characteristic clinical features of the syndrome, these changes cannot be demonstrated and only nonspecific inflammation can be detected. Although the presence of granulomas in the setting of orofacial swelling confirms the disease, when they are absent, a clinical diagnosis can be established based on the constellation of findings.

Patients with histologic features demonstrating granulomatous inflammation should be evaluated for systemic diseases that display identical histologic features, namely sarcoid and Crohn's disease. Although the oral manifestations of these diseases are also characterized by intraoral and labial swelling, they usually coincide with systemic symptoms. Rarely, they precede systemic involvement; accordingly, their presence necessitates a careful and complete systemic evaluation. Furthermore, oral granulomatous inflammation may result from identifiable hypersensitivity reactions to metals and foods, although this also is uncommon.

The multiple therapies for Melkersson-Rosenthal syndrome reflect the inadequacy of any individual agent to control the disease. Occasionally, a dental focus of infection is identified, which, when corrected, results in marked improvement. Intralesional and systemic corticosteroids are most frequently used but with limited success. Clofazimine, minocycline, and hydroxychloroquine are also beneficial and may be used to control the symptoms.

Wegener's Granulomatosis

Wegener's granulomatosis is characterized by necrotizing granulomas of the upper and lower respiratory tracts, a generalized necrotizing vasculitis of the small arteries and veins, and focal necrotizing glomerulonephritis. Clinical symptoms commonly include intractable sinusitis, nasal obstruction, serous otitis media, hemoptysis, and pleurisy. Fever, weight loss, myalgias, and neuropathy may also occur. Early recognition of the disease and initiation of therapy are essential in preventing renal failure, facial mutilation, and death.

Oral cavity involvement is common and occurs in more than 50% of patients. Furthermore, the oral cavity may be the initial manifestation of the disease in as many as 7% of patients. Buccal mu-

FIG. 12-25 Painful, bleeding, hyperplastic, friable gingivae with a "strawberry" appearance are characteristic of Wegener's granulomatosis.

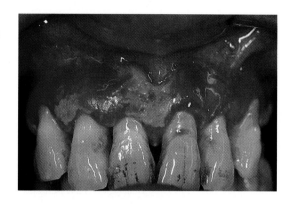

FIG. 12-26 Necrotic ulcerations of the tongue are commonly observed during active stages in Wegener's granulomatosis.

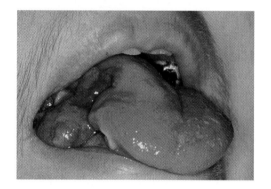

cosal ulcerations resembling large aphthae are the most consistent findings, although these are nonspecific in their appearance. A less common but pathognomonic feature of oral Wegener's granulomatosis is the gingivitis that occurs in the early stages of the disease. The gingivitis first develops in the interdental papillae and progresses into a painful, bleeding, hyperplastic, friable, and highly characteristic petechial and granular gingivitis (Fig. 12-25). The "strawberry" appearance of the gingiva is observed segmentally, and usually it does not involve all of the gingiva. Additional oral manifestations of the disease include large and necrotic tongue ulcerations (Fig. 12-26), nonhealing tooth extraction sockets, and palatal ulcerations as a result of direct extension of the disease from the nose through the nasal septum.

Microscopic examination of oral ulcerations and inflamed gingivae shows a nonspecific inflammatory infiltrate with scattered giant cells that may be accompanied by microabscesses and necrosis. Vasculitis is not observed.

A positive antineutrophil cytoplasmic antibody (c-ANCA) result provides strong circumstantial evidence for the diagnosis of Wegener's granulomatosis in patients with compatible symptoms.

The oral lesions generally do not respond well to topical agents, and the unique gingivitis is refractory to conventional oral hygiene measures. As the activity of oral disease usually parallels that of the systemic disease, resolution occurs with systemic therapy using immunosuppressive agents.

Lethal Midline Granuloma

Lethal midline granuloma is the term used to describe the clinical features of progressive and often fatal ulceration and destruction of the nasal cavity, the paranasal sinuses, the palate, and the midline segment of the face. A variety of disorders including infections, autoimmune diseases, and neoplasms may result in midline defects; however, the term *lethal midline granuloma* is reserved for cases caused by non-Hodgkin's lymphoma or polymorphic reticulosis (T-cell lymphoma).

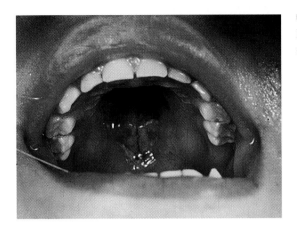

FIG. 12-27   Palatal ulceration with perforation into the nasal cavity is characteristic of lethal midline granuloma.

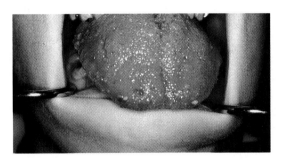

FIG. 12-28   Macroglossia with nodules and bullae on the tongue in amyloidosis.

Lethal midline granuloma is characterized by a prodromal stage with symptoms of nasal stuffiness and obstruction or palatal pain resulting from an ulceration. Lethal midline granuloma may originate in the nasal structures or in the oral cavity. As the disease progresses, the oral palatal ulceration enlarges, undergoes necrosis, and eventually perforates into the nasal cavity (Fig. 12-27). The disease may result in the total destruction of the entire palate and severe facial mutilation.

The aggressive nature of the lethal midline granuloma mimics malignancy, and repeated biopsies are often necessary to establish the diagnosis. In addition to demonstrating infiltration of lymphocytes in biopsy specimens, immunohistochemistry and cytophotometric studies are needed to define the associated lymphoma.

The prognosis is poor, with a high fatality rate despite radiation therapy.

Amyloidosis

Amyloidosis represents a heterogenous group of disorders characterized by the deposition of amyloid, an insoluble proteinaceous fibrillar material, in various organs of the body. There are many subtypes of amyloidosis whose classification is based on the chemical origin, etiologic factors, and the sites of deposition of the amyloid. Primary systemic amyloidosis and myeloma-associated amyloidosis are similar in their clinical presentation, with amyloid being deposited most commonly in the heart, nerves, skin, gastrointestinal tract, and oral cavity. The oral lesions, which predominantly affect the tongue, can often represent the initial manifestation of the disease. The initial amyloid deposition causes diffuse enlargement as evidenced by serrated indentations along the lateral borders of the tongue. As the disease progresses, the tongue becomes indurated with the development of nodules, ulcerations, and hemorrhagic bullae on the dorsal and lateral surfaces (Fig. 12-28). The macroglossia, which occurs in approximately 30% to 50% of patients with systemic amyloidosis, is associated with a poor prognosis compared with patients who do not exhibit oral involvement. Ad-

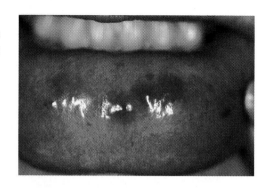

FIG. 12-29 Purpura of the oral mucous membranes are identical to lesions that develop around the eyes in amyloidosis.

ditional oral features of systemic amyloidosis include the presence of diffuse petechiae and ecchymosis, which are also encountered on the cutaneous surfaces (Fig. 12-29).

Secondary amyloidosis is more common than the primary form and is preceded by chronic inflammatory diseases such as rheumatoid arthritis, chronic infectious diseases, and Mediterranean fever. Amyloid deposition occurs most frequently in the kidneys, liver, and spleen. Oral involvement is identical in all forms of amyloidosis but occurs infrequently in the secondary type.

A tongue biopsy should be performed in patients displaying macroglossia who are suspected of having amyloidosis. Congo red staining will identify amyloid in the tissues, revealing apple-green birefringence when viewed using polarized microscopy. Immunofluorescence is diagnostic and demonstrates strong reactivity of the basement membrane with light chain antisera, as well as diffuse staining of the thickened vessel walls. Even when oral involvement is absent, a labial salivary gland biopsy for the diagnosis of both primary and secondary amyloidosis is highly sensitive and specific. When combined with immunodetection of amyloid by anti-SAP antibody, the labial salivary gland biopsy is a more sensitive test for the diagnosis of amyloidosis than the traditional methods, including biopsy of the rectal submucosa or abdominal fat aspiration.

Surgery to correct the macroglossia is infrequently performed because patients die of their underlying disease within months after diagnosis.

SUGGESTED READINGS

Gastrointestinal diseases

Crohn's disease

Halme L et al: Oral findings in patients with active or inactive Crohn's disease, *Oral Surg Oral Med Oral Pathol* 76:175, 1993.

Plauth M, Jenss H, Meyle J: Oral manifestations of Crohn's disease: an analysis of 79 cases, *J Clin Gastroenterol* 13:29, 1991.

Williams AJK, Wray D, Ferguson A: The clinical entity of orofacial Crohn's disease, *QJM* 79:451, 1991.

Ulcerative colitis and pyostomatitis vegetans

Calobrisi SD, Mutasim DF, McDonald JS: Pyostomatitis vegetans associated with ulcerative colitis, *Oral Surg Oral Med Oral Pathol Oral Radiol Endod* 79:452, 1995.

Chan SWY et al: Pyostomatitis vegetans: oral manifestation of ulcerative colitis, *Oral Surg Oral Med Oral Pathol* 72:689, 1991.

Healy CM et al: Pyostomatitis vegetans and associated systemic disease, *Oral Surg Oral Med Oral Pathol* 78:32, 1994.

Hepatitis and other liver diseases

Bagan JV et al: Oral lichen planus and chronic liver disease: a clinical and morphometric study of the oral lesions in relation to transaminase elevation, *Oral Surg Oral Med Oral Pathol* 78:337, 1994.

Gandolfo S et al: Oral lichen planus and hepatitis C virus (HCV) infection: is there a relationship? A report of 10 cases, *J Oral Pathol Med* 23:119, 1994.

Cutaneous diseases

Psoriasis

Dawson TAJ: Tongue lesions in generalized pustular psoriasis, *Br J Dermatol* 91:419, 1974.

Morris LF et al: Oral lesions in patients with psoriasis: a controlled study, *Cutis* 49:339, 1992.

Pogrel MA, Cram D: Intraoral findings in patients with psoriasis with a special reference to ectopic geographic tongue (erythema circinata), *Oral Surg Oral Med Oral Pathol* 66:184, 1988.

Ulmansky M, Michelle R, Azaz B: Oral psoriasis: report of six new cases, *J Oral Pathol Med* 24:42, 1995.

Pityriasis rosea

Kay MH, Rapini RP, Fritz KA: Oral lesions in pityriasis rosea, *Arch Dermatol* 121:1449, 1985.

Kestel JL: Oral lesions in pityriasis rosea, *JAMA* 105:597, 1968.

Acanthosis nigricans

Bang G: Acanthosis nigricans: paraneoplasia with oral manifestations, *Oral Surg Oral Med Oral Pathol* 29:370, 1970.

Hall JM et al: Oral acanthosis nigricans: report of a case and comparison of oral and cutaneous pathology, *Am J Dermatopathol* 10:68, 1988.

Schwartz RA: Acanthosis nigricans, *J Am Acad Dermatol* 31:1, 1994.

Sedano HO, Gorlin RJ: Acanthosis nigricans, *Oral Surg Oral Med Oral Pathol* 63:462, 1987.

Tyler TT et al: Malignant acanthosis nigricans with florid papillary oral lesions, *Oral Surg Oral Med Oral Pathol Oral Radiol Endod* 81:445, 1996.

Hematologic diseases

Disorders of red blood cells

Baird IM et al: The tongue and esophagus in iron deficiency anemia and effect of iron therapy, *J Clin Pathol* 14:603, 1961.

Berlin NJ: Diagnosis and classification of the polycythemias, *Semin Hematol* 12:339, 1976.

Cullen CL: Erythroblastosis fetalis produced by Kell immunization: dental findings, *Pediatr Dent* 12:393, 1990.

Grannum PA, Copel JA: Prevention of Rh isoimmunization and treatment of the compromised fetus, *Semin Perinatol* 12:324, 1988.

Greenberg MS: Clinical and histologic changes of the oral mucosa in pernicious anemia, *Oral Surg* 52:38, 1981.

Millard HD, Gobetti JP: Nonspecific stomatitis—a presenting sign in pernicious anemia, *Oral Surg* 29:562, 1975.

Schmitt RJ, Sheridan PJ, Rogers RS: Pernicious anemia with associated glossodynia, *J Am Diet Assoc* 117:838, 1988.

Van Dis ML, Langlais RP: The thalassemias: oral manifestations and complications, *Oral Surg* 62:229, 1986.

Disorders of platelets

James WD, Guiry CC, Grote WR: Acute idiopathic thrombocytopenic purpura, *Oral Surg* 57:149, 1984.

Stasi R et al: Long-term observation of 208 adults with chronic idiopathic thrombocytopenic purpura, *Am J Med* 98:436, 1995.

Disorders of white blood cells

Barrett AP: Gingival lesions in leukemia: a classification, *J Periodontol* 55:585, 1984.

Bennett JH, Shankar S: Gingival bleeding as the presenting feature of multiple myeloma, *Br Dent J* 157:101, 1984.

Dale DC, Hammond WP: Cyclic neutropenia: a clinical review, *Blood Rev* 2:178, 1988.

Declerck D, Vinckier F: Oral complications of leukemia, *Quintessence Int* 19:575, 1988.

Epstein JB, Voss NJS, Stevenson-Moore P: Maxillofacial manifestations of multiple myeloma, *Oral Surg Oral Med Oral Pathol* 57:267, 1984.

Ferguson MM et al: The presentation and management of oral lesions in leukemia, *J Dent* 6:201, 1978.

Heussner P et al: G-CSF in the long term treatment of cyclic neutropenia and chronic idiopathic neutropenia in adults, *Int J Hematol* 62:225, 1995.

Michaud M et al: Oral manifestations of acute leukemia in children, *J Am Diet Assoc* 95:1145, 1977.

Souid AK: Congenital cyclic neutropenia, *Clin Pediatr* 34:151, 1995.

Tabachnick TT, Levine B: Multiple myeloma involving the jaws and oral soft tissues, *J Oral Surg* 34:931, 1976.

Weckx LLM, Tabacow LB, Marucci G: Oral manifestations of leukemia, *Ear Nose Throat J* 69:341, 1990.

Wright DG et al: Human cyclic neutropenia: clinical review and long term follow-up of patients, *Medicine (Baltimore)* 60:1, 1981.

Langerhans cell histiocytosis

Broadbent V et al: Histiocytosis syndromes in children. II. Approach to the clinical and laboratory evaluation of children with Langerhans cell histiocytosis, *Med Pediatr Oncol* 17:492, 1989.

Hartman KS: Histiocytosis X: a review of 114 cases with oral involvement, *Oral Surg* 49:38, 1980.

Shea CR, McNutt NS: Langerhans cell histiocytosis. In Arndt KA et al, editors: *Cutaneous medicine and surgery: an integrated program in dermatology,* Philadelphia, 1996, WB Saunders.

Nutritional disorders

Dreizen S: The mouth as an indicator of internal nutritional problems, *Pediatrics* 16:139, 1989.

Huber MA, Hall EH: Glossodynia in patients with nutritional deficiencies, *Ear Nose Throat J* 68:771, 1989.

Nizel AE: Nutrition and oral problems, *World Rev Nutr Diet* 16:226, 1973.

Rosenblum LA, Jolliffe N: The oral manifestations of vitamin deficiencies, *JAMA* 117:2245, 1941.

Stein G, Spencer H: Changes of the human tongue in protein and vitamin depletion and repletion, *Ann N Y Acad Sci* 85:368, 1960.

Tuovinen V et al: Oral mucosal changes related to plasma ascorbic acid levels, *Proc Finn Dent Soc* 88:117, 1992.

Wolbach SB, Bessey OA: Tissue changes in vitamin deficiencies, *Physiol Rev* 22:233, 1942.

Connective tissue disorders

Alfaro-Giner A, Penarrocha-Diago M, Bagan-Sebastian JV: Orofacial manifestations of mixed connective tissue disease with an uncommon serologic evolution, *Oral Surg Oral Med Oral Pathol* 73:441, 1992.

Barton DH, Henderson HZ: Oral-facial characteristics of circumscribed scleroderma: case report, *J Clin Pediatr Dent* 17:239, 1993.

Nagy G et al: Analysis of the oral manifestations of systemic sclerosis, *Oral Surg Oral Med Oral Pathol* 77:141, 1994.

Wood RE, Lee P: Analysis of the oral manifestations of systemic sclerosis, *Oral Surg Oral Med Oral Pathol* 65:172, 1988.

Sjögren's syndrome

Bohuslavizki KH et al: Value of quantitative salivary gland scintigraphy in the early stage of Sjögren's syndrome, *Nucl Med Commun* 16:917, 1995.

Daniels TE, Fox PC: Salivary and oral components of Sjögren's syndrome, *Rheum Dis Clin North Am* 18:571, 1992.

Fox RI, Kang H I: Pathogenesis of Sjögren's syndrome, *Rheum Dis Clin North Am* 18:517, 1992.

Lindvall AM, Jonsson R: The salivary gland component of Sjögren's syndrome: an evaluation of diagnostic methods, *Oral Surg Oral Med Oral Pathol* 62:32, 1986.

Oxholm P: Primary Sjögren's syndrome—clinical and laboratory markers of disease activity, *Semin Arthritis Rheum* 22:114, 1992.

Price EJ, Venables PJ: The etiopathogenesis of Sjögren's syndrome, *Semin Arthritis Rheum* 25:117, 1995.

Risheim H, Arneberg P, Birkhed D: Oral sugar clearance and root caries prevalence in rheumatic patients with dry mouth symptoms, *Caries Res* 26:439, 1992.

s'Gravenmade EJ, Vissink A: Management of the oral features of Sjögren's syndrome, *Neth J Med* 40:117, 1992.

van der Reijden WA et al: Treatment of xerostomia with polymer-based saliva substitutes in patients with Sjögren's syndrome, *Arthritis Rheum* 39:57, 1996.

Wise CM, Woodruff RD: Minor salivary gland biopsies in patients investigated for primary Sjögren's syndrome: a review of 187 patients, *J Rheumatol* 20:151, 1993.

Multisystem diseases

Melkersson-Rosenthal syndrome

Allen CM et al: Cheilitis granulomatosa: report of six cases and review of the literature, *J Am Acad Dermatol* 23:444, 1990.

Oliver AJ et al: Monosodium glutamate-related orofacial granulomatosis, *Oral Surg Oral Med Oral Pathol* 71:560, 1991.

Williams PM, Greenberg MS: Management of cheilitis granulomatosa, *Oral Surg Oral Med Oral Pathol* 72:436, 1991.

Worsaae N et al: Melkersson-Rosenthal syndrome and cheilitis granulomatosa: a clinical pathologic study of thirty-three patients with special reference to their oral lesions, *Oral Surg Oral Med Oral Pathol* 54:404, 1982.

Zimmer WM et al: Orofacial manifestations of Melkersson-Rosenthal syndrome, *Oral Surg Oral Med Oral Pathol* 74:610, 1992.

Wegener's granulomatosis

Hoffman GS et al: Wegener's granulomatosis: an analysis of 158 patients, *Ann Intern Med* 116:488, 1992.

Napier SS et al: "Strawberry gums"—a case of Wegener's granulomatosis, *Br Dent J* 175:327, 1993.

Patten SF, Tomecki KJ: Wegener's granulomatosis: cutaneous and oral mucosal disease, *J Am Acad Dermatol* 28:710, 1993.

Rao JK et al: A prospective study of antineutrophil cytoplasmic antibody (c-ANCA) and clinical criteria in diagnosing Wegener's granulomatosis, *Lancet* 346:926, 1995.

Scott J, Finch L: Wegener's granulomatosis presenting as gingivitis: review of the clinical and pathologic features and report of a case, *Oral Surg Oral Med Oral Pathol* 34:920, 1972.

Lethal midline granuloma

Anonymous: Wegener's granulomatosis and lethal midline granuloma, *Rhinology* 14:269, 1992.

Grange C et al: Centrofacial malignant granulomas: clinicopathologic study of 40 cases and review of the literature, *Medicine (Baltimore)* 71:179, 1992.

Kojya S et al: Lethal midline granuloma in Okinawa with special emphasis on polymorphic reticulosis, *Jpn J Cancer Res* 85:384, 1994.

Maxymiw WG et al: B-cell lymphoma presenting as a midfacial necrotizing lesion, *Oral Surg Oral Med Oral Pathol* 74:343, 1992.

Amyloidosis

Geist JR, Geist SR, Wesley RK: Diagnostic procedures in oral amyloidosis, *Compendium* 14:924, 1993.

Hachulla E et al: Labial salivary gland biopsy is a reliable test for the diagnosis of primary and secondary amyloidosis, *Arthritis Rheum* 36:691, 1993.

Reinish EI et al: Tongue, primary amyloidosis, and multiple myeloma, *Oral Surg Oral Med Oral Pathol* 77:121, 1994.

Salisbury PS, Jacoway JR: Oral amyloidosis: a late complication of multiple myeloma, *Oral Surg Oral Med Oral Pathol* 56:48, 1983.

Smith A, Speculand B: Amyloidosis with oral involvement, *Br J Oral Maxillofac Surg* 23:435, 1985.

CHAPTER 13

Oral Manifestations of Human Immunodeficiency Virus Infection

EPIDEMIOLOGY

Since the initial description of its effects in 1981, the human immunodeficiency virus (HIV) has dominated the biomedical, political, and public arenas. Whereas approximately 17 million individuals throughout the world are estimated to be infected with HIV, more than 4 million persons worldwide in nearly 200 nations have been diagnosed with acquired immunodeficiency syndrome (AIDS). In the United States an estimated 1.5 million people have been infected with HIV, and more than 500,000 cases of AIDS have been recorded, with approximately 1500 new cases reported each week. In persons between the ages of 25 and 44 years in the United States, AIDS is the leading cause of death in men and the second most frequent cause in women.

Although initially described in homosexual and bisexual men and subsequently in injecting drug users, HIV is currently spreading in the United States and worldwide most rapidly in heterosexuals. Approximately 20% of new cases of AIDS in the United States afflict women, and it is estimated that by the turn of the century, HIV infection in women will account for nearly 50% of all newly reported cases.

The identification of the oral manifestations of HIV infection is of great significance because they may be the first signs of the disease and, furthermore, are highly predictive markers of severe immune deterioration and disease progression. In addition to reflecting the status of HIV immunosuppression, oral lesions are key elements in the staging and classification of AIDS patients and, if not properly recognized and treated, may contribute to the overall deterioration of the patient.

The oral manifestations of AIDS are divided into three groups (Box, p. 238). Group 1 lesions are strongly associated with HIV infection and include candidiasis, hairy leukoplakia, HIV-associated periodontal diseases, Kaposi's sarcoma, and non-Hodgkin's lymphoma. Group 2 lesions are less commonly associated with HIV infection and include a variety of bacterial and viral infections, salivary gland dysfunction, and oral mucosal disorders. Group 3 lesions are composed of conditions that have been reported in HIV-infected patients but are not strongly linked to either HIV infection or AIDS. With the adoption of the most recent classification system for AIDS in 1993, more than two dozen AIDS-defining diseases or conditions, including several involving the oral cavity, have been identified.

GROUP ONE LESIONS
Candidiasis

Oral candidiasis, described in detail in Chapter 8, develops in as many as 90% of HIV-infected patients. Although not included as an AIDS-defining disease, oral candidiasis may be initially observed during the primary HIV infection and in the early stages of AIDS. Persistent oral candidiasis, even in the presence of CD4 counts up to 700 cells/mm^3, should arouse suspicion of HIV infection. With advanced immunosuppression, the frequency and severity of oral candidiasis increase, and its presence may serve as a marker for other serious opportunistic infections and neoplasms. In infants with AIDS, chronic refractory oral candidal infections are indicative of severe immunosuppression.

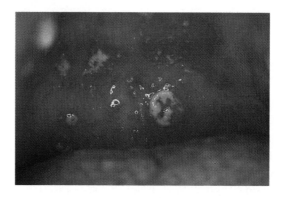

FIG. 13-1   Mixed patterns of oral candidiasis, as on the soft palate in this patient with erythematous and pseudomembranous candidiasis, are common in patients with acquired immunodeficiency syndrome.

ORAL MANIFESTATIONS OF HUMAN IMMUNODEFICIENCY VIRUS (HIV) INFECTION

GROUP 1 LESIONS

Strongly Associated with HIV Infection
Candidiasis
    Erythematous
    Pseudomembranous
    Angular cheilitis
Hairy leukoplakia
Periodontal disease
    Linear gingival erythema
    Necrotizing gingivostomatitis
    Necrotizing ulcerative periodontitis
Kaposi's sarcoma
Non-Hodgkin's lymphoma

GROUP 2 LESIONS

Less Strongly Associated with HIV Infection
Bacterial infections
    Mycobacterium avium
    Mycobacterium tuberculosis
Melanotic hyperpigmentation
Necrotizing ulcerative stomatitis
Salivary gland disease
    Xerostomia
    Major salivary gland enlargement
Thrombocytopenic purpura
Viral infections
    Herpes simplex virus
    Human papillomavirus
        Condyloma acuminatum
        Multifocal papillomavirus epithelial
            hyperplasia
        Verruca vulgaris

Varicella-zoster virus
    Varicella
    Herpes zoster

GROUP 3 LESIONS

Weakly Associated with HIV Infection
Bacterial infections
    Actinomyces israelii
    Escherichia coli
    Klebsiella pneumoniae
    Mycobacterium kansasii
Epithelioid (bacillary) angiomatosis
Drug reactions
    Ulcerative
    Erythema multiforme
    Lichenoid
    Toxic epidermolysis
Opportunistic fungal infections (other than
    candidiasis)
Neurologic disturbances
    Facial palsy
    Trigeminal neuralgia
Recurrent aphthous stomatitis
Viral infections
    Cytomegalovirus
    Molluscum contagiosum
Miscellaneous
    Squamous cell carcinoma
    Atypical oral ulcers (not otherwise specified)
    Delayed wound healing
    Reiter's syndrome
    Granuloma annulare

Modified from EC Clearinghouse on oral problems related to HIV infection and WHO collaborating centre on oral manifestations of the human immunodeficiency virus: *J Oral Pathol Med* 22:289, 1993.

Oral candidiasis in HIV-infected patients may appear in one or more forms and often at multiple oral sites (Fig. 13-1). Pseudomembranous candidiasis (thrush) develops most frequently on the tongue, hard palate, and soft palate and is the most common variant in AIDS patients. Affected individuals may also present with ill-defined, irregular erythematous patches (erythematous candidiasis) or infrequently with adherent hyperkeratotic white patches (candidal leukoplakia). Angular cheilitis (perlèche), a disease of multifactorial etiology including infection with *Candida* species, develops in as many as 10% of HIV-infected patients, commonly in association with intraoral candidiasis. All forms may be asymptomatic, although some patients may experience burning, pain, and taste alterations.

A presumptive diagnosis of oral candidiasis can often be made based on the clinical appearance of the lesions, although when there is uncertainty regarding the etiology of the clinical signs and symptoms, smears and cultures may be required. Although *Candida albicans* is the most frequently isolated pathogen in oral candidiasis, a variety of *Candida* species have been identified. Hyperplastic candidiasis must be diagnosed by biopsy to differentiate it from other oral white lesions such as oral hairy leukoplakia (OHL).

Management of patients with oral candidiasis includes the use of topical polyenes such as nystatin and amphotericin or imidazoles including clotrimazole (see Chapters 8 and 15). In HIV-infected patients the response to topical treatment is transient and recurrences are common, requiring the use of systemic therapy with either fluconazole or itraconazole. Early, successful treatment of oral candidiasis may prevent local and esophageal extension.

Oral Hairy Leukoplakia

Since its initial description in the mid-1980s, OHL has become the most specific oral manifestation of HIV infection, developing in up to one third of HIV-seropositive individuals. Although initially described in HIV-seropositive homosexual men and subsequently in all HIV risk groups, OHL is now regarded as a marker of immunosuppression, having been reported after transplantation and immunosuppressive drug therapy. Several case reports, however, have documented the presence of OHL in HIV-negative immunocompetent patients.

OHL is currently thought to be caused by repeated direct infection of differentiated superficial epithelial cells with Epstein-Barr virus (EBV), rather than reactivation of latent EBV. Under immunocompromised conditions the replication of EBV is facilitated, resulting in continuous viral shedding in saliva and subsequent accumulation of the virus in lesions of OHL.

OHL develops most commonly on the lateral borders of the tongue and, most often, bilaterally. The lesions arise much less frequently on the dorsal and ventral surfaces of the tongue, buccal mucosa, and soft palate and rarely elsewhere. Clinically, OHL is characterized by white adherent plaques with a corrugated or "hairy" texture. The lesions may range in size from several millimeters to several centimeters and appear in a variety of morphologic patterns including well-defined plaques and poorly delineated, coalescing papules. When OHL involves the dorsal or lateral surfaces of the tongue, the lesion assumes a "hairy" appearance; lesions on the ventral tongue and floor of the mouth appear more plaquelike (Figs. 13-2 and 13-3). A number of other mucosal diseases and conditions may mimic oral hairy leukoplakia including candidiasis, lichen planus, frictional keratoses, and idiopathic and tobacco-related leukoplakia.

OHL has a distinctive histopathologic appearance characterized by epithelial hyperplasia, immature surface keratin, and vacuolated squamous cells resembling koilocytes. A mild inflammatory infiltrate may be present in the lamina propria, although this feature is often absent. The diagnosis of OHL may be confirmed by the use of *in situ* hybridization, which reveals the presence of EBV deoxyribonucleic acid in the keratinocytic nuclei of the upper epithelium. This technique can be used in both incisional biopsy specimens and exfoliative cytologic smears; it is especially valuable to rule out the diagnosis of OHL patients who are not HIV infected but have clinically similar oral changes.

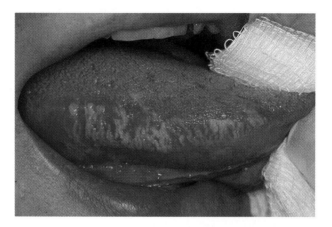

FIG. 13-2 Oral hairy leukoplakia arises most frequently on the lateral borders of the tongue as a vertically corrugated white patch.

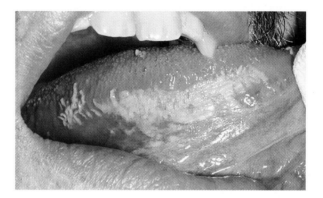

FIG. 13-3 Oral hairy leukoplakia assumes a flat, plaquelike appearance when it develops on the ventral tongue. (From Weinert M, Grimes RM, Lynch DP: *Ann Intern Med* 125:485, 1996.)

The majority of patients with OHL are asymptomatic, although the lesions may occasionally result in burning and discomfort. Secondary infection with candidiasis occurs in almost all cases and may be responsible for symptoms in some patients. Persistent symptoms may be treated with short-contact applications of podophyllin or continuous use of tretinoin gel. As with systemic therapy using acyclovir, azidothymidine, ganciclovir, or foscarnet, resolution of the lesions is usually followed by recurrences when therapy is discontinued.

The accurate diagnosis of OHL has significant implications. Although the lesion itself is benign, OHL is the first clinical sign of HIV infection in more than 5% of cases. Furthermore, the presence of OHL in HIV-infected patients, even when CD4 counts exceed 300 cells/mm^3, is highly predictive of advanced immunodeficiency and disease progression to AIDS and death within several years.

HIV-Associated Periodontal Diseases

Patients with various forms of immunosuppression are at risk for severe periodontal diseases, as illustrated by the high rate of periodontal involvement in those infected with HIV. The gingival and periodontal manifestations of HIV infection, present in up to 50% of patients, may be divided into three categories. Linear gingival erythema, formerly known as HIV-associated gingivitis, is charac-

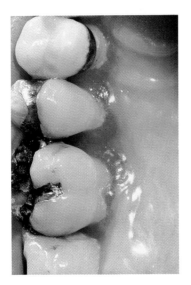

FIG. 13-4   Linear gingival erythema is characterized by intense erythema of the marginal gingiva and failure to respond to conventional oral hygiene measures.

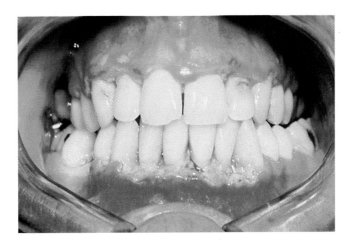

FIG. 13-5   Necrotizing ulcerative gingivitis is a bacterial infection of the gingiva that results in loss of the interdental papillae, sparing underlying supporting periodontal structures.

terized by an intensely erythematous, linear band up to several millimeters wide that affects the marginal and coronal attached gingivae (Fig. 13-4). The gingivitis is diffuse, involving all four quadrants of the oral cavity, and frequently painful. In addition, gingival petechiae, which characteristically appear as punctate and speckled areas of erythema and diffuse erythematous patches on the vestibular and buccal mucosa, may also develop. Ulcerations and erosions are generally absent, and periodontal destruction resulting in gingival attachment loss does not occur; however, the intensity of gingival erythema is disproportionate to the degree of dental plaque accumulation. The diagnosis of linear gingival erythema should always be suspected when intensive oral hygiene measures including plaque control, dental scaling, and root planing fail to alleviate the inflammation.

Patients who are HIV-infected are also at increased risk for developing necrotizing gingivo-stomatitis (see Chapter 6), which is characterized by ulceration and necrosis, primarily of the interproximal gingiva, accompanied by mucosal sloughing (Fig. 13-5). Although this bacterial infection occurs in healthy, immunocompetent patients and is amenable to treatment with antibiotics, it is often refractory to therapy and may infiltrate and involve adjacent mucosa and bone in AIDS patients.

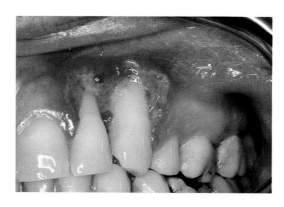

FIG. 13-6 Necrotizing ulcerative periodontitis results in rapid destruction of the periodontal attachment and underlying alveolar bone, potentially leading to spontaneous exfoliation of teeth.

Necrotizing ulcerative periodontitis, which may precede or follow necrotizing gingivostomatitis, is the most severe form of the HIV-associated periodontal diseases. Its development has been strongly correlated with low peripheral CD4 cell counts and may serve as a marker for systemic disease progression. The condition manifests with severe pain, spontaneous gingival bleeding, extensive soft tissue necrosis, and rapid destruction of the periodontal attachment apparatus, frequently exposing underlying alveolar bone (Fig. 13-6). The pain is often perceived deeply in the bone and may precede the development of visible lesions. A striking, characteristic feature of necrotizing ulcerative periodontitis is the swift loss of periodontal attachment. More than 90% of attachment may be destroyed in less than 6 months, and the necrosis may result in spontaneous exodontia. Initial lesions may reveal few radiographic abnormalities, but bone loss is evident in advanced lesions. Although necrotizing ulcerative periodontitis may be generalized, it more commonly affects localized gingival regions in a random fashion.

The exact pathogenesis of HIV-associated periodontal diseases remains controversial, although mixed aerobic and anaerobic bacteria are often isolated from lesions. Although the qualitative microbiologic profiles of linear gingival erythema and necrotizing ulcerative periodontitis are similar to each other and to conventional periodontitis, including gram-negative organisms, they are significantly different from conventional gingivitis. Additionally, because the two conditions share similar patterns of gingival inflammation and are resistant to conventional therapeutic measures, they may represent different stages of one disease process. Therefore early diagnosis and therapeutic intervention may prevent progression and serious sequelae.

Standard treatment of gingivitis and periodontitis is relatively ineffective for HIV-associated periodontal diseases. Aggressive intervention by removal of plaque and calculus from the teeth and root surfaces, as well as débridement of the soft tissues, using povidone-iodine irrigation, is paramount in controlling the infection. Chlorhexidine 0.12% (Peridex), a broad-spectrum antimicrobial rinse used twice daily, is valuable in alleviating pain and inflammation during the early phase of therapy and for long-term maintenance. Systemic antibiotics, specifically metronidazole (Flagyl), 250 mg four times a day, should be reserved for severe infections that are accompanied by systemic symptoms. Secondary candidiasis often develops as a result of antibiotic therapy and, when identified, requires treatment. It is essential that patients maintain an optimal oral hygiene home regimen supplemented with frequent dental visits to prevent recurrences. Otherwise, recurrences invariably develop, leading to continued destruction of the soft tissues and bone.

Kaposi's Sarcoma

Kaposi's sarcoma is a cardinal feature of AIDS and is the most common malignancy associated with HIV infection. As described in Chapter 5, a variety of viral infections have been implicated as etio-

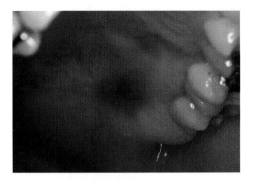

FIG. 13-7   In the early stage of oral Kaposi's sarcoma, the lesions appear as reddish-purple macules.

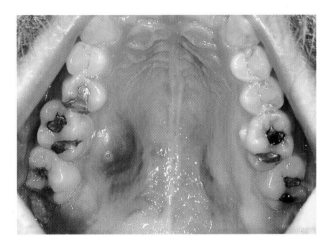

FIG. 13-8   Kaposi's sarcoma most commonly affects the hard palate and, in the nodular stage, is prone to ulceration and bleeding. (From Anneroth G, Anneroth I, Lynch DP: *J Oral Maxillofac Surg* 44:956, 1986.)

logic agents. Overall, in the United States approximately 15% of AIDS patients develop Kaposi's sarcoma, which is an AIDS-defining disease. Among patients with AIDS, the frequency of Kaposi's sarcoma is highest in homosexual and bisexual men. Although the malignancy may develop in the oral cavity in any of the four major groups at risk for Kaposi's sarcoma including intravenous drug users, kidney transplantation recipients, and immunocompromised patients who are not HIV-infected, almost all cases occur in association with AIDS. The oral cavity may be the initial site of the malignancy in as many as 50% of patients with AIDS and the only site of involvement in some individuals. Oral lesions develop concomitantly with skin or visceral involvement in approximately 50% of cases and subsequent to the appearance of skin lesions in one third of cases.

Oral Kaposi's sarcoma may develop on any mucosal surface, although the palate is most commonly involved, followed by the gingiva. Multiple oral sites of involvement are noted in approximately one third of patients. Early lesions of oral Kaposi's sarcoma appear innocuously as asymptomatic, reddish-purple macules (Fig. 13-7). Eventually the lesions progress to painful papules and nodules that may ulcerate and bleed (Figs. 13-8 to 13-10). The presence of oral lesions is associated with low CD4 cell counts, and transformation from macular to papular and nodular forms may be indicative of progressive immunosuppression.

A biopsy is often required to differentiate oral Kaposi's sarcoma from other clinically similar-appearing conditions including coagulation disorders, vascular neoplasms, and various focal inflam-

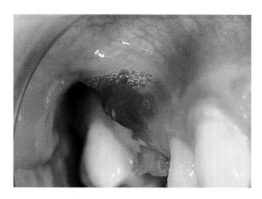

FIG. 13-9   Kaposi's sarcoma of the gingiva may be confused with periapical dental infections, abscesses, and benign vascular neoplasms. (From Weinert M, Grimes RM, Lynch DP: *Ann Intern Med* 125:485, 1996.)

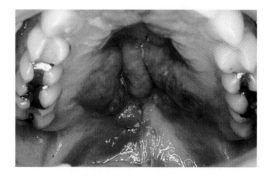

FIG. 13-10   In the advanced stages, Kaposi's sarcoma may be extensive and interfere with normal oral functions.

matory diseases. Furthermore, in dark-skinned individuals, physiologic pigmentation and macular lesions of oral Kaposi's sarcoma can appear clinically identical. A unique vascular proliferation caused by *Rochalimaea* species, bacillary angiomatosis, may affect the oral cavity and mimic Kaposi's sarcoma both clinically and microscopically. Additionally, nonpigmented tumors of oral Kaposi's sarcoma and other atypical presentations complicate the clinical diagnosis. Tissue biopsy and fine needle aspiration cytology are necessary to confirm the clinical suspicion of Kaposi's sarcoma.

Microscopically, early macular oral lesions are comprised of inconspicuous patches of spindle cells containing ill-defined vascular spaces. Late nodular and infiltrative lesions in the oral cavity are dominated by spindle cells lining vascular slits and bizarre-shaped vessels. Extravasated red blood cells are almost always evident, and hemosiderin deposits and hyaline globules are frequently observed in both the early and late lesions.

Treatment of oral Kaposi's sarcoma may not affect the prognosis of AIDS patients but often improves their quality of life. Palliative treatment improves the cosmetic appearance of visible gingival lesions and reduces pain, which may lead to improved oral intake.

Tumors confined to the oral cavity may be successfully treated by injection with a sclerosing agent, 3% sodium tetradecyl sulfate. Intralesional therapy with vinblastine (0.1 mg/ml) is also beneficial, but, as with tetradecyl sulfate, large lesions require multiple treatments. Intralesional injection with interferon-α 2b produces similar results. All of these local treatments may result in pain and ulceration, although the adverse effects are transient. Accessible exophytic and pedunculated le-

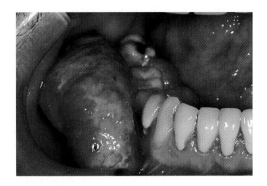

FIG. 13-11   Non-Hodgkin's lymphoma is the second most common malignancy in patients with acquired immunodeficiency syndrome and is associated with a poor prognosis.

sions can be surgically excised or treated by laser surgery or cryotherapy. Widespread and progressive Kaposi's sarcoma may require the use of systemic chemotherapy or radiotherapy. Regression may be observed with single and multiagent cytotoxic chemotherapy including interferon-α, azidothymidine, etoposide, vincristine, and liposomal doxorubicin. Extensive oral Kaposi's sarcoma responds most favorably to low-dose radiation. To minimize the possibility of radiation-induced mucositis, therapy should be delivered in fractionated doses of 2 to 3 cGy administered 10 to 15 times.

Non-Hodgkin's Lymphoma

Non-Hodgkin's lymphoma is the second most common malignancy in AIDS patients (see Chapter 5). The increasing incidence of lymphoma in AIDS patients may be caused by, in part, the fact that the malignancy, unlike Kaposi's sarcoma, primarily develops in heterosexuals or intravenous drug users infected with HIV, groups that are increasing in number. Also, longer survival of AIDS patients may be responsible for the reported increased incidence on non-Hodgkin's lymphoma.

As with Kaposi's sarcoma, viruses, specifically EBV, have been implicated as etiologic agents in the development of non-Hodgkin's lymphoma.

Oral non-Hodgkin's lymphomas are predominantly of B-cell origin, although T-cell lymphoma and Hodgkin's disease have also been reported. The oral features may be the initial manifestation of lymphoma and of AIDS. The tumors present as extranodal soft tissue masses, frequently with secondary ulceration, although in the early stages non-Hodgkin's lymphoma can mimic a variety of oral soft tissue neoplasms and reactive processes (Fig. 13-11). Because the tumors occur most frequently on the palate and gingiva and often appear vascular, non-Hodgkin's lymphoma may clinically resemble Kaposi's sarcoma. Even with aggressive therapeutic intervention including chemotherapy and radiotherapy, the prognosis of patients with non-Hodgkin's lymphoma is poor, with survival rates of less than 25%.

GROUP TWO LESIONS
Tuberculosis

A growing number of atypical bacterial infections including those caused by *Mycobacterium avium* and *Mycobacterium tuberculosis* develop more frequently in HIV-seropositive individuals and patients with AIDS. The dramatic resurgence of tuberculosis in immunocompromised patients, including those infected with HIV, has been of great concern to health care workers. Especially worrisome is the emergence of multidrug-resistant tuberculosis, which is associated with a high rate of mortality. Oral manifestations of tuberculosis (see Chapter 6), although uncommon, are important to

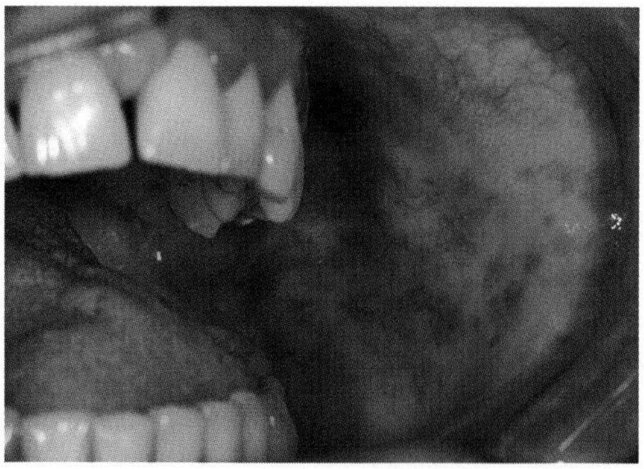

FIG. 13-12   Mucosal hyperpigmentation in human immunodeficiency virus infection may be precipitated by drugs, adrenal insufficiency, and infections, but in the majority of cases the cause is unknown.

recognize. The lesions most frequently appear as chronic, asymptomatic, indurated ulcers with surrounding erythema, although oral tuberculosis may present as nodules, patches, plaques, or vesicles. Oral lesions usually are accompanied by pulmonary symptoms and are the result of contact with infected sputum.

Melanotic Hyperpigmentation

Alterations in pigmentation of the skin, nails, and oral mucous membranes can be observed in patients infected with HIV. Although in some instances hyperpigmentation may result from the administration of pharmacologic agents such as ketoconazole, clofazimine, and azidothymidine, in the majority of cases the cause is unknown. It is probable that some cases represent postinflammatory hyperpigmentation similar to that occurring on the skin after trauma or infection. Clinically, the oral lesions appear as well-defined or diffuse, brownish-black macules most commonly arising on the tongue, buccal mucosa, gingiva, and palate (Fig 13-12). Underlying systemic causes of oral hyperpigmentation such as adrenal insufficiency should be excluded. Microscopically, the findings are nonspecific and include increased melanin deposition in the basal cell layer and mucosal melanophages. The pigmented lesions require no therapy and their significance remains unknown.

Necrotizing Ulcerative Stomatitis

Necrotizing ulcerative stomatitis is characterized by an acute, massively destructive infection of the gingiva that progresses and extends to adjacent mucosal surfaces, soft tissues, and underlying alveolar bone (Fig. 13-13). The disease uncommonly develops as a complication of necrotizing ulcerative periodontitis and is life threatening. As with the HIV-associated periodontal diseases, treatment consists of surgical débridement followed by topical and systemic antimicrobial therapy.

Salivary Gland Disease

HIV-associated salivary gland disease is characterized by xerostomia or generalized enlargement of the major salivary glands (most commonly the parotid glands) or both. The cause remains unknown; however, the condition may be caused by lymphoid proliferation in response to HIV infection or other viral infections. The disease occurs in all groups at risk for HIV infection and is observed frequently in children with AIDS. The clinical presentation is similar to that seen in Sjögren's syndrome with bilateral swelling of the parotids more common than unilateral swelling. Decreased stimulated parotid flow rates may be demonstrated, and these changes appear identical to those observed in Sjögren's syndrome. Serologic markers such as anti-SS-A, anti-SS-B, and rheumatoid factor that are

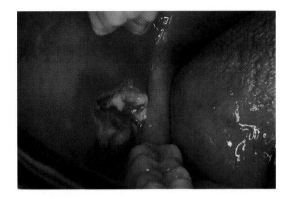

FIG. 13-13   Necrotizing ulcerative stomatitis is a potentially life-threatening complication of necrotizing ulcerative periodontitis, although it may develop *de novo*. (From Weinert M, Grimes RM, Lynch DP: *Ann Intern Med* 125:485, 1996.)

positive in Sjögren's syndrome are absent in HIV-associated salivary gland disease. Characteristic multicentric cysts or large unilocular cysts may be detected by computed tomography and magnetic resonance imaging studies. Fine needle aspiration may be used to exclude neoplasms as the cause of salivary gland swelling.

Microscopically, affected minor and major salivary glands exhibit a diffuse lymphocytic infiltration dominated by CD8+ cells as seen in Sjögren's syndrome. The parotid glands reveal large cystic cavities lined with nonkeratinized squamous epithelium surrounded by germinal centers.

The degree of salivary gland swelling varies considerably among patients. Surgical intervention may be required for expanding cystic lesions. Treatment of xerostomia is primarily symptomatic and includes the use of sialogogues and cholinergic medications (pilocarpine or bethanechol) to increase saliva production. The increased incidence of dental caries in xerostomic patients necessitates scrupulous oral hygiene habits supplemented with the application of topical fluoride and chlorhexidine mouth rinses. Thus far HIV-associated salivary gland enlargement has not been associated with an increased risk for extranodal lymphoma, as is the case in Sjögren's syndrome.

Thrombocytopenic Purpura

Thrombocytopenia is a noteworthy complication in patients with AIDS, both in the early and late stages, and has an incidence approximating 10% of reported cases. Increased platelet destruction and a reduced production of megakaryocytes and platelets may be a result of the deposition of immune complexes on platelet receptors and direct infection of platelets by HIV. Orally, thrombocytopenic purpura manifests as petechiae, ecchymosis, and spontaneous submucosal hemorrhages, most often of the gingiva. Dental and oral surgical procedures may result in significant bleeding. As with classic autoimmune thrombocytopenic purpura, patients with HIV-associated thrombocytopenia respond to platelet transfusions, prednisone, and splenectomy.

Viral Infections

Herpes simplex virus. Human herpesvirus infections, most commonly caused by herpes simplex virus (HSV), types 1 and 2 (see Chapter 7) are seen with increased frequency in HIV-positive individuals. In contrast to infections that occur in immunocompetent individuals, HSV infections in HIV-seropositive and AIDS patients are dramatically altered and are generally more widespread, aggressive, prolonged, and atypically distributed. Recurrent oral herpetic infections may involve not only the typical sites such as the attached gingiva and hard palate but also other oral mucosal surfaces, extending even to the esophagus. Vesicles and erosions in the oral cavity often persist for extended periods, and their diffuse pattern may resemble primary herpetic gingivostomatitis. Other atypical presentations include herpetic geometric glossitis characterized by extremely painful, cross-hatched, branched, or linear fissures on the dorsal aspect of the tongue. Severe perioral ulcerations, which often coalesce with weeping crusts, are also commonly encountered (Fig. 13-14). Long-standing herpetic infections in the oral cavity persisting for more than 3 weeks are associated with CD4 cell counts below 100 cells/mm^3.

The diagnosis of recurrent intraoral HSV infections should always be suspected in AIDS patients with persistent oral ulcerations. Biopsy may be required for diagnosis because cultures may be falsely negative. Treatment of identified intraoral HSV infections depends on the extent of the infection and the immunologic status of the patient. Systemic antiviral therapy should be initiated with either oral doses of acyclovir (1000 to 3000 mg/day) or intravenous doses (5 mg/kg every 8 hours). Prophylactic maintenance doses of acyclovir may be required to suppress recurrences. In patients with acyclovir-resistant HSV, foscarnet (50 mg/kg every 8 hours) may be administered intravenously.

Human papillomaviruses. Warts in the oral cavity caused by human papillomaviruses (HPVs) occur with increased frequency in HIV-seropositive patients (see Chapter 7). Typically, the warts are larger, spread to multiple sites, and are refractory to therapy. Unusual genotypes including HPV 7, 72, and 73 have been isolated from oral warts in HIV-seropositive patients, the latter types associated with cytologic atypia.

Condyloma acuminata (venereal warts) occurs intraorally, usually in association with anogenital condylomata. Clinically, the lesions have a typical warty appearance, although they may also manifest as smooth-surfaced, flesh-colored papules that may be clinically confused with other benign neoplasms and reactive mucosal processes. HPV types most frequently identified are 6, 11, 16, and 18.

Multifocal papillomavirus epithelial hyperplasia (Heck's disease) caused by HPV types 13 and 32 is also observed with increased frequency in HIV-seropositive patients. Additional genotypes in HIV-infected patients include HPV 11 and 18. Widespread, flesh-colored mucosal papules and plaques may affect all oral mucosal surfaces.

The frequency of oral verruca vulgaris is also increased in HIV-positive patients. The lesions may be papillary, sessile, or pedunculated and may develop on multiple mucosal sites.

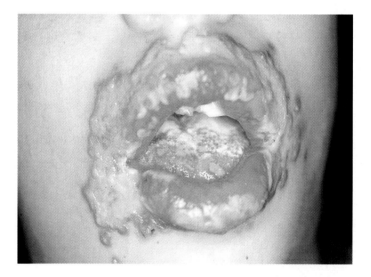

FIG. 13-14   Recurrent herpes simplex virus infections in human immunodeficiency virus-positive patients are often severe, involving intraoral and perioral structures.

The treatment of oral warts consists of surgical excision or destructive modalities including cryosurgery and electrodesiccation. Recurrences are especially common in HIV-infected patients.

Varicella-zoster virus. Chronic and persistent primary varicella infections occur with increased frequency in perinatal AIDS. The incidence of herpes zoster infections is also significantly increased in HIV-seropositive patients. As with other viral infections in patients with AIDS, clinical signs and symptoms are more severe and prolonged. Dissemination beyond the dermatomal distribution may occur, and visceral involvement may be life threatening. Recurrent episodes of herpes zoster have also been reported in HIV-seropositive and AIDS patients. Oral involvement is exquisitely painful, and ulcerations often persist for extended periods. Treatment of varicella-zoster infections consists of acyclovir, usually administered intravenously (30 mg/kg/day). Acyclovir-resistant strains may be treated with intravenous foscarnet.

GROUP THREE LESIONS

Bacterial Infections (see Chapter 6)

In addition to the HIV-associated periodontal diseases, several unusual bacterial infections occur intraorally in HIV-seropositive and AIDS patients. These infections usually result in chronic and persistent ulcerations without any distinctive clinical features. Diverse organisms such as *Actinomyces israelii, Escherichia coli, Enterobacter cloacae, Klebsiella pneumoniae,* and *Mycobacterium kansasii* have been isolated from the oral cavity. As with any atypical or persistent oral ulceration or mass, especially in HIV-infected patients, biopsy and culture are mandatory. Bacillary angiomatosis, an unusual vascular proliferation caused by infection with *Rochalimaea* species, can resemble Kaposi's sarcoma. When the disease is widespread, oral lesions are more likely to be encountered, although isolated intraoral lesions may also occur. Biopsy is necessary for confirmation of the disease.

The frequency of syphilis is increased in AIDS and, because oral manifestations are prominent in all stages, the diagnosis should be considered when oral ulcerations or plaques are observed in HIV-infected patients. The diagnosis should be established by serology and, if necessary, biopsy.

Adverse Drug Reactions

The large number of medications administered to HIV-seropositive and AIDS patients predisposes them to a diverse group of drug reactions, many with prominent oral manifestations. For example, oral ulcerations may infrequently occur as a result of foscarnet and interferon but develop in more than 50% of patients treated with dideoxy-cytidine. In addition to these nonspecific oral ulcerative lesions, erythema multiforme, lichenoid drug reactions, Stevens-Johnson syndrome, and toxic epidermolysis affecting the oral cavity have been reported in HIV-infected individuals.

Fungal Infections (Other than Candidiasis)

A number of opportunistic systemic fungal infections with oral manifestations (see Chapter 8) may develop in immunocompromised patients, especially in HIV-seropositive and AIDS patients. The oral lesions generally represent dissemination, although they may be the initial and sole feature of the disease. Clinically, they all manifest as persistent ulcerations or masses and are diagnosed by biopsy and culture. Systemic infections by these organisms are life threatening and require aggressive antifungal therapy.

Neurologic Disturbances

Neurologic abnormalities commonly develop during the course of AIDS. Potential causes include opportunistic central nervous system infections, tumors, and HIV-associated diseases. Peripheral neuropathies eventually develop in almost all HIV-seropositive patients. Trigeminal and facial nerve involvement with accompanying facial and oral dysfunction have also been reported in HIV-seropositive patients.

Recurrent Aphthous Stomatitis

Recurrent aphthous stomatitis, an immunologically mediated condition that affects up to 40% of the general population, may occur with greater frequency in HIV-seropositive patients (see Chapter 9). The severity and chronicity of the lesions are undoubtedly greater and of the three types described (minor, major, and herpetiform), major ulcerations are most often encountered and cause the greatest morbidity. Ulcerations are typically large (greater than 1 cm), affect the posterior portion of the oral cavity, and often do not respond to topical medications. Clinically, they may resemble infectious and neoplastic processes, requiring culture and biopsy for confirmation. The presence of major aphthous ulcerations in HIV-seropositive patients is a marker for deterioration and severe immune suppression.

In addition to the use of topical anesthetics, corticosteroids, ointments, elixirs, and other palliative measures, short-term, high-dose systemic corticosteroids (prednisone, 50 to 80 mg for 7 to 10 days) should be used for patients with significant discomfort. Patients with recurrent, multiple, and severe lesions may respond to 100 to 200 mg of thalidomide per day. Such patients require monitoring for peripheral neuropathy and teratogenicity.

Viral Infections

Cytomegalovirus. Cytomegalovirus (CMV) exposure is ubiquitous, as evidenced by the high rate of positive serology to the virus in more than 60% of the general population. Not surprisingly, antibodies to CMV are almost always detected in HIV-seropositive individuals, and the virus can also be frequently cultured from the oral cavity. In AIDS patients CMV infection results in serious sequelae, most commonly retinitis, which may lead to blindness and adrenal gland involvement.

Oral infections with CMV are probably more common than have been reported in the literature and may develop in any immunocompromised patient (see Chapter 7). These manifest most frequently as painful, large, sharply demarcated, nonspecific ulcerations and usually represent dissemination of CMV (Fig. 13-15). The ulcers may arise on both keratinized and nonkeratinized mucosa, but their clinical appearance cannot be differentiated from large aphthae. A number of nonspecific, atypical, aphthouslike ulcerations undiagnosed in AIDS patients probably represent CMV infections. The definitive diagnosis must be established by biopsy, although CMV inclusions may not always be detectable on routine light microscopy, thus resulting in misdiagnosis. Adjunctive techniques that may be used to firmly establish the diagnosis include the use of immunohistochemistry, *in situ* hybridization, and electron microscopy. The oral infections may be responsive to treatment with either foscarnet or ganciclovir.

Molluscum contagiosum. The frequency and severity of molluscum contagiosum, which is caused by a poxvirus, are increased in HIV-infected patients. Although the lesions are frequently wide-

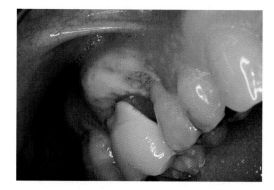

FIG. 13-15   Oral mucosal ulcers caused by cytomegalovirus infection are painful and persistent, clinically resembling recurrent aphthous stomatitis and other oral aphthae. (From Weinert M, Grimes RM, Lynch DP: *Ann Intern Med* 125:485, 1996.)

spread on the skin and involve the face and perioral regions, intraoral lesions occur infrequently. They display the same morphologic pattern as skin lesions and are treated by cryotherapy or excision.

Miscellaneous

A diverse group of oral lesions and diseases have been reported in association with HIV infection and AIDS. For example, younger than expected, HIV-seropositive patients without other risk factors have been reported to develop oropharyngeal squamous cell carcinomas. Atypical oral ulcerations that are not caused by fungal, bacterial, or viral infection; neoplasms; or medications have been identified with greater frequency in HIV-infected patients. These ulcers do not clinically resemble recognized patterns of recurrent aphthous stomatitis and microscopically reveal nonspecific features. Although a trial of topical and intralesional corticosteroids may be attempted, persistent lesions should always be biopsied to exclude potentially treatable entities. Delayed wound healing in the oral cavity is frequently observed in AIDS patients after an oral surgical procedure or dental extraction and may be caused by impaired cellular immunity caused by HIV. HIV-infected patients with Reiter's syndrome have been described, with almost all patients exhibiting painless oral ulcerations. Granuloma annulare, which is commonly observed on the skin, has been reported to occur in the oral cavity of an AIDS patient. As treatments for AIDS become more effective and survival is prolonged, the likelihood for development of unusual oral abnormalities never before observed will significantly increase.

SUGGESTED READINGS

General

Glick M et al: Oral manifestations associated with HIV-related disease as markers for immune suppression in AIDS, *Oral Surg Oral Med Oral Pathol* 77:344, 1994.

Greenberg MS: HIV-associated lesions, *Dermatol Clin* 14:319, 1996.

Greenspan JS, Greenspan D: *Oral manifestations of HIV infection,* Chicago, 1995, Quintessence.

Revised classification for HIV infection and expanded surveillance case definition for AIDS among adolescents and adults, *MMWR* 41:RR-17, 1993.

Schulten EA, Ten Kate RW, van der Waal I: Oral findings in HIV-infected patients attending a department of internal medicine: the contribution of intraoral examination towards the clinical management of HIV disease, *QJM* 76:741, 1990.

Silverman S Jr: *Color atlas of oral manifestations of AIDS,* ed 2, St Louis, 1996, Mosby.

Weinert M, Grimes RM, Lynch DP: Oral manifestations of HIV infection, *Ann Intern Med* 125:485, 1996.

Epidemiology

Centers for Disease Control and Prevention: Update: AIDS among women—United States, 1994, *MMWR* 44:81, 1995.

de Vincenzi I: A longitudinal study of human immunodeficiency virus transmission by heterosexual partners, *N Engl J Med* 331:341, 1994.

EC Clearinghouse on Oral Problems Related to HIV Infection and WHO Collaborating Centre on Oral Manifestations of the Human Immunodeficiency Virus: Classification and diagnostic criteria for oral lesions and HIV Infection, *J Oral Pathol Med* 22:289, 1993.

Group one lesions

Candidiasis

Como JA, Dismukes WE: Oral azole drugs as systemic antifungal therapy, *N Engl J Med* 330:263, 1994.

McCarthy G: Host factors associated with HIV-positive–related oral candidiasis, *Oral Surg Oral Med Oral Pathol* 73:181, 1992.

Muzyka BC, Glick M: A review of oral fungal infections and appropriate therapy, *J Am Dent Assoc* 126:63, 1995.

Oral hairy leukoplakia

Fisher DA, Daniels TE, Greenspan JS: Oral hairy leukoplakia unassociated with human immunodeficiency virus: pseudo oral hairy leukoplakia, *J Am Acad Dermatol* 27:257, 1992.

Green TL et al: Oral lesions mimicking hairy leukoplakia: a diagnostic dilemma, *Oral Surg Oral Med Oral Pathol* 67:422, 1989.

Greenspan D, Greenspan JS, Overby G: Risk factors for rapid progression from hairy leukoplakia to AIDS: a nested case-control study, *J Acquir Immune Defic Syndr* 4:652, 1991.

Greenspan D et al: Relation of oral hairy leukoplakia to infection with the human immunodeficiency virus and the risk of developing AIDS, *J Infect Dis* 155:475, 1987.

Greenspan JS, Greenspan D: Oral hairy leukoplakia: diagnosis and management, *Oral Surg Oral Med Oral Pathol* 67:396, 1989.

Husak R, Garbe C, Orfanos CE: Oral hairy leukoplakia in 71 HIV-seropositive patients: clinical symptoms, relation to immunologic status, and prognostic significance, *J Am Acad Dermatol* 35:928, 1996.

Schiodt M, Norgaard T, Greenspan JS: Oral hairy leukoplakia in an HIV-negative woman with Behçet's syndrome, *Oral Surg Oral Med Oral Pathol Oral Radiol Endod* 79:53, 1995.

HIV-associated periodontal diseases

Barr CE: Periodontal problems related to HIV-1 infection, *Adv Dent Res* 9:147, 1995.

Grbic JT et al: The relationship of candidiasis to linear gingival erythema in HIV-infected homosexual men and potential drug users, *J Periodontol* 66:30, 1995.

Holmstrup P, Westergaard J: Periodontal diseases in HIV-infected patients, *J Clin Periodontol* 21:270, 1994.

Klein RS, Quart AM, Small CB: Periodontal disease in heterosexuals with acquired immunodeficiency syndrome, *J Periodontol* 62:535, 1991.

Robinson PG et al: The diagnosis of periodontal conditions associated with HIV infection, *J Periodontol* 65:236, 1994.

Smith GL, Cross DL, Ray D: Comparison of periodontal disease in HIV seropositive subjects and controls (1). Clinical features, *J Clin Periodontol* 22:558, 1995.

Winkler JR et al: Diagnosis and management of HIV-associated periodontal lesions, *J Am Dent Assoc* Suppl:255, 1989.

Zambon JJ, Reynolds HS, Genco RJ: Studies of the subgingival microflora in patients with acquired immunodeficiency syndrome, *J Peridontol* 61:699, 1990.

Kaposi's sarcoma

Epstein JB: Treatment of oral Kaposi's sarcoma with intralesional vinblastine, *Cancer* 71:1722, 1993.

Epstein JB, Scully C: HIV infection: clinical features and treatment of thirty-three homosexual men with Kaposi's sarcoma, *Oral Surg Oral Med Oral Pathol* 71:38, 1991.

Langford A et al: Regression of oral Kaposi's sarcoma in a case of AIDS on zidovudine (AZT), *Br J Dermatol* 120:709, 1989.

Le-Bourgeois JP et al: Radiotherapy in the management of epidemic Kaposi's sarcoma of the oral cavity, the eyelids, and the genitals, *Radiother Oncol* 30:263, 1994.

Lucatorto FM, Sapp JP: Treatment of oral Kaposi's sarcoma with a sclerosing agent in AIDS patients, *Oral Surg Oral Med Oral Pathol* 75:192, 1993.

Moore PS, Chang Y: Detection of herpesvirus-like DNA sequences in Kaposi's sarcoma in patients with and those without HIV infection, *N Engl J Med* 332:1181, 1995.

Schweitzer VG, Visscher D: Photodynamic therapy for treatment of AIDS-related oral Kaposi's sarcoma, *Otolaryngol Head Neck Surg* 102:639, 1990.

Sulis E et al: Interferon administered intralesionally in skin and oral cavity lesions in heterosexual drug addicted patients with AIDS-related Kaposi's sarcoma, *Eur J Cancer* 25:759, 1989.

Non-Hodgkin's lymphoma

Armitage JO: Treatment of non-Hodgkin's lymphoma, *N Engl J Med* 328:1023, 1993.

Epstein J, Silverman S Jr: HIV-associated malignancies, *Oral Surg Oral Med Oral Pathol* 73:193, 1992.

Ficarra G, Eversole LE: HIV-related tumors of the oral cavity, *Crit Rev Oral Biol Med* 5:159, 1994.

Green TL, Eversole LR: Oral lymphomas in HIV-infected patients: associated with Epstein-Barr virus DNA, *Oral Surg Oral Med Oral Pathol* 67:437, 1989.

Hicks MJ et al: Intraoral presentation of anaplastic large-cell Ki-1 lymphoma in association with HIV infection, *Oral Surg Oral Med Oral Pathol* 76:73, 1993.

Sparano JA et al: Infusional cyclophosphamide, doxorubicin and etoposide in HIV-related non-Hodgkin's lymphoma: a follow-up report of the highly active regimen, *Leuk Lymphoma* 14:263, 1994.

Group two lesions

Tuberculosis

Eng HL et al: Oral tuberculosis, *Oral Surg Oral Med Oral Pathol Oral Radiol Endod* 81:415, 1996.

Jawad DJ, El-Zuebi F: Primary lingual tuberculosis: a case report, *J Laryngol Otol* 110:177, 1996.

Laskaris G: Oral manifestations of infectious diseases, *Dent Clin North Am* 40:395, 1996.

Phelan JA, Jimenez V, Tompkins DC: Tuberculosis, *Dent Clin North Am* 40:327, 1996.

Weiner GM, Pahor AL: Tuberculosis parotitis: the limited role of surgery, *J Laryngol Otol* 110:96, 1996.

Melanotic hyperpigmentation

Langford A et al: Oral hyperpigmentation in HIV-infected patients, *Oral Surg Oral Med Oral Pathol* 67:301, 1989.

Porter SR, Glover S, Scully C: Oral hyperpigmentation and adrenocortical hypofunction in a patient with acquired immunodeficiency syndrome, *Oral Surg Oral Med Oral Pathol* 70:59, 1990.

Tal A, Gaggel RF: The diagnostic dilemma of hyperpigmentation in patients with acquired immunodeficiency syndrome, *Cutis* 48:153, 1991.

Necrotizing ulcerative stomatitis

Horning GM, Cohen ME: Necrotizing ulcerative gingivitis, periodontitis, and stomatitis; clinical staging and predisposing factors, *J Periodontol* 66:990, 1995.

Liang GS et al: An evaluation of oral ulcers in patients with AIDS and AIDS-related complex, *J Am Acad Dermatol* 29:563, 1993.

Muzyka BC, Glick M: HIV infection and necrotizing stomatitis, *Gen Dent* 42:66, 1994.

William CA et al: HIV-associated periodontitis complicated by necrotizing stomatitis, *Oral Surg Oral Med Oral Pathol* 69:351, 1990.

Salivary gland disease

Itescu S et al: A diffuse infiltrative CD8 lymphocytosis syndrome in human immunodeficiency virus (HIV) infection: a host immune response associated with HLA-DR5, *Ann Intern Med* 112:3, 1990.

Schiodt M: HIV-associated salivary gland disease: a review, *Oral Surg Oral Med Oral Pathol* 73:164, 1992.

Schiodt M et al: Parotid gland enlargement and xerostomia associated with labial sialoadenitis in HIV-infected patients, *J Autoimmun* 2:415, 1989.

Schiodt M et al: Natural history of HIV-associated salivary gland disease, *Oral Surg Oral Med Oral Pathol* 74:326, 1992.

Terry JH et al: Major salivary gland lymphoepithelial lesions and the acquired immunodeficiency syndrome, *Am J Surg* 162:324, 1991.

Thrombocytopenic purpura

Riguad M et al: Thrombocytopenia in children infected with human immunodeficiency virus: long-term follow-up and therapeutic considerations, *J Acquir Immun Defic Syndr* 5:450, 1992.

Viral infections

Bagdades EK, Pillay D, Squire SB: Relationship between herpes simplex virus ulceration and CD4+ cell counts in patients with HIV infection, *AIDS* 6:1317, 1992.

Balfour HH Jr, Benson C, Braun J: Management of acyclovir-resistant herpes simplex and varicella-zoster virus infections, *J Acquir Immun Defic Syndr* 7:254, 1994.

Barone R et al: Prevalence of oral lesions among HIV-infected intravenous drug abusers and other risk groups, *Oral Surg Oral Med Oral Pathol* 69:169, 1990.

De Clercq E: Antivirals for the treatment of herpesvirus infections, *J Antimicrob Chemother* 32:121, 1993.

Eversole LR: Viral infections of the head and neck among HIV-seropositive patients, *Oral Surg Oral Med Oral Pathol* 73:155, 1992.

Greenspan D et al: Unusual HPV types in oral warts in association with HIV infection, *J Oral Pathol* 17:482, 1988.

Grossman ME, Stevens AW, Cohen PR: Brief report: herpetic geometric glossitis, *N Engl J Med* 329:1859, 1993.

Jacobson MA et al: Acyclovir-resistant varicella zoster virus infection after chronic oral acyclovir therapy in patients with the acquired immunodeficiency syndrome (AIDS), *Ann Intern Med* 112:187, 1990.

Linnemann CC Jr et al: Emergence of acyclovir-resistant varicella zoster virus in an AIDS patient on prolonged acyclovir therapy, *AIDS* 4:577, 1990.

Vilmer C et al: Focal epithelial hyperplasia and multifocal human papillomavirus infection in an HIV-seropositive man, *J Am Acad Dermatol* 30:497, 1994.

Zunt SL, Tomich CE: Oral condyloma acuminatum, *J Dermatol Surg Oncol* 15:591, 1989.

Group three lesions

Bacterial infections

Glick M, Cleveland DB: Oral mucosal bacillary epithelioid angiomatosis in a patient with AIDS associated with rapid alveolar bone loss: case report, *J Oral Pathol Med* 22:235, 1993.

Levell NJ et al: Bacillary angiomatosis with cutaneous and oral lesions in an HIV-infected patient from the U.K, *Br J Dermatol* 132:113, 1995.

Manders SM: Bacillary angiomatosis, *Clin Dermatol* 14:295, 1996.

Nuesch R et al: Oral manifestation of disseminated *Mycobacterium kansasii* infection in a patient with AIDS, *Dermatology* 192:183, 1996.

Fungal infections (other than candidiasis)

Berger TG: Treatment of bacterial, fungal, and parasitic infections in the HIV-infected host, *Semin Dermatol* 12:296, 1993.

Chinn H et al: Oral histoplasmosis in HIV-infected patients: a report of two cases, *Oral Surg Oral Med Oral Pathol Oral Radiol Endod* 79:710, 1995.

Drew RH: Pharmacotherapy of disseminated histoplasmosis in patients with AIDS, *Ann Pharmacother* 27:1510, 1993.

Hay RJ: Antifungal therapy and the new azole compounds, *J Antimicrob Chemother* 28:35, 1991.

Heinic GS et al: Oral *Histoplasma capsulatum* infection in association with HIV infection: a case report, *J Oral Pathol Med* 21:85, 1992.

Kuruvilla A, Humphrey DM, Emko P: Coexistent oral cryptococcosis and Kaposi's sarcoma in acquired immunodeficiency syndrome, *Cutis* 49:260, 1992.

Lynch DP, Naftolin LZ: Oral *Cryptococcus neoformans* infection in AIDS, *Oral Surg Oral Med Oral Pathol* 64:449, 1987.

Swindells S, Durham T, Johansson SL: Oral histoplasmosis in a patient infected with HIV: a case report, *Oral Surg Oral Med Oral Pathol* 72:126, 1994.

Neurologic disturbances

Belec L et al: Peripheral facial paralysis in HIV infection: a report of four African cases and review of the literature, *J Neurol* 236:411, 1989.

Brown MM et al: Bell's palsy in HIV infection, *J Neurol Neurosurg Psychiatry* 51:425, 1988.

Recurrent aphthous stomatitis

Anneroth G, Anneroth I, Lynch DP: Acquired immunodeficiency syndrome (AIDS) in the United States in 1986: etiology, epidemiology, clinical manifestations, and dental implications, *J Oral Maxillofac Surg* 44:956, 1986.

Friedman MN, Brenski A, Taylor L: Treatment of aphthous ulcers in AIDS patients, *Laryngoscope* 104:566, 1994.

MacPhail LA, Greenspan D, Greenspan JS: Recurrent aphthous ulcers in association with HIV infection, *Oral Surg Oral Med Oral Pathol* 73:283, 1992.

Manders SM et al: Thalidomide-resistant HIV-associated aphthae successfully treated with granulocyte colony-stimulating factor, *J Am Acad Dermatol* 33:380, 1995.

Radeff B, Kuffer R, Samson J: Recurrent aphthous ulcer in patient infected with human immunodeficiency virus: successful treatment with thalidomide, *J Am Acad Dermatol* 23:523, 1990.

Viral infections

Epstein JB, Shurlock CH, Wolber RA: Oral manifestations of cytomegalovirus infection, *Oral Surg Oral Med Oral Pathol* 75:443, 1993.

Flaitz CM, Nichols CM, Hicks MJ: Herpesviridae-associated persistent mucocutaneous ulcers in acquired immunodeficiency syndrome: a clinical pathologic study, *Oral Surg Oral Med Oral Pathol Oral Radiol Endod* 81:433, 1996.

Jones AC et al: Cytomegalovirus infections of the oral cavity, *Oral Surg Oral Med Oral Pathol* 75:76, 1993.

Langford A et al: Cytomegalovirus associated oral ulcerations in HIV-infected patients, *J Oral Pathol Med* 19:71, 1990.

Laskaris G, Sklavounou A: Molluscum contagiosum of the oral mucosa, *Oral Surg Oral Med Oral Pathol* 58:688, 1984.

Leimola-Virtanen R, Happonen RP, Syrjanen S: Cytomegalovirus (CMV) and *Helicobacter pylori* (HP) found in oral mucosal ulcers, *J Oral Pathol Med* 24:14, 1995.

Schubert MM et al: Oral infections due to cytomegalovirus in immunocompromised patients, *J Oral Pathol Med* 22:268, 1993.

Sugihara K, Reichart PA, Gelderbolm HR: Molluscum contagiosum associated with AIDS: a case report with ultrastructural study, *J Oral Pathol Med* 19:235, 1990.

Whitaker SB, Weigand SE, Budnick SD: Intraoral molluscum contagiosum, *Oral Surg Oral Med Oral Pathol* 72:344, 1991.

CHAPTER 14

Salivary Gland Diseases

NONNEOPLASTIC SALIVARY GLAND DISEASES

The nonneoplastic salivary gland diseases include a group of entities with diverse causes. Many of the conditions are clinically characterized by swelling and enlargement of the salivary glands without other oral manifestations. By contrast, disruption of salivary gland flow, disorders of saliva production, and infarction and trauma of the salivary glands often result in distinctive oral conditions.

Sialadenosis

Sialadenosis is an uncommon, nonneoplastic, noninflammatory enlargement of the salivary glands. The cause of the glandular enlargement is unknown, but the condition is associated with a number of systemic abnormalities including diabetes mellitus, malnutrition, alcoholism, anorexia nervosa and bulimia, and drug reactions. The parotid glands are most frequently involved, usually with bilateral painless enlargement. The swelling may be intermittent with frequent recurrences. Treatment of the associated systemic disorder generally results in resolution of the salivary gland swelling.

Benign Lymphoepithelial Lesion and Sjögren's Syndrome

Another cause of salivary gland enlargement is the benign lymphoepithelial lesion, or Mikulicz's syndrome. In this condition patients present with bilateral enlargement of the salivary and lacrimal glands in association with various entities such as lymphoma, tuberculosis, and sarcoidosis. Many cases of Mikulicz's disease may actually represent Sjögren's syndrome with potential widespread involvement of other organ systems.

Sjögren's syndrome is most commonly seen in older adults, and more than two thirds of cases are in women (see Chapter 12). The parotid gland is involved in the majority of cases, although any of the major or minor salivary glands may be affected. Clinically, the parotid gland is asymptomatic, firm, and diffusely swollen. Microscopically, there is an intense lymphocytic infiltrate and widespread destruction of salivary gland acini. Characteristic residual ductal epithelium and myoepithelial cells remain as "epimyoepithelial islands." Affected individuals are at an increased risk for lymphoma, both within the affected gland and in extraglandular sites. A rare malignant counterpart, lymphoepithelial carcinoma, has been reported to develop primarily in Inuits, Eskimos, and Asians. Epstein-Barr virus has been implicated in the pathogenesis of this condition.

Adenomatoid Hyperplasia of Salivary Glands

Occasionally, lobules of minor salivary glands undergo hyperplasia, mimicking the clinical appearance of salivary gland neoplasms. This process most often involves the minor salivary glands of the palate, although minor salivary glands in other anatomic sites may be affected. Adenomatoid hyperplasia most commonly occurs in adults and is characterized by a painless, well-circumscribed, soft tissue nodule (Fig. 14-1). The high incidence of tobacco use and dentures in patients with these lesions suggests that chronic, local trauma to the minor salivary glands may be important in their development. A biopsy is required to exclude a salivary gland neoplasm, although once the nature of the process has been identified, no further treatment is necessary.

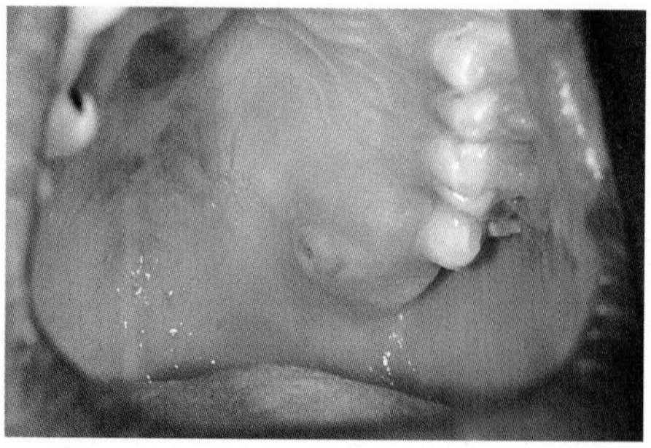

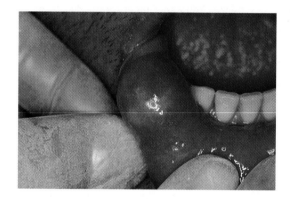

FIG. 14-1   Minor salivary gland hyperplasia resembling a salivary gland neoplasm.

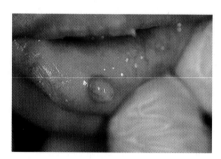

FIG. 14-2   Superficial mucoceles are blue, translucent, and soft in consistency.

FIG. 14-3   Deep-seated mucoceles are mucosa-colored and firm in consistency.

Mucocele (Mucus Retention Phenomenon)

Mucoceles are common, traumatically induced, cystic-appearing lesions of the oral cavity that arise from obstruction or rupture of the minor salivary gland. A recent hypothesis suggests that some mucoceles develop intraglandularly as a result of continuous secretion from the residual acini after traumatic destruction of the glandular parenchyma. In contrast to the much less common mucus retention cyst, mucoceles lack a true epithelial lining and represent a reactive process.

Mucoceles develop most frequently in children and adolescents, although they can occur in all age groups. Clinically, mucoceles appear as painless, dome-shaped, fluctuant masses, which may range in size from several millimeters to several centimeters. Superficial lesions are translucent and soft with a bluish hue (Fig. 14-2), whereas deep lesions are of normal mucosal color and firm in consistency (Fig. 14-3). Mucoceles frequently fluctuate in size as a result of rupture and release of saliva with subsequent reorganization of the lesion.

More than three fourths of all mucoceles involve the mucosal surface of the lower lip, usually lateral to the midline. Their occurrence on other mucosal surfaces where minor salivary glands are found (the buccal mucosa, ventral tongue, floor of the mouth, and soft palate) is infrequent. Rarely, multiple mucoceles may develop. Mucoceles are characteristically uncommon on the upper lip despite the abundance of minor salivary glands in this location. The majority of nodules detected on

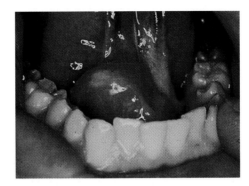

FIG. 14-4   Ranulas represent mucoceles on the floor of the mouth.

the upper lip represent true neoplastic salivary gland tumors, which, unlike mucoceles, are exceedingly rare on the lower lip.

Microscopically, mucoceles consist of a collection of mucus surrounded by fibrosis, foamy macrophages, and neutrophils. The associated minor salivary glands may show degeneration and squamous metaplasia.

Although mucoceles may spontaneously rupture, reestablish drainage, and heal without complication, the majority of lesions require surgical excision. At the time of removal, care should be taken to also excise adjacent minor salivary glands to decrease the possibility of inducing an iatrogenic mucocele secondary to surgical trauma. Alternatively, treatment of superficial mucoceles with cryosurgery has been reported to yield excellent results and a low recurrence rate.

Ranula

The ranula is a unique clinical variant of mucocele that occurs only in the floor of the mouth in association with submandibular and sublingual glands (Fig. 14-4). Clinically, the lesions are unilateral, smooth, dome-shaped elevations that resemble a frog's belly (*rana,* Latin for frog). Ranulas develop lateral to the lingual frenum and are typically larger than mucoceles, often resulting in elevation of the tongue and affecting speech and swallowing. The plunging ranula is an uncommon variant in which the lesion dissects through the mylohyoid muscle, resulting in a swelling of the anterior neck. The ranula may resemble other masses that develop in the floor of the mouth, including dermoid cysts and cystic hygromas, although the latter are usually not unilateral.

Marsupialization of ranulas, consisting of excising the entire roof of the lesion and permitting the area to heal by secondary intention, is frequently attempted because of ease of the procedure and minimal associated morbidity to the patient. Unfortunately, recurrences are common after this procedure and require more aggressive treatment that includes removal of the involved salivary gland.

Mucus Retention Cyst (Salivary Duct Cyst)

The mucous retention cyst is an uncommon, epithelial-lined cyst of the salivary glands that has historically been confused and grouped with mucoceles and ranulas. Obstruction of the salivary gland duct by infection, calculus, or sialoliths, resulting in ductal dilatation, appears to be important in the pathogenesis of these lesions.

In contrast to mucoceles, mucus retention cysts develop more commonly in adults and occur in association with both major and minor salivary glands. The parotid gland is the most frequent major salivary gland to be affected, whereas minor salivary glands of the lip, buccal mucosa, and floor of the mouth may also develop mucus retention cysts. Clinically, the lesions are indistinguishable from mucoceles, and their differentiation must be made on the basis of their microscopic features (i.e., a

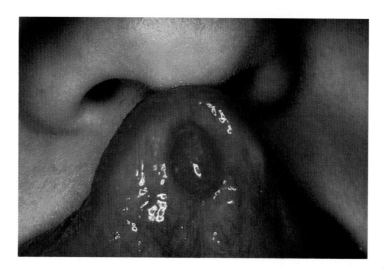

FIG. 14-5 Mucus retention cysts are lined by ductal epithelium and are true cysts. They are clinically indistinguishable from mucoceles.

true epithelial lining arising from ductal epithelium) (Fig. 14-5). Mucus retention cysts are treated in the same fashion as mucoceles.

Sialolithiasis (Salivary Gland Stone)

Sialoliths are calcified structures that occur within salivary glands or their ducts. They are thought to arise from the deposition of calcium salts in either inspissated mucus, exfoliated ductal luminal cells, or other debris in the lumen of the salivary gland duct. There is no relationship between the development of sialoliths and alterations in calcium-phosphorus metabolism.

Sialoliths are most commonly found in adults and usually affect the submandibular gland. The propensity for involvement of the submandibular gland is a result of several factors, including the high level of calcium in submandibular saliva, the high proportion of mucus relative to serous saliva produced by the submandibular gland, and the anatomic configuration of Wharton's duct, which contains several acute bends. Sialoliths, however, may arise in any of the major or minor salivary glands.

Patients with sialolithiasis of the major salivary gland frequently complain of pain and swelling, especially at mealtime. Large salivary stones are often palpable, especially those in the distal portion of the duct. The diagnosis may be aided by the fact that many sialoliths contain a sufficient amount of calcium to be visible radiographically. Minor salivary gland stones are frequently asymptomatic but may cause a focal swelling that appears clinically as a dome-shaped nodule identical to a mucocele. Unlike mucoceles, however, sialoliths in minor salivary glands arise most frequently on the buccal mucosa and upper lip.

Frequently, small sialoliths in the major salivary glands can be expelled if the patient increases water intake and uses sialogogues such as sugar-free lemon drops. Moist heat and gentle massaging of the salivary gland may expedite the process. Small stones in the terminal portion of the duct may be expelled more rapidly if the duct is dilated with lacrimal probes of progressively increasing diameter. Large stones require surgical removal, which occasionally necessitates excision of the associated salivary gland. Minor salivary gland stones generally require surgical removal of the entire gland. Extracorporeal shock wave lithotripsy used in the treatment of renal and gallbladder stones, has been successfully employed for salivary stones in select patients. Endoscopy can also be used in the exploration and extraction of calculi from the salivary duct system.

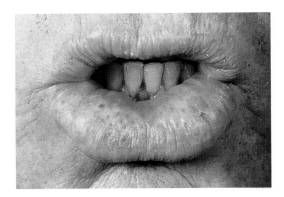

FIG. 14-6   Cheilitis glandularis is characterized by swelling of the lip, dilated orifices of the minor salivary gland, and ectropion of the lip.

Sialadenitis

Sialadenitis refers to a diverse group of nonspecific inflammatory conditions of salivary glands caused by both infectious and noninfectious agents. Several viral infections may result in sialadenitis, including mumps, coxsackievirus, echovirus, and cytomegalovirus. Mild sialadenitis is a common finding in patients with hepatitis C virus infection. Alterations in salivary gland flow caused by ductal obstruction may occur from bacterial infections, salivary gland stones, or scar formation secondary to trauma. The subsequent decrease in salivary flow facilitates a retrograde infection. Medications such as atropine and conditions of dehydration and debilitation may all cause decreased saliva production and subsequent sialadenitis.

Sialadenitis most frequently involves the parotid gland and is, in the majority of cases, caused by an acute bacterial infection with *Staphylococcus aureus.* Up to one fourth of cases may be bilateral. The involved gland is tender and enlarged, and in severe cases the overlying facial skin may be erythematous and warm. Palpation of the gland may result in the expression of purulent exudate from the duct orifice.

Chronic sialadenitis is most frequently the result of chronic obstruction resulting from the presence of a salivary stone, either intraglandularly or in the salivary gland duct. Increased saliva production at mealtime often results in episodic pain and swelling. A sialogram may disclose whether the salivary gland duct is patent or occluded.

Acute bacterial sialadenitis responds well to antibiotics, rehydration, and the use of sialogogues. Focal abscess formation may require incision and drainage. Chronic sialadenitis normally resolves after reestablishment of normal salivary gland flow following the removal of the underlying source of obstruction. Secondary scar formation may result in severe stricture of the duct, necessitating surgical removal of the gland.

Cheilitis Glandularis

Cheilitis glandularis is an uncommon inflammatory condition of minor salivary glands, most often affecting the lower lip. The condition affects elderly men and, rarely, women and children. Actinic damage from ultraviolet radiation, bacterial infections, use of tobacco products, and poor oral hygiene have all been implicated as causes, although the precise cause remains obscure.

Clinically, cheilitis glandularis has been subdivided into three stages. The initial stage is characterized by pronounced, painless swelling of the lower lip secondary to hypertrophy and inflammation of the minor salivary glands. In the subsequent superficial suppurative stage (also known as Baelz's disease), induration, crusting, and ulcerations of the lower lip may develop. Excessive mucus secretion of the glands occurs, and the ductal orifices appear dilated, swollen, and inflamed (Fig. 14-6). Occasionally, purulent exudate can be expressed from the glands. The final deep suppurative stage (cheilitis glandularis apostematosa) represents advanced disease with widespread lip involvement.

The lip is painful and may become permanently enlarged. Erosions and repeated bacterial infections heal with scarring, which may result in ectropion of the lower lip. Microscopic features include duct ectasia with inflammation of the minor salivary glands and adjacent tissue. The overlying mucosa may exhibit intracellular and extracellular edema with reticular degeneration.

Cheilitis glandularis is a premalignant condition, with approximately one third of cases eventually developing squamous cell carcinomas. The high incidence of malignant degeneration occurs predominantly in association with the deep suppurative stage and is thought to be related to eversion of the lower lip, which results in increased actinic exposure. Intralesional corticosteroids may be helpful in the management of the condition, especially in the early stages. If actinic damage is present, a vermilionectomy should be performed.

Sialorrhea (Ptyalism)

Sialorrhea, or increased salivation, is a clinical phenomenon that may result from a variety of causes. Historically, sialorrhea was associated with both heavy metal intoxication and rabies. Any chronic irritation in the mouth can result in some degree of increased saliva production. In addition, patients with new complete dentures frequently complain of increased saliva during the initial adjustment phase. In recent years the most common cause of sialorrhea is the administration of cholinergic and psychotropic medications such as clozapine. Clozapine paradoxically results in sialorrhea in approximately 25% of patients, although it is unclear why this occurs, because it has potent anticholinergic effects. Patients who are pregnant or who have hiatal hernia commonly develop gastroesophageal reflux, which in turn results in a marked increase in salivary flow. Sialorrhea is also typically observed in children with cerebral palsy and mental retardation, although this may result from the inability to control swallowing rather than excess saliva production.

For most individuals sialorrhea is more of an annoyance than a significant health problem, although infrequent reports of gagging on excessive saliva have been noted. The treatment of sialorrhea depends on the severity of symptoms. Mild cases require no treatment. Anticholinergic drugs such as atropine may be effective in decreasing saliva production, but the dosage must be titrated to avoid adverse effects. More recently, scopolamine dermal patches have been used successfully. Surgical intervention including salivary duct repositioning, duct ligation, and tympanic neurectomy have all been tried with varying degrees of success. Parasympathectomy, although effective, inherently results in the loss of taste to the anterior two thirds of the tongue.

Xerostomia

Xerostomia, or dry mouth, is a common symptom of reduced or absent salivary secretion, which may be caused by a variety of etiologic factors. It is most frequently observed as a side effect of various medications including antihistamines, decongestants, tricyclic antidepressants, antipsychotics, antihypertensives, and various anticholinergic drugs. In addition, individuals may experience xerostomia as a result of mouth breathing, autoimmune destruction of salivary gland acini (i.e., Sjögren's syndrome) (see Chapter 12), congenital salivary gland anomalies, neurologic diseases, radiation therapy to the head and neck, and human immunodeficiency virus infection.

Xerostomia is more common in women than in men and is also more frequently noted in aging populations. Clinically, patients with xerostomia have decreased salivary secretions, resulting in saliva that is thick, stringy, mucoid, and sometimes foamy. The oral mucosal surfaces are dry and adherent to the touch, whereas the dorsal tongue is frequently fissured and atrophic. Xerostomia may result in impairment of mastication, swallowing, and speech, although some patients who complain of a dry mouth have a completely normal oral examination. Conversely, patients who appear to have clinical features of xerostomia may have no oral complaints. Quantitative salivary gland flow rates, sialography, and microscopic examination may reveal the severity of salivary gland dysfunction.

The dry oral environment predisposes patients with xerostomia to the development of recurrent episodes of candidiasis. Affected individuals also have an increased incidence of dental caries.

Dental caries secondary to xerostomia is atypically located on the facial aspect of the gingival one third of the teeth and on the root surfaces rather than on the occlusal and interproximal surfaces of teeth. Historically, this type of decay was termed *radiation caries* because it frequently occurred as a complication of radiation therapy. This decay pattern may develop in all patients with severe xerostomia regardless of the cause. Poor oral hygiene contributes significantly to the development of xerostomia-related caries.

The management of xerostomia must be tailored to the individual, and identifiable causes should be definitively treated. Mucin-containing lozenges, polymer-based saliva substitutes, and xanthan gum-based saliva substitutes have all been tried with variable success. Many patients simply sip water periodically to achieve the same results. Various sialogogues, such as sugar-free lemon drops, are helpful in stimulating saliva from residual functional acini. Pilocarpine may be prescribed to stimulate salivation, although the dosage must be titrated to avoid side effects. In patients who develop xerostomia as a result of medications, altering the dosage may result in resolution of the dry mouth. In some cases a change in medications may be required and, frequently, there will be a significant improvement, even if the new medication has anticholinergic properties. To prevent cervical and root-surface dental caries, patients with xerostomia should have frequent dental visits and maintain an optimal oral hygiene program. Topical fluoride applied with customized vinyl carriers and chlorhexidine-based mouth rinses may be helpful in reducing the incidence of xerostomia-related caries.

Necrotizing Sialometaplasia

Necrotizing sialometaplasia is an uncommon, self-limiting lesion of salivary glands. The precise cause of necrotizing sialometaplasia is unknown, although it is believed that a traumatic episode results in a compromised blood supply to salivary gland lobules with subsequent ischemic necrosis and infarction. Precipitating traumatic events include dental injections, ill-fitting dentures, and prior surgical intervention, although not all reported cases have been associated with predisposing traumatic events.

Necrotizing sialometaplasia occurs primarily in adults, most commonly in the fifth decade of life. It is twice as common in men as in women. Clinically, necrotizing sialometaplasia usually presents initially as a relatively asymptomatic palatal swelling, although some patients may experience pain or paresthesia. As the infarction progresses, the lesion becomes necrotic, sloughs, and evolves into an ulceration that frequently exceeds several centimeters in diameter (Fig. 14-7). Lesions that were initially painful become asymptomatic during this stage. Necrotizing sialometaplasia may involve any mucosal site including the parotid gland, nasal cavity, maxillary sinus, and larynx. Nearly 80% of all cases involve minor salivary glands of the palate, most frequently at the junction of the hard and soft palates. Approximately two thirds of palatal lesions are unilateral.

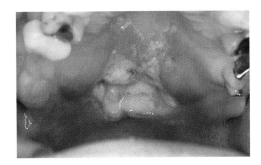

FIG. 14-7   Necrotizing sialometaplasia is characterized by a large necrotic ulceration caused by infarction and ischemic necrosis.

Although a history of trauma supports the clinical diagnosis, the appearance of necrotizing sialometaplasia resembles malignant salivary gland tumors such as mucoepidermoid carcinoma and adenoid cystic carcinoma. A biopsy is always indicated to exclude these entities. Microscopically, a spectrum of histologic findings has been reported. Characteristic features include acinar necrosis and squamous metaplasia of the minor salivary gland ducts that frequently coalesce with overlying epithelium. These changes may mimic the histopathologic appearance of both squamous cell carcinoma and high-grade mucoepidermoid carcinoma. The overall architecture of the affected minor salivary glands, however, remains intact. Extravasated mucin may result in an overlying patchy, inflammatory infiltrate.

Despite the ominous clinical appearance of the lesion and often confusing histopathologic appearance, once the diagnosis of necrotizing sialometaplasia has been established, no further treatment is necessary. The condition is benign and heals spontaneously within 5 to 6 weeks.

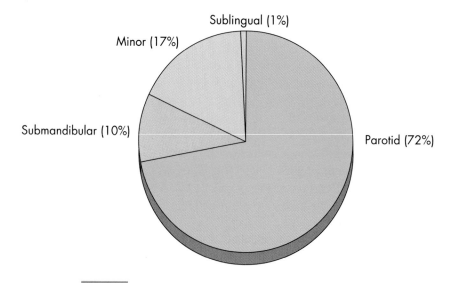

FIG. 14-8   Site of occurrence of salivary gland neoplasms.

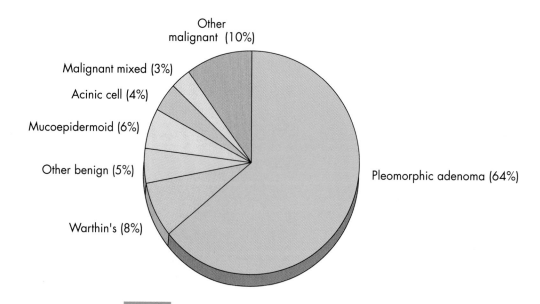

FIG. 14-9   Frequency of occurrence of parotid neoplasms.

NEOPLASTIC SALIVARY GLAND DISEASES

Salivary gland neoplasms are not uncommon occurrences in the oral cavity, with an annual incidence of approximately 6/100,000 individuals. The majority of all salivary gland neoplasms occur in the parotid gland (Fig. 14-8). The most common salivary gland neoplasm is the pleomorphic adenoma, which comprises approximately two thirds of all parotid neoplasms followed by Warthin's tumor (papillary cystadenoma lymphomatosum), which accounts for an additional 10% of parotid neoplasms. Malignant tumors of salivary glands most frequently affect the parotid gland, comprising nearly one fourth of all parotid gland neoplasms, with mucoepidermoid carcinoma diagnosed most commonly (Fig. 14-9).

Although salivary gland tumors arise in the submandibular gland much less frequently than the parotid gland, approximately 40% of those that develop are malignant. The pleomorphic adenoma is also the most common neoplasm in the submandibular gland and accounts for approximately one half of all neoplasms in this anatomic location. The most common malignancy in the submandibular gland is the adenoid cystic carcinoma, which comprises over one third of all submandibular malignancies (Fig. 14-10). Sublingual gland neoplasms are relatively uncommon, although when they do develop, the vast majority are malignant (Fig. 14-11).

Minor salivary glands are the second most frequent site of salivary gland neoplasms, comprising approximately 20% of all reported cases. Nearly one half of all minor salivary gland tumors are malignant, the most common of which is mucoepidermoid carcinoma. The pleomorphic adenoma is the most frequently observed benign neoplasm (Fig. 14-12). In general, oral benign minor salivary gland tumors present as asymptomatic nodules. The presence of pain, ulceration, and radiographic alterations is more frequently associated with malignant lesions. Approximately 50% of minor salivary gland tumors occur in the palate, followed by the lips (21%) and buccal mucosa (13%) (Fig. 14-13). Almost all salivary gland neoplasms involving the lips occur in the upper lip. Site specificity is also significant in predicting the benign and malignant nature of the tumors. For example, 90% of all minor salivary gland tumors of the retromolar pad area are malignant as are minor salivary gland tumors of the tongue and the floor of the mouth (Fig. 14-14). Almost 50% of salivary gland tumors of the palate and buccal mucosa are malignant, whereas 75% in the upper lip are benign. Although minor salivary gland tumors are distinctly uncommon in the lower lip, when they develop, approximately 75% are malignant and are usually mucoepidermoid carcinomas. In the diagnosis of oral salivary

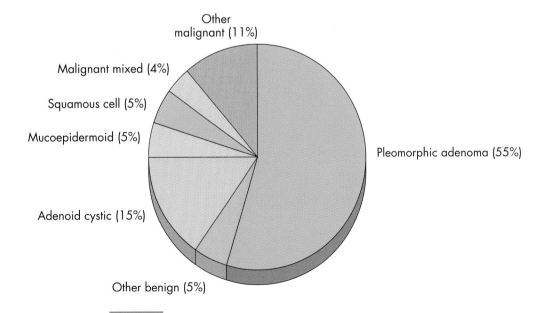

FIG. 14-10   Frequency of occurrence of submandibular neoplasms.

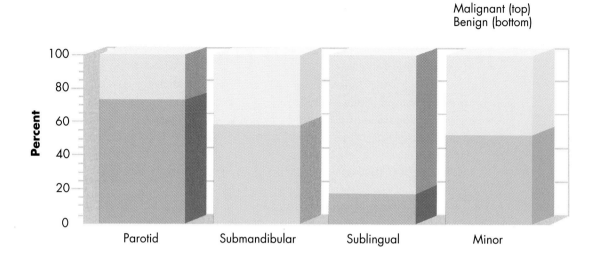

FIG. 14-11 Frequency of malignancy of salivary gland neoplasms.

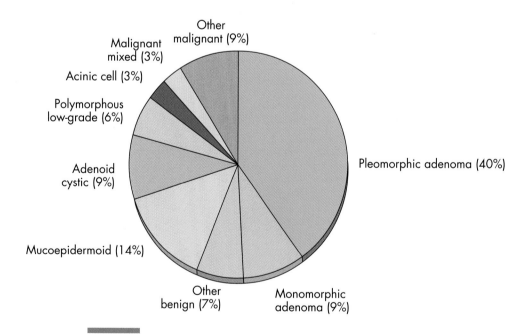

FIG. 14-12 Frequency of occurrence of minor salivary gland neoplasms.

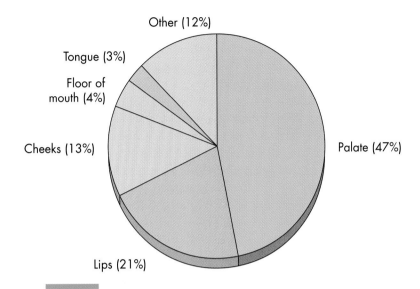

FIG. 14-13   Site of occurrence of minor salivary gland neoplasms.

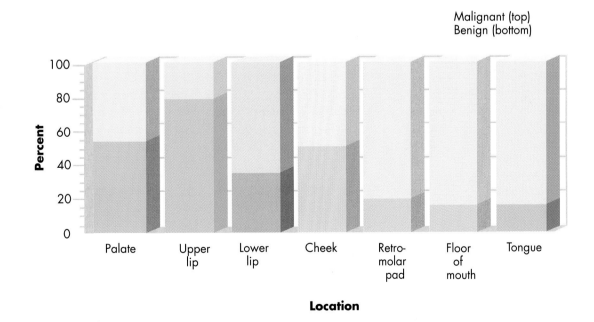

FIG. 14-14   Frequency of malignancy of minor salivary gland neoplasms.

gland neoplasms, fine needle aspiration may be useful for masses that are not accessible to routine surgical biopsy. Unsatisfactory aspirates necessitate an incisional biopsy for definitive diagnosis.

Salivary gland tumors display allelic loss patterns that are different from other tumor types, suggesting that distinct genetic pathways are important in the progression of these lesions.

Benign Salivary Gland Neoplasms

Pleomorphic adenoma (benign mixed tumor). Pleomorphic adenomas or benign mixed tumors are the most common salivary gland neoplasm, accounting for nearly three fourths of all parotid neoplasms, more than one half of all submandibular neoplasms, and more than one third of all minor salivary gland neoplasms. The term *pleomorphic* refers to the variable histologic pattern of the tumor and not cellular atypia. Additionally, the tumor does not arise from more than one germ layer and is not truly "mixed."

Pleomorphic adenomas develop most commonly in young and middle-aged adults and are slightly more prevalent in women than in men. When they involve the parotid gland, pleomorphic adenomas arise most commonly in the superficial lobe and appear as a preauricular swelling. When they arise in the minor salivary glands, the palate is the most common site of occurrence. Such lesions comprise approximately 60% of all intraoral salivary gland neoplasms. Palatal tumors arise in the site of the highest concentration of minor salivary glands, namely, the posterior lateral palate. The lesions are asymptomatic, firm, and slow growing, appearing as smooth, dome-shaped masses (Fig. 14-15). The overlying mucosa generally remains intact, although large lesions may become ulcerated secondary to trauma. Unlike lesions of the parotid gland and buccal mucosa, palatal pleomorphic adenomas are fixed to the underlying surface and are not freely moveable. Pleomorphic adenomas of minor salivary glands in the upper lip and buccal mucosa appear as firm masses that resemble palatal lesions in their growth pattern and behavior.

Microscopically, pleomorphic adenomas are well circumscribed and encapsulated, although infiltration of the capsule occasionally occurs with subsequent local spread of the lesion. The lesion is comprised of epithelial and mesenchymal elements that most likely have a common single-cell origin. Diverse histologic stromal components may be observed, including loose myxoid material, hyalinized collagen, cartilage, and bone.

Pleomorphic adenomas are treated by aggressive surgical excision rather than simple enucleation. Pleomorphic adenomas of the submandibular, sublingual, and minor salivary glands are treated by extirpation of the entire gland to minimize the risk of recurrence. When the tumors develop in the superficial lobe of the parotid gland, a lobectomy is normally performed. Involvement of the deep lobe of the parotid usually requires total parotidectomy. The cure rate for pleomorphic adenomas

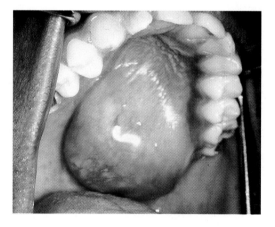

FIG. 14-15   Pleomorphic adenomas are slow-growing, palatal masses that are smooth and dome-shaped.

treated by excision is more than 95%. Malignant degeneration does occur, but the incidence is less than 5% of reported cases.

Monomorphic adenoma. Monomorphic adenomas consist of a group of benign salivary gland neoplasms that characteristically demonstrate a uniform histopathologic pattern throughout the tumor. Tumors included in this category include canalicular adenoma, basal cell adenoma, and oncocytoma.

CANALICULAR ADENOMA. The canalicular adenoma is an uncommon neoplasm. The majority of lesions occur on the upper lip (Fig. 14-16), although they may also develop in the minor salivary glands of the buccal mucosa and other intraoral sites. Canalicular adenomas rarely occur in the major salivary glands. They arise most frequently in the elderly and are twice as prevalent in women as men. Clinically, they are asymptomatic, slow-growing masses that may achieve a diameter of several centimeters. The treatment of choice is excision.

BASAL CELL ADENOMA. The basal cell adenoma is an uncommon benign salivary gland neoplasm, developing predominantly in the parotid gland and involving the superficial lobe. Basal cell adenomas may also occur in the minor salivary glands of the upper lip and buccal mucosa. Like canalicular adenomas, basal cell adenomas occur more commonly in the elderly and in women. The lesions present as relatively small, freely movable, soft tissue masses. Membranous basal cell adenomas are a variant of these tumors, which have a hereditary tendency and occur in association with trichoepitheliomas and cylindromas of the skin. Up to one third of membranous basal cell adenomas recur, but malignant transformation is rare. Basal cell adenomas are treated by surgical excision.

ONCOCYTOMA. Oncocytomas comprise less than 1% of all salivary gland neoplasms and occur in the elderly, with only a slight female predilection. They typically develop in the parotid gland (approximately 80%) and rarely develop in the minor salivary glands. Clinically, oncocytomas present as firm, asymptomatic, slowly-growing soft tissue masses that attain a maximum size of 3 to 4 cm. Parotid lesions are normally found in the superficial lobe. Oncocytomas are best treated by aggressive surgical excision (i.e., superficial parotid lobectomy or total removal of the salivary gland). Simple enucleation should be avoided because of the subsequent high rate of recurrence. Malignant oncocytomas have been reported, although their occurrence is rare.

Warthin's tumor (papillary cystadenoma lymphomatosum). Warthin's tumor or papillary cystadenoma lymphomatosum is the second most common parotid neoplasm. The older term *adenolymphoma* has been abandoned. Clinically, Warthin's tumor presents as an asymptomatic, slow-growing parotid mass that occurs most frequently in elderly men; however, minor salivary gland involvement has been reported. The tumor is unique in that over 10% of reported cases occur bilaterally in the parotid glands, although not simultaneously. Warthin's tumor is treated by surgical excision and requires a superficial parotid lobectomy. Approximately 10% of surgically treated cases recur, possibly because of the multicentricity of the tumor rather than inadequate surgical removal.

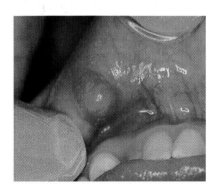

FIG. 14-16   Monomorphic adenomas develop most frequently in the minor salivary glands of the upper lip.

Ductal papillomas (sialadenoma papilliferum, intraductal papilloma, and inverted ductal papilloma). In addition to Warthin's tumor, several benign salivary gland neoplasms, collectively termed *ductal papillomas,* are characterized by a papillomatous microscopic pattern. Sialadenoma papilliferum occurs most frequently on the palate, usually in older adults, in association with the minor salivary glands. They are reported twice as frequently in women as in men. The intraductal papilloma arises from the minor salivary glands of the lips and presents as a submucosal mass with nonspecific clinical features. The inverted ductal papilloma is exceedingly uncommon and develops in the minor salivary glands of the lower lip and mandibular vestibule as a nonspecific soft tissue mass. All ductal papillomas are treated by conservative surgical excision.

Malignant Salivary Gland Neoplasms

Mucoepidermoid carcinoma (mucoepidermoid tumor). Mucoepidermoid carcinoma is the most common salivary gland malignancy, comprising approximately 10% of all major salivary gland neoplasms and 20% of minor salivary gland neoplasms in the United States. The term *mucoepidermoid tumor* was once used to describe a subset of mucoepidermoid carcinomas that behaved in a benign fashion. It is now recognized that even these low-grade lesions may metastasize and, as such, the term *mucoepidermoid tumor* should not be used.

Mucoepidermoid carcinomas develop most frequently in adulthood. Despite their rarity in children, they remain the most common salivary gland malignancy in this age group. The lesions are slightly more prevalent in women than in men.

Clinically, mucoepidermoid carcinomas usually present as an asymptomatic mass of the parotid gland. Aggressive tumors frequently involve underlying nerves, which may result in pain or facial nerve palsy. Patients often report the presence of lesions for months to years before seeking medical attention.

Intraorally, mucoepidermoid carcinomas most often arise from minor salivary glands of the palate. These lesions present as asymptomatic, occasionally fluctuant, submucosal masses that may be mucosal-colored or bluish, resembling mucoceles (Fig. 14-17). Occasionally the lesions ulcerate or develop small cystic blebs. The tumors may also develop in minor salivary glands of the lower lip, tongue, floor of mouth, and retromolar pad. Although uncommon in these locations, the mucoepidermoid carcinoma is still the most frequent salivary gland tumor to arise in each of these sites. Intraosseous tumors have also been reported.

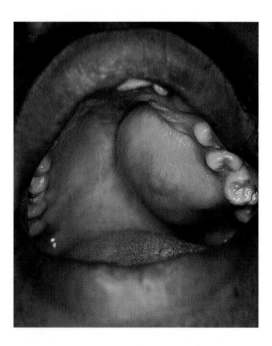

FIG. 14-17 Mucoepidermoid carcinomas are the most common malignant salivary gland neoplasms and present most frequently as asymptomatic palatal masses.

The clinical behavior of mucoepidermoid carcinomas varies significantly. Some tumors grow slowly, are minimally invasive, and metastasize late, whereas others rapidly enlarge and metastasize early. Their clinical behavior is reflected in the microscopic appearance of the lesions. Low-grade mucoepidermoid carcinomas exhibit a high percentage of mucous cells with prominent cyst formation and minimal atypia. By contrast, high-grade mucoepidermoid carcinomas have significant squamous and intermediate cell components, with prominent pleomorphism and cellular mitoses. Extremely high-grade mucoepidermoid carcinomas may sometimes be microscopically indistinguishable from squamous cell carcinoma. Intermediate grade mucoepidermoid carcinomas have clinical and histopathologic features of both low- and high-grade tumors and exhibit intermediate cells, mucous-secreting cells, and epidermoid cells.

The treatment of mucoepidermoid carcinoma varies greatly, depending on the location of the lesion, its histopathologic grade, and the clinical stage. Small, low-grade tumors can be successfully treated by lobectomy (for parotid lesions), extirpation of the gland (for other major salivary glands), or wide local excision (for minor salivary gland lesions). High-grade tumors require a more radical excision with regional lymph node dissection and postsurgical radiation therapy for patients with metastatic disease. The long-term survival of patients with mucoepidermoid carcinoma depends on the histopathologic grade and clinical stage of the disease. Patients with low-grade lesions without metastatic disease have a cure rate greater than 90%. In contrast, fewer than one third of patients with high-grade mucoepidermoid carcinomas survive for more than 5 years.

Adenoid Cystic Carcinoma (Cylindroma)

The adenoid cystic carcinoma is a common malignancy of salivary glands. The historical synonym, *cylindroma,* describes its distinctive microscopic appearance. This term should be reserved, however, for adnexal cutaneous lesions with similar histologic features, which have a dramatically different clinical presentation and prognosis.

Adenoid cystic carcinomas develop most commonly in the fifth to sixth decades of life and are distinctly uncommon in children and young adults. The lesions arise equally in men and women. Almost one half of all adenoid cystic carcinomas occur in minor salivary glands, most frequently in the palate, followed by the buccal mucosa and lips. These lesions constitute nearly 15% of all tumors in the palate. Adenoid cystic carcinomas typically develop in the submandibular gland and much less frequently in the parotid gland. They account for nearly one fifth of all submandibular gland neoplasms and represent the most common malignancy of this major salivary gland.

Clinically, adenoid cystic carcinomas present as slow-growing masses covered with normal mucosa that commonly ulcerates (Fig. 14-18). Although the initial discomfort may be minimal, symp-

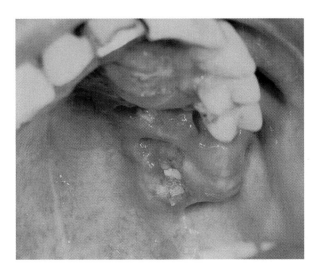

FIG. 14-18 Adenoid cystic carcinomas commonly spread by neural invasion and present as ulcerated masses on the palate.

toms increase proportionately to the growth of the lesions. Parotid tumors may involve the facial nerve and result in paralysis.

Microscopically, adenoid cystic carcinomas have a characteristic cribriform pattern, although a solid variant and other histologic patterns have also been described. Perineural invasion by tumor cells is common; however, this finding is not unique to adenoid cystic carcinomas.

The adenoid cystic carcinoma is a slowly progressive tumor. The overall survival rate is extremely low because of the propensity of adenoid cystic carcinomas to spread by perineural invasion, commonly to the base of the brain. The 5-year survival rate is approximately 65%, although the rate decreases to 20% after 20 years. The lesions uncommonly metastasize, most frequently to the lungs and bone. Although surgical excision is the treatment of choice, adjunctive radiation therapy may be beneficial and improve long-term survival. The measurement of carcinoembryonic antigen, an oncofetal glycoprotein used as a marker for colon carcinoma, may play a role in the management of patients with adenoid cystic carcinomas. Because these tumors bear remarkable similarity to adenoid cystic carcinomas of the breast, progesterone receptor expression may also be a useful prognostic or therapeutic marker for salivary gland lesions. Deoxyribonucleic acid ploidy pattern, as detected by flow cytometry, has also been demonstrated to be an important prognostic factor in predicting recurrences.

Malignant Mixed Tumor (Carcinoma Ex Pleomorphic Adenoma, Carcinosarcoma, and Metastasizing Mixed Tumor)

The malignant mixed tumors represent approximately 5% of all salivary gland tumors. The most common malignant mixed tumor is carcinoma ex pleomorphic adenoma in which the epithelial component of a pleomorphic adenoma undergoes malignant degeneration. The role of p53 gene mutation in the malignant transformation of pleomorphic adenomas has been demonstrated by immunohistochemistry. The metastasizing mixed tumor is a rare entity that displays histopathologic features of a pleomorphic adenoma but behaves in a malignant fashion by metastasizing. Carcinosarcoma is a truly "mixed" malignancy, involving both epithelial and mesenchymal components.

Carcinoma ex pleomorphic adenoma develops most frequently in the sixth to eighth decades of life. A preexisting mass, presumably representing a pleomorphic adenoma, is commonly noted by patients before the onset of sudden growth of the tumor and pain. The vast majority of carcinoma ex pleomorphic adenomas arise in the parotid gland. Intraoral lesions involving minor salivary glands are most common on the palate (Fig. 14-19). The lesions may ulcerate, although this clinical feature

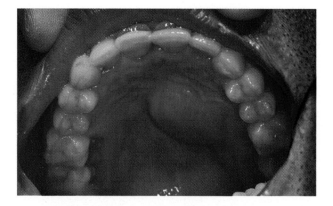

FIG. 14-19   Malignant mixed tumor of the palate developing from a long-standing lesion that was probably a pleomorphic adenoma initially.

is also observed with benign tumors. Carcinosarcoma and metastasizing mixed tumor are both extremely rare and have no distinctive clinical features.

The treatment of choice for malignant mixed tumors consists of wide surgical excision, frequently supplemented by adjunctive radiation therapy and lymph node dissection. With the exception of encapsulated carcinoma ex pleomorphic adenomas, which have a survival rate similar to pleomorphic adenomas, the long-term survival rate in patients with malignant mixed tumors is approximately 50%.

Acinic Cell Carcinoma (Acinic Cell Tumor)

Acinic cell carcinomas are uncommon, well-differentiated malignancies that arise most frequently in the parotid gland. Because of their slow growth pattern and infrequent rate of metastasis, they were historically referred to as *acinic cell tumors,* although this term should be avoided.

Acinic cell carcinomas constitute approximately 2% of all parotid tumors. The lesions have been reported in the major salivary glands and the minor salivary glands of the buccal mucosa, lips, and palate. They are reported more commonly in women than men and generally occur in the fifth decade, although they have been reported in all age groups. Clinically, acinic cell carcinomas present as asymptomatic, slow-growing masses. Intraoral lesions are firm and relatively fixed to the underlying tissue and occasionally ulcerate (Fig. 14-20). With advanced disease, pain and facial paralysis may ensue. Microscopically, acinic cell carcinomas display serous differentiation of neoplastic cells, and a variety of tissue antigens may be demonstrated in the tubuloglandular components, the cyst lining cells, and the acinic cells.

Acinic cell carcinomas are treated by wide local excision. The long-term survival of patients with acinic cell carcinoma ranges from 60% to 80% of cases. The presence of a predominantly solid architecture microscopically is strongly associated with a poor prognosis. Large tumors greater than 2.75 cm and cervical node disease with parotid lesions are also negative prognostic indicators. Immunohistochemical staining demonstrating high levels of MIB-1 antibody is the most predictive indicator of tumor recurrence, even in cases with bland histologic features and low mitotic rates. Overall, 30% of cases recur locally after treatment and 15% metastasize.

Polymorphous Low-Grade Adenocarcinoma (Terminal Duct Carcinoma)

Polymorphous low-grade adenocarcinoma is a recently defined salivary gland malignancy that was previously classified inappropriately as atypical pleomorphic adenoma, adenoid cystic carcinoma,

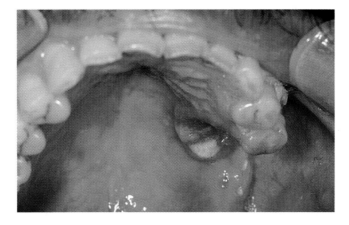

FIG. 14-20   Acinic cell carcinomas are typically firm, fixed, ulcerated masses on the palate.

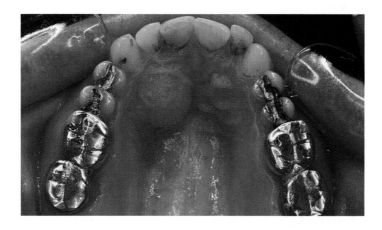

FIG. 14-21   Polymorphous low-grade adenocarcinomas are slow-growing, asymptomatic masses that develop predominantly on the palate.

or unclassified adenocarcinoma. Polymorphous low-grade adenocarcinomas occur primarily in the minor salivary glands, with approximately two thirds of reported cases developing in the palate and followed in frequency by the buccal mucosa and upper lip. The lesion arises most commonly in older adults and twice as often in women as in men.

Polymorphous low-grade adenocarcinomas present as asymptomatic, slow-growing masses with an intact overlying mucosa (Fig. 14-21). The lesions are generally larger than 1 cm. Microscopically, they exhibit infiltrative growth by small uniform cells in single-layered ducts. A syncytium of tumor cells is characteristic, although solid and cribriform patterns may also be observed. Treatment includes wide surgical excision. Recurrences develop in fewer than 20% of cases. Regional and distant metastases are uncommon, and the prognosis is favorable.

SUGGESTED READINGS

Nonneoplastic salivary gland diseases
General
Daley TD, Lovas JG: Diseases of the salivary glands: a review, *J Can Dent Assoc* 57: 411, 1991.
Sialadenosis
Batsakis JG. Sialadenosis, *Ann Otol Rhinol Laryngol* 97:94, 1988.
Ino C et al: Approach to the diagnosis of sialadenosis using sialography, *Acta Otolaryngol Suppl* 500:121, 1993.
Pape SA et al: Sialadenosis of the salivary glands, *Br J Plast Surg* 48:419, 1995.
Vavrina J, Muller W, Gebbers JO: Enlargement of salivary glands in bulimia, *J Laryngol Otol* 108:516, 1994.
Benign lymphoepithelial lesion and Sjögren's syndrome
Bridges AJ, England DM: Benign lymphoepithelial lesion: relationship to Sjögren's syndrome and evolving malignant lymphoma, *Semin Arthritis Rheum* 19:201, 1989.

Penfold CN: Mikulicz syndrome, *J Oral Maxillofac Surg* 43:900, 1985.
Schiodt M, Thorn J: Criteria for the salivary component of Sjögren's syndrome: a review, *Clin Exp Rheumatol* 7:119, 1989.
Shaha AR et al: Benign lymphoepithelial lesions of the parotid, *Am J Surg* 166:403, 1993.
Adenomatoid hyperplasia of salivary glands
Barrett AW, Speight PM: Adenomatoid hyperplasia of oral minor salivary glands, *Oral Surg Oral Med Oral Pathol Oral Radiol Endod* 79:482, 1995.
Buchner A et al: Adenomatoid hyperplasia of minor salivary glands, *Oral Surg Oral Med Oral Pathol* 71:583, 1991.
Scully C, Eveson JW, Richards A: Adenomatoid hyperplasia in the palate: another sheep in wolf's clothing, *Br Dent J* 173:141, 1992.
Mucocele (mucus retention phenomenon)
Eveson JW: Superficial mucoceles: pitfall in clinical and microscopic diagnosis, *Oral Surg Oral Med Oral Pathol* 66:318, 1988.

Jensen JL: Superficial mucoceles of the oral mucosa, *Am J Dermatopathol* 12:88, 1990.

Toida M, Ishimaru JI, Hobo N: A simple cryosurgical method for treatment of oral mucous cysts, *Int J Oral Maxillofac Surg* 22:353, 1993.

Yamasoba T et al: Clinicostatistical study of lower lip mucoceles, *Head Neck* 12:316, 1990.

Ranula

Baurmash HD: Marsupialization for treatment of oral ranula: a second look at the procedure, *J Oral Maxillofac Surg* 50:1274, 1992.

Crysdale WS, Mendelsohn JD, Conley S: Ranulas mucoceles of the oral cavity: experience in 26 children, *Laryngoscope* 98:296, 1988.

Galloway RH et al: Pathogenesis and treatment of ranula: report of three cases, *J Oral Maxillofac Surg* 47:299, 1989.

Langlois NE, Kolhe P: Plunging ranula: a case report and a literature review, *Hum Pathol* 23:1306, 1992.

Yoshimura Y et al: A comparison of three methods used for treatment of ranula, *J Oral Maxillofac Surg* 53:280, 1995.

Mucus retention cyst (salivary duct cyst)

Bodner L, Tal H: Salivary gland cysts of the oral cavity: clinical observation and surgical management, *Compendium* 12:150, 1991.

Eversole LR: Oral sialocysts, *Arch Otolaryngol* 113:51, 1987.

Praetorius F, Hammarstrom L: A new concept of the pathogenesis of oral mucous cysts based on a study of 200 cases, *J Dent Assoc S Afr* 47:226, 1992.

Sialolithiasis (salivary gland stone)

Bodner L: Salivary gland calculi: diagnostic imaging and surgical management, *Compendium* 14:572, 1993.

Bodner L, Fliss DM: Parotid and submandibular calculi in children, *Int J Pediatr Otorhinolaryngol* 31:35, 1995.

Ho V, Currie WJ, Walker A: Sialolithiasis of minor salivary glands, *Br J Oral Maxillofac Surg* 30:273, 1992.

Lustmann J, Regev E, Melamed Y: Sialolithiasis: a survey on 245 patients and a review of the literature, *Int J Oral Maxillofac Surg* 19:135, 1990.

Nahlieli O, Neder A, Baruchin AM: Salivary gland endoscopy: a new technique for diagnosis and treatment of sialolithiasis, *J Oral Maxillofac Surg* 52:1240, 1994.

Yoshizaki T et al: Clinical evaluation of extracorporeal shock wave lithotripsy for salivary stones, *Ann Otol Rhinol Laryngol* 105:63, 1996.

Zou ZJ et al: Chronic obstructive parotitis: report of ninety-two cases, *Oral Surg Oral Med Oral Pathol* 73:434, 1992.

Sialadenitis

Blitzer A: Inflammatory and obstructive disorders of salivary glands, *J Dent Res* 66:675, 1987.

Johnson A: Inflammatory conditions of the major salivary glands, *Ear Nose Throat J* 68:94, 1989.

Pirisi M et al: Mild sialoadenitis: a common finding in patients with hepatitis C virus infection, *Scand J Gastroenterol* 29:940, 1994.

Werning JT, Waterhouse JP, Mooney JW: Subacute necrotizing sialadenitis, *Oral Surg Oral Med Oral Pathol* 70:756, 1990.

Cheilitis glandularis

Doku HC, Shklar G, McCarthy PL: Cheilitis glandularis, *Oral Surg Oral Med Oral Pathol* 20:563, 1965.

Lederman DA: Suppurative stomatitis glandularis, *Oral Surg Oral Med Oral Pathol* 78:319, 1994.

Rada DC, Koranda FC, Katz FS: Cheilitis glandularis: a disorder of ductal ectasia, *J Dermatol Surg Oncol* 11:372, 1985.

Swerlick RA, Cooper PH: Cheilitis glandularis: a re-evaluation, *J Am Acad Dermatol* 10:466, 1984.

Sialorrhea (ptyalism)

Crysdale WS: Drooling: experience with team assessment and management, *Clin Pediatr* 31:77, 1992.

Finkelstein DM, Crysdale WS: Evaluation and management of the drooling patient, *J Otolaryngol* 21:414, 1992.

Lew KM, Younis RT, Lazar RH: The current management of sialorrhea, *Ear Nose Throat J* 70:99, 1991.

Mandel L, Tamari K: Sialorrhea and gastroesophageal reflux, *J Am Dent Assoc* 126:1537, 1995.

Talmi YP, Finkelstein Y, Zohar Y: Reduction of salivary flow with transdermal scopolamine: a four-year experience, *Otolaryngol Head Neck Surg* 103:615, 1990.

Vasile JS, Steingard S: Clozapine and the development of salivary gland swelling: a case study, *J Clin Psychiatry* 56:511, 1995.

Xerostomia

Atkinson JC, Fox PC: Salivary gland dysfunction, *Clin Geriatr Med* 8:499, 1992.

Atkinson JC, Wu AJ: Salivary gland dysfunction: causes, symptoms, treatment, *J Am Dent Assoc* 125:409, 1994.

Epstein JB, Scully CS: The role of saliva in oral health and the causes and effects of xerostomia, *J Can Dent Assoc* 58:217, 1992.

Epstein JB, Stevenson-Moore P, Scully C: Management of xerostomia, *J Can Dent Assoc* 58:140, 1992.

Ferguson MM: Pilocarpine and other cholinergic drugs in the management of salivary gland dysfunction, *Oral Surg Oral Med Oral Pathol* 75:186, 1993.

Fox PC et al: Pilocarpine treatment of salivary gland hypofunction and dry mouth (xerostomia), *Arch Intern Med* 151:1149, 1991.

Johnson JT et al: Oral pilocarpine for post-irradiation xerostomia in patients with head and neck cancer, *N Engl J Med* 329:390, 1993.

Locker D: Xerostomia in older adults: a longitudinal study, *Gerontology* 12:18, 1995.

Navazesh M, Christensen C, Brightman V: Clinical criteria for the diagnosis of salivary gland hypofunction, *J Dent Res* 71:1363, 1992.

Semba SE, Mealey BL, Hallmon WW: The head and neck radiotherapy patient: Part 1. Oral manifestations of radiation therapy, *Compendium* 15:250, 1994.

Smith RG, Burtner AP: Oral side-effects of the most frequently prescribed drugs, *Spec Care Dentist* 14:96, 1994.

van der Reijden WA et al: Treatment of xerostomia with polymer-based saliva substitutes in patients with Sjögren's syndrome, *Arthritis Rheum* 6:57, 1996.

Wiseman LR, Faulds D: Oral pilocarpine: a review of its pharmacological properties and clinical potential in xerostomia, *Drugs* 49:143, 1995.

Necrotizing sialometaplasia

Brannon RB, Fowler CB, Hartman KS: Necrotizing sialometaplasia: a clinicopathologic study of sixty-nine cases and review of the literature, *Oral Surg Oral Med Oral Pathol* 72:317, 1991.

Jainkittivong A, Sookasam M, Philipsen HP: Necrotizing sialometaplasia: review of 127 cases, *J Dent Assoc Thai* 39:11, 1989.

Lynch DP, Crago CR, Martinez MG: Necrotizing sialometaplasia: a review of the literature and report of two additional cases, *Oral Surg Oral Med Oral Pathol* 47:63, 1979.

Mesa ML, Gertler RS, Schneider LC: Necrotizing sialometaplasia: frequency of histologic misdiagnosis, *Oral Surg Oral Med Oral Pathol* 57:71, 1984.

van der Wal JE, van der Waal I: Necrotizing sialometaplasia: report of 12 new cases, *Br J Oral Maxillofac Surg* 28:326, 1990.

Neoplastic salivary gland diseases

General

Beckhardt RN et al: Minor salivary gland tumors of the palate: clinical and pathologic correlates of outcome, *Laryngoscope* 105:1155, 1995.

Chidzonga MM, Lopez Perez VM, Portilla Alvarez AL: A clinicopathologic study of parotid gland tumors, *J Oral Maxillofac Surg* 52:1253, 1994.

Cramer H, Lampe H, Downing P: Intraoral and transoral fine needle aspiration: a review of 25 cases, *Acta Cytol* 39:683, 1995.

Ellis GL, Auclair PL, Gnepp DR: *Surgical pathology of the salivary glands,* Philadelphia, 1991, WB Saunders.

Eveson JW, Cawson RA: Salivary gland tumours: a review of 2410 cases with particular reference to histological types, site, age, and sex distribution, *J Pathol* 146:51, 1985.

Eveson JW, Cawson RA: Tumours of the minor (oropharyngeal) salivary glands: a demographic study of 336 cases, *J Oral Pathol* 14:500, 1985.

Illes RW, Brian MB: A review of the tumors of the salivary gland, *Surg Gynecol Obstet* 163:399, 1986.

Neville BW et al: Labial salivary gland tumors, *Cancer* 61:2113, 1988.

Ogata H, Ebihara S, Mukai K: Salivary gland neoplasms in children, *Jpn J Clin Oncol* 24:88, 1994.

Seifert G et al: WHO International Histological Classification of Tumours. Tentative Histological Classification of Salivary Gland Tumours, *Pathol Res Pract* 186:555, 1990.

Spiro RH: Salivary neoplasms: overview of a thirty-five year experience with 2,807 patients, *Head Neck Surg* 8:177, 1986.

Waldron CA, el Mofty SK, Gnepp DR: Tumors of the intraoral minor salivary glands: a demographic and histologic study of 426 cases, *Oral Surg Oral Med Oral Pathol* 66:323, 1988.

Benign salivary gland neoplasms

Abrams AM, Finck FM: Sialadenoma papilliferum: a previously unreported salivary gland tumor, *Cancer* 24:1057, 1969.

Batsakis JG, Luna MA, el Naggar AK: Basaloid monomorphic adenomas, *Ann Otol Rhinol Laryngol* 100:687, 1991.

Brandwein MS, Huvos AG: Oncocytic tumors of major salivary glands: a study of 68 cases with follow-up of 44 patients, *Am J Surg Pathol* 15:514, 1991.

Chau MNY, Radden BG: A clinical-pathological study of 53 intra-oral pleomorphic adenomas, *Int J Oral Maxillofac Surg* 18:158, 1989.

Chidzonga MM, Lopez Perez VM, Portilla Alvarez AL: Pleomorphic adenoma of the salivary glands: clinicopathologic study of 206 cases in Zimbabwe, *Oral Surg Oral Med Oral Pathol Oral Radiol Endod* 79:747, 1995.

Cleary KR, Batsakis JG: Sialadenoma papilliferum, *Ann Otol Rhinol Laryngol* 99:756, 1990.

Daley TD: The canalicular adenoma: considerations on differential diagnosis and treatment, *J Oral Maxillofac Surg* 42:728, 1984.

Daley TD, Gardner DG, Smout MS: Canalicular adenoma: not a basal cell adenoma, *Oral Surg Oral Med Oral Pathol* 57:181, 1984.

Damm DD et al: Benign solid oncocytoma of intraoral minor salivary glands, *Oral Surg Oral Med Oral Pathol* 67:84, 1989.

Dietert SE: Papillary cystadenoma lymphomatosum (Warthin's tumor) in patients in a general hospital over a 24-year period, *Am J Clin Pathol* 63:866, 1975.

Ellis GL, Wiskovitch JG: Basal cell adenocarcinomas of the major salivary glands, *Oral Surg Oral Med Oral Pathol* 69:461, 1990.

Fantasia JE, Miller AS: Papillary cystadenoma lymphomatosum arising in minor salivary glands, *Oral Surg Oral Med Oral Pathol* 52:411, 1981.

Fantasia JE, Neville BW: Basal cell adenomas of the minor salivary glands, *Oral Surg Oral Med Oral Pathol* 50:433, 1980.

Gardner DG, Daley D: The use of the terms monomorphic adenoma, basal cell adenoma, and canalicular adenoma as applied to salivary gland tumors, *Oral Surg Oral Med Oral Pathol* 56:608, 1983.

Goode RK, Corio RL: Oncocytic adenocarcinoma of salivary glands, *Oral Surg Oral Med Oral Pathol* 65:61, 1988.

Hegarty DJ, Hopper C, Speight PM: Inverted ductal papilloma of minor salivary glands, *J Oral Pathol Med* 23:334, 1994.

Maurizi M et al: Monomorphic adenomas of the major salivary glands: clinicopathological study of 44 cases, *J Laryngol Otol* 104:790, 1990.

Maynard JD: Management of pleomorphic adenoma of the parotid, *Br J Surg* 75:305, 1988.

Myssiorek D, Ruah CB, Hybels RL: Recurrent pleomorphic adenomas of the parotid glands, *Head Neck* 12:332, 1990.

Nagao K et al: Histopathologic studies of basal cell adenoma of the parotid gland, *Cancer* 50:736, 1982.

Nelson JF, Jacoway JR: Monomorphic adenoma (canalicular type): report of 29 cases, *Cancer* 31:1151, 1973.

Palmer TJ et al: Oncocytic adenomas and oncocytic hyperplasia of salivary glands: a clinicopathological study of 26 cases, *Histopathology* 16:487, 1990.

Phillips PP, Olsen KD: Recurrent pleomorphic adenoma of the parotid gland: report of 126 cases and a review of the literature, *Ann Otol Rhinol Laryngol* 104:100, 1995.

van der Wal JE, Davids JJ, van der Waal I: Extraparotid Warthin's tumours: report of 10 cases, *Br J Oral Maxillofac Surg* 31:43, 1993.

van der Wal JE, van der Waal I: The rare sialadenoma papilliferum: report of a case and review of the literature, *Int J Oral Maxillofac Surg* 21:104, 1992.

White DK et al: Inverted ductal papilloma: a distinctive lesion of minor salivary gland, *Cancer* 49:519, 1982.

Zappia JJ, Sullivan MJ, McClatchey KD: Unilateral multicentric Warthin's tumors, *J Otolaryngol* 20:93, 1991.

Malignant salivary gland neoplasms

Auclair PL, Goode RK, Ellis GL: Mucoepidermoid carcinoma of intraoral salivary glands, *Cancer* 69:2021, 1992.

Barnes L et al: Salivary duct carcinoma. Part I. A clinicopathologic evaluation and DNA image analysis of 13 cases with review of the literature, *Oral Surg Oral Med Oral Pathol* 78:64, 1994.

Batsakis JG, Luna MA: Histopathologic grading of salivary gland neoplasms. I. Mucoepidermoid carcinomas, *Ann Otol Rhinol Laryngol* 99:835, 1990.

Brookstone MS, Huvos AG: Central salivary gland tumors of the maxilla and mandible: a clinicopathologic study of 11 cases with an analysis of the literature, *J Oral Maxillofac Surg* 50:229, 1992.

Chou C et al: Carcinoma of the minor salivary glands: results of surgery and combined therapy, *J Oral Maxillofac Surg* 54:448, 1996.

de Vries EJ et al: Base of tongue salivary gland tumors, *Head Neck Surg* 9:329, 1987.

Eneroth CM: Salivary tumors in the parotid gland, submandibular gland, and the palate region, *Cancer* 27:1415, 1971.

Epivatianos A, Dimitrakopoulos J, Trigonidis G: Intraoral salivary duct carcinoma: a clinicopathological study of four cases and review of the literature, *Ann Dent* 54:36, 1995.

Hicks MJ et al: Prognostic factors in mucoepidermoid carcinomas of major salivary glands: a clinicopathologic and flow cytometric study, *Eur J Cancer B Oral Oncol* 30: 329, 1994.

Hunter RM et al: Primary malignant tumors of salivary gland origin: a 52-year review, *Am Surg* 49:82, 1983.

Lack EE, Upton MP: Histopathologic review of salivary gland tumors in childhood, *Arch Otolaryngol Head Neck Surg* 114:898, 1988.

Shikhani AH, Johns ME: Tumors of the major salivary glands in children, *Head Neck Surg* 10:257, 1988.

Spiro RH et al: Mucoepidermoid carcinoma of salivary gland origin: a clinicopathologic study of 367 cases, *Am J Surg* 136:461, 1978.

Adenoid cystic carcinoma (cylindroma)

Batsakis JG, Luna MA, el Naggar A: Histopathologic grading of salivary gland neoplasms. III. Adenoid cystic carcinomas, *Ann Otol Rhinol Laryngol* 99:1007, 1990.

Hamper K et al: Prognostic factors for adenoid cystic carcinoma of the head and neck: a retrospective evaluation of 96 cases, *J Oral Pathol Med* 19:101, 1990.

Kuhel WI et al: Elevated carcinoembryonic antigen levels correlating with disease recurrence in a patient with adenoid cystic carcinoma, *Head Neck* 17:431, 1995.

Matsuba HM et al: Adenoid cystic salivary gland carcinoma: a clinicopathologic correlation, *Head Neck Surg* 8:200, 1986.

Shick PC, Riordan GP, Foss RD: Estrogen and progesterone receptors in salivary gland adenoid cystic carcinoma, *Oral Surg Oral Med Oral Pathol* 80:440, 1995.

van der Wal JE, van der Waal I: Intraoral adenoid cystic carcinoma: the presence of perineural spread in relation to site, size, local extension, and metastatic spread in 22 cases, *Cancer* 66:2031, 1990.

Malignant mixed tumor (carcinoma ex pleomorphic adenoma, carcinosarcoma, and metastasizing mixed tumor)

Garner SL et al: Salivary gland carcinosarcoma: true malignant mixed tumor, *Ann Otol Rhinol Laryngol* 98:611, 1989.

LiVolsi VA, Perzin KH: Malignant mixed tumors arising in salivary glands. I. Carcinomas arising in benign mixed tumor: a clinicopathologic study, *Cancer* 39:2209, 1977.

Righi PD et al: The role of p53 gene in the malignant transformation of pleomorphic adenomas of the parotid gland, *Anticancer Res* 14:2253, 1994.

Stephen J et al: True malignant mixed tumors (carcinosarcoma) of salivary glands, *Oral Surg Oral Med Oral Pathol* 61:597, 1986.

Takeda Y: True malignant mixed tumor (carcinosarcoma) of palatal minor salivary gland origin, *Ann Dent* 50:33, 1991.

Tortoledo ME, Luna MA, Batsakis JG: Carcinomas ex pleomorphic adenoma and malignant mixed tumors, *Arch Otolaryngol* 110:172, 1984.

Acinic cell carcinoma (acinic cell tumor)

Anavi Y et al: Intraoral acinic cell carcinoma, *Ann Dent* 52:26, 1993.

Batsakis JG, Luna MA, el Naggar AK: Histopathologic grading of salivary gland neoplasms. II. Acinic cell carcinomas, *Ann Otol Rhinol Laryngol* 99:929, 1990.

Colmenero C, Patron M, Sierra I: Acinic cell carcinoma of the salivary glands: a review of 20 new cases, *J Craniomaxillofac Surg* 19:260, 1991.

Ellis GL, Corio RL: Acinic cell adenocarcinoma: a clinicopathologic analysis of 294 cases, *Cancer* 52:542, 1983.

Lewis JE, Olsen KD, Weiland LH: Acinic cell carcinoma: clinicopathologic review, *Cancer* 67:172, 1991.

Timon CI et al: Clinico-pathological predictors of recurrence for acinic cell carcinoma, *Clin Otolaryngol* 20:396, 1995.

Zbaeren P, Lehmann W, Widgren S: Acinic cell carcinoma of minor salivary gland origin, *J Laryngol Otol* 105:782, 1991.

Polymorphous low-grade adenocarcinoma (terminal duct carcinoma)

Aberle AM et al: Lobular (polymorphous low-grade) carcinoma of minor salivary gland: a clinicopathologic study of 20 cases, *Oral Surg Oral Med Oral Pathol* 60:387, 1985.

Anderson C et al: Polymorphous low grade adenocarcinoma of minor salivary gland: a clinicopathologic and comparative immunohistochemical study, *Mod Pathol* 3:76, 1990.

Colmenero CM et al: Polymorphous low-grade adenocarcinoma of the oral cavity: a report of 14 cases, *J Oral Maxillofac Surg* 50:595, 1992.

Levine SB, Potsic WP: The need for clinical awareness of polymorphous low-grade adenocarcinoma: a review, *J Otolaryngol* 21:149, 1992.

Vincent SD, Hammond HL, Finkelstein MW: Clinical and therapeutic features of polymorphous low-grade adenocarcinoma, *Oral Surg Oral Med Oral Pathol* 77:41, 1994.

Therapy of Oral Diseases

GENERAL PRINCIPLES

The identification and treatment of oral manifestations of systemic diseases require close collaboration with appropriate medical and dental specialists in the fields of dermatology, infectious disease, rheumatology, endocrinology, and hematology, as well as the dental specialties of oral and maxillofacial pathology, oral and maxillofacial surgery, and periodontology. For example, the recognition of oral manifestations of systemic malignancy in patients with Cowden disease or multiple endocrine neoplasia should prompt a referral to a genetic clinic for counseling and to an internist for a complete general evaluation. Likewise, the therapy of oral cancers requires a team approach in which the team consists of a surgeon, medical oncologist, radiation oncologist, and dentist.

After a definitive diagnosis has been established, appropriate therapy should be instituted by practitioners who are most skilled in that particular aspect of patient care. The comprehensive treatment of oral diseases, however, often requires a multidisciplinary approach to achieve maximum therapeutic benefit. For example, many of the vesiculoerosive diseases involve cutaneous manifestations that require treatment with systemic immunosuppressant agents most appropriately prescribed by dermatologists. Because the status of patients' oral hygiene, especially gingival health, is significantly influenced by these diseases, the dentist must also be actively involved in the treatment of their oral manifestations. Additionally, consultation with gynecologists and ophthalmologists is often required because these diseases frequently involve the genital and ocular mucosa. Although small oral neoplasms may be surgically excised by most dentists and physicians, large lesions should be referred to oral and maxillofacial surgeons or otolaryngologists who are most proficient in these complicated procedures.

Regardless of the clinical acuity of the practitioner and the ability to arrive at a presumptive diagnosis, the accuracy of histopathologic interpretation of oral biopsy specimens is paramount in the identification of oral abnormalities. Therefore oral specimens should preferentially be interpreted by oral and maxillofacial pathologists and the microscopic findings correlated with the clinical features of the disease.

TREATMENT OF ORAL PAIN

The oral mucosa, in addition to providing a protective barrier, provides significant neurosensory input. The diverse number of receptors in the oral cavity for touch, pain, pressure, and temperature illustrates the various sensations that may be perceived.

Of these, oral discomfort is most often associated with significant anxiety and morbidity, as reflected by the adverse effects on normal oral functions. Oral pain may result from a myriad of causes including infection, neoplasia, trauma, and inflammation. Appropriate management depends on identifying the underlying cause.

Nonopioid Analgesics

Regardless of the cause, the sensation of oral pain results from the liberation of one or more biochemical mediators including histamine, bradykinin, and various prostaglandins. The vast majority of peripherally acting analgesics such as aspirin act as cyclooxygenase inhibitors to prevent the production of prostaglandins. In double-blind controlled studies, two aspirin tablets (650 mg) were shown to be as effective as 60 mg of codeine in alleviating pain after third molar extraction. In addition to its analgesic effects, aspirin possesses potent antiinflammatory and antipyretic properties, which may be beneficial in the treatment of inflammatory oral diseases.

The efficacy of acetaminophen in controlling oral pain is equivalent to aspirin. Although acetaminophen also functions as a cyclooxygenase inhibitor, its antiinflammatory effects are significantly less than those of aspirin. Whereas aspirin exerts its maximum therapeutic efficacy at doses of 650 mg, an increasing level of analgesia may be achieved with acetaminophen in doses up to 1000 mg.

Alternatives to aspirin and acetaminophen include phenylpropionic acid derivatives such as ibuprofen and sodium naproxen. Both ibuprofen (600 mg every 4 hours) and sodium naproxen (550 mg loading dose followed by 275 mg every 6 hours) appear to be superior in controlling oral pain when compared with aspirin (650 mg), even when supplemented with codeine (60 mg). Other phenylpropionic acid derivatives have essentially equivalent analgesic properties.

Diflunisal, administered as a loading dose of 1000 mg followed by 500 mg every 8 to 12 hours, is another nonsteroidal agent that may be used in the management of oral pain. Advantages include an extended period of analgesia that may last up to 12 hours. Anthranilic acid derivatives such as sodium meclofenamate (100 mg every 6 hours) and mefenamic acid (500 mg loading dose followed by 250 mg every 6 hours) may also be used as analgesics for oral discomfort. Both exert greater analgesic effects than therapeutic doses of either aspirin or acetaminophen with codeine.

Opioid Analgesics

Severe dental and oral pain may require the use of opioid analgesics, either alone or in combination with peripherally acting nonopioid analgesics. Agents most commonly used for oral pain include codeine, oxycodone, propoxyphene, and pentazocine. Because these drugs do not possess antiinflammatory effects, they are frequently combined with aspirin or other peripherally acting analgesic agents.

Palliative Therapy

Topical agents are frequently used for the sole purpose of alleviating oral discomfort even though they are largely ineffective in modifying the underlying disease process. A variety of topical anesthetics that are available by prescription and over the counter (OTC) can be used effectively. Lidocaine viscous (2% to 10%) is beneficial for rapid pain relief of both localized and widespread oral ulcerations, but the effects, as with all topical anesthetics, are short-lived. Patients should be advised to apply topical lidocaine using a cotton-tipped applicator and maintain contact of the lidocaine with the mucosa for at least 1 minute. Patients using lidocaine viscous or spray as a mouth rinse should be cautioned to expectorate the medication as thoroughly as possible to prevent anesthesia of the pharynx, which may result in difficulty with breathing and deglutition. Prolonged use in patients with extensive inflammation and ulcerations may result in increased absorption and potential systemic toxicity.

Benzocaine 20% and dyclonine 1% are topical anesthetic agents that temporarily relieve oral pain and are incorporated into a number of OTC medications. Both diphenhydramine elixir and promethazine syrup possess topical anesthetic properties, although promethazine is only available by prescription. Commonly, these and other anesthetics and antiinflammatory agents such as corticosteroid solutions and antibiotics are mixed in varying proportions and used as mouth rinses. Kaopectate, Milk of Magnesia, and solutions of sucralfate (Carafate) may be used as bases for these mixtures because they provide a coating barrier for the mucosa. Medications that can be applied in top-

Table 15-1   Selected Agents for the Palliation of Oral Mucosal Pain

MEDICATION	FORMULATION	COMMENTS
Benzocaine	6.3% liquid 20% gels and ointments	OTC products in various forms (Zilactin-B, Orajel Mouth-Aid, Tanac No Sting)
Benzyl alcohol	10% gel	OTC analgesic (Zilactin Medicated Gel)
Carbamide peroxide	10%-15% liquid	OTC wound healing promoter (Gly-Oxide, Orajel Perioseptic Liquid)
Capsaicin	0.25% cream	Prescription analgesic (Zostrix), use sparingly, may result in severe burning
Dexamethasone	Elixir (0.5 mg/5ml)	Prescription corticosteroid (Decadron), used alone both topically and systemically, used topically mixed with other agents
Diphenhydramine	Elixir (12.5 mg/5 ml)	OTC antihistamine (Benadryl), topical anesthetic effects, mixed with other agents (e.g., Milk of Magnesia)
	1.25% ointment	OTC topical analgesic (Mouthkote Ointment)
Dyclonine	0.5%-1% solution	Prescription anesthetic (Dyclone)
Hydrocortisone	1%-2.5% suspension	Prescription corticosteroid (Solu-Cortef), mixed with other agents (Miles mixture)
Lidocaine	2% viscous 2.5%-5% ointment 4% solution 10% spray	Prescription anesthetic (Xylocaine), OTC when mixed with other agents (Zilactin-L)
Promethazine	Syrup (6.25 mg/ml)	Prescription antiemetic (Phenergan), topical anesthetic effects, mixed with other agents (e.g., Kaopectate)
Tetracaine	2% spray with 14% benzocaine	Prescription anesthetic (Cetacaine)
Tetracycline	Suspension (250 mg/5 ml)	Antibiotic (Sumycin), antiinflammatory action, mixed with other agents (Miles mixture)
Triamcinolone	Suspension (10 mg/ml)	Prescription corticosteroid (Kenalog-10), intralesional injection, mixed with other agents (Kenalog in Orabase)

OTC, Over the counter.

ical form to oral mucous membranes may also be incorporated into occlusive dressings such as Orabase and Zilactin. One of the most common extemporaneously compounded mouth rinses known as Miles mixture (typically consisting of tetracycline [1 g], hydrocortisone [20 mg], and nystatin [2 million U] in 4 oz of water or diphenhydramine elixir) has many ingredient variations and palliative uses. Stability and efficacy of this product and similar concoctions have not been carefully evaluated, but adverse effects are equally uncommon. Topical agents used in commercial products or incorporated into mouth rinse formulations are outlined in Table 15-1, and selected bases for these formulations are listed in Table 15-2.

Table 15-2   Rinses, Therapeutic Bases, and Occlusive Dressings

AGENTS	COMMENTS
Kaopectate	Mix with other analgesics and antiinflammatory agents, oral rinse that coats mucosa
Milk of Magnesia	Mix with other analgesics and antiinflammatory agents, oral rinse that coats mucosa
Orabase	May be used alone as an occlusive dressing or as a base for the incorporation of corticosteroids and analgesics
Sucralfate suspension (1 gm/10cc)	May be used alone or mixed with other agents, oral rinse that coats mucosa
Zilactin and Zilactin-B	May be used alone as an occlusive dressing or to occlude mucosa after application of corticosteroids and analgesics

Occlusive Dressings

A variety of occlusive OTC dressings may be of value for patients with vesiculoerosive diseases of the mouth such as recurrent aphthous stomatitis. For example, Orabase and Zilactin act as oral mucosal occlusive dressings that may be used alone, formulated, or in combination with topical anesthetics and antiinflammatory agents. In addition to providing a protective barrier between ulcerated mucosa and the oral environment, these occlusive dressings help sustain high levels of active agents such as corticosteroids at the site of application.

TOPICAL TREATMENT OF INFLAMMATORY ORAL DISEASES

Corticosteroids

Topical corticosteroids remain the most effective and frequently used form of therapy for inflammatory and erosive diseases affecting the oral mucosa. With the exception of triamcinolone acetonide, which is marketed for use in the oral cavity, all topical corticosteroids used in the treatment of inflammatory oral mucosal diseases are manufactured and approved by the Food and Drug Administration for cutaneous application. Nevertheless, their widespread use in the treatment of oral inflammatory and vesiculoerosive conditions and lack of adverse effects confirm the therapeutic benefits and margin of safety of such medications. In general, intermediate strength corticosteroids such as fluocinonide (Lidex) are the drugs of first choice for active vesiculoerosive disease; however, superpotent topical preparations such as clobetasol propionate (Temovate) and halobetasol propionate (Ultravate) can be used initially for more severe disease. Patients with erosive lichen planus, recurrent aphthous stomatitis, pemphigus, pemphigoid, erythema multiforme, lupus erythematosus, linear IgA disease, and other potentially painful oral diseases benefit from topical corticosteroids, even when systemic therapy is administered concomitantly.

Ointments cause the least irritation when compared with other topical delivery preparations but adhere poorly to the oral mucosa. Creams and gels taste bitter and may burn on contact with irritated mucosa but are generally well tolerated. Corticosteroid inhalers intended for the treatment of asthma may be used when widespread oral disease is present.

Patients should be instructed to apply topical corticosteroids to involved areas using a finger cot or a cotton-tipped applicator, gently massage the medication into the affected mucosa if possible, and maintain contact of the preparation with the mucosa for at least 30 seconds. To maximize efficacy, patients should not eat or drink for 30 minutes after application of the medication and should reapply it several times daily. When inflammatory and vesiculoerosive diseases result in a desquamative gingivitis characterized by erythema and ulcerations of the gingiva, the use of a custom-fabricated vinyl appliance as a means of delivering and occluding the topical corticosteroid against the gingiva greatly increases the efficacy of the topical preparation.

Atrophy, commonly observed in skin exposed to prolonged use of potent topical corticosteroids, rarely occurs in the mouth. Systemic absorption resulting in hypothalamic-pituitary-adrenal axis suppression is of concern when potent topical corticosteroids are administered chronically to mucous membranes. Therefore when patients who have been prescribed superpotent topical steroids for severe oral disease improve and the mucosal erythema and erosions resolve, a weaker preparation such as triamcinolone acetonide or fluocinonide acetonide should be substituted. These less-potent corticosteroids may also be administered as initial agents when the disease is of mild or moderate severity. Therapy should be temporarily discontinued when the disease is inactive and should not be prescribed prophylactically.

Topical corticosteroids may result in secondary candidal infections when applied in the oral cavity. Antifungal therapy with either topical or systemic medications may be administered empirically and intermittently during chronic corticosteroid treatment, or candidiasis may be monitored by repeated cultures and treated when identified.

Intralesional corticosteroid injection using 0.5 ml of triamcinolone acetonide suspension, 10 mg/ml, (Kenalog-10), often results in rapid resolution of inflammatory oral ulcers. This procedure may be repeated every 3 to 4 weeks as necessary.

Antibiotics

Topical antibiotics may be of value in the treatment of recurrent aphthous ulcerations by inhibiting bacterial colonization or by their antiinflammatory properties. Tetracycline inhibits collagenase activity, and rinses with a suspension of tetracycline may alleviate the discomfort caused by recurrent aphthae. The contents of a 250-mg capsule of tetracycline may be dissolved in a cup of water and swished and expectorated several times a day. More concentrated solutions may be made, but to avoid cosmetic staining of the teeth, the solution should be applied directly to the ulceration with gauze or a cotton-tipped applicator. Prolonged contact of the antibiotic with the mucosa appears to improve efficacy. Erythromycin and cephalexin have been used in a similar fashion with some success.

Retinoids

Topical preparations using tretinoin (Retin-A) as a 0.01% gel or as a 0.1% cream have been reported to improve oral lichen planus, although their use is based on results from a small number of studies and patients. When administered, retinoids should be alternated with topical corticosteroids to minimize the irritation that commonly results when these preparations are used in the mouth. Gingival lesions seem to respond most favorably, whereas erosive lesions on the buccal mucosa are often paradoxically worsened by the use of tretinoin. Retinoids do not appear to be of any significant value in the treatment of any of the other vesiculoerosive diseases.

Cyclosporine

Although used as a potent systemic immunosuppressant for patients undergoing organ transplantation, cyclosporine (Sandimmune), 100 mg/ml, has been demonstrated in open and double-blind studies as an effective oral rinse to treat erosive oral lichen planus. Patients should hold 2 to 5 ml of the undiluted solution in their mouth for approximately 5 minutes and then expectorate. As with all other topical preparations used in the mouth, eating and drinking should be avoided for at least 30 minutes after use. The medication should be administered three times a day and the regimen maintained for 8 weeks or longer, depending on the response.

Large and thus expensive volumes of cyclosporine are needed to achieve a clinical response. The high cost of cyclosporine has limited its long-term use for chronic oral diseases such as lichen planus. To maximize savings, topical corticosteroids, which greatly hasten resolution of erythema and ulcerations, can be used concomitantly. Abnormal laboratory studies have not been reported in patients using cyclosporine solution as an oral rinse in the treatment of oral mucosal lichen planus, even when cyclosporine blood levels were detectable by high performance liquid chromatography. Topical cyclosporine may also be used as a mouthwash in patients with oral chronic graft-versus-host (GVH) disease and may be useful as an adjuvant therapy for patients with oral pemphigus and pemphigoid.

SYSTEMIC TREATMENT OF INFLAMMATORY ORAL DISEASES

A large number of antiinflammatory, immunosuppressive, and cytotoxic agents have been identified as being effective in the treatment of a variety of oral diseases. Their use has achieved great importance, primarily in alleviating inflammatory and erosive diseases. Such drugs control rather than cure these disease processes, thus chronic administration or intermittent dosing for exacerbations is required to attain benefits. Topical therapy with the same or a complementary drug should always be instituted simultaneously in an attempt to minimize the dose of the systemic agent and hasten clinical improvement. All of these agents should be used judiciously, with careful consideration of the risk/benefit ratio in all cases. Acute and chronic toxicities of these drugs necessitate careful monitoring by practitioners familiar with their adverse effects. Topical and systemic therapeutic agents used in the treatment of the oral vesiculoerosive diseases are summarized in Table 15-3.

Corticosteroids

The administration of systemic corticosteroids generally produces the most rapid response in patients with oral vesiculoerosive diseases. Disorders such as lichen planus should be treated with short courses of corticosteroids and only during periods of acute exacerbation that do not respond to topical therapy. Uninterrupted administration of systemic corticosteroids for this chronic disorder is limited by drug toxicity. Daily prednisone doses of 40 to 60 mg are sufficient to control most flare-ups; however, higher doses may be necessary. Similarly, acute and limited reactive processes in the oral cavity, such as contact stomatitis and erythema multiforme, respond equally well to this regimen.

In contrast, the more severe oral eruptions such as pemphigus, cicatricial pemphigoid, and linear IgA disease usually require higher doses and chronic administration of prednisone often combined with other systemic agents. Corticosteroid-sparing agents, including dapsone for cicatricial pemphigoid and linear IgA disease and azathioprine for pemphigus and cicatricial pemphigoid, should be considered when the disease is severe or necessitates chronic corticosteroid use for maintaining remission. Alternate day therapy of corticosteroids, which minimizes deleterious side effects, is usually effective for most of the oral erosive diseases that require chronic administration. As with topical corticosteroids, the chronic administration of prednisone predisposes patients toward secondary oral candidiasis.

Dapsone

Dapsone, a sulfone drug normally prescribed for the primary treatment of dermatitis herpetiformis and as an antibacterial drug for leprosy, possesses potent antiinflammatory effects. The mechanism of action of dapsone is, in part, caused by its inhibition of neutrophil migration, which accounts for its benefit in the treatment of a variety of inflammatory oral diseases. Dapsone is an effective agent in patients with cicatricial pemphigoid and linear IgA disease and should be used when topical agents are ineffective in achieving resolution of the inflammation. Although its use in oral lichen planus has been reported, its value appears limited for this disorder. Patients with oral manifestations of Behçet's

Table 15-3   Treatment of Vesiculoerosive Diseases of the Oral Mucosa

DISEASES	RECOMMENDED THERAPEUTIC AGENTS
Recurrent aphthous stomatitis, Behçet's disease, other disorders with aphthae	Palliative agents: mouth rinses and occlusive dressings (see Tables 15-1 and 15-2) Topical corticosteroids: clobetasol (Temovate), halobetasol (Ultravate), betamethasone (Diprolene), fluocinonide (Lidex), triamcinolone (Aristocort) Systemic therapy: colchicine 0.6 mg 2-3 times per day, dapsone 50-150 mg/day, pentoxifylline 400 mg 3 times per day, thalidomide 100-200 mg/day, prednisone 20-60 mg/day
Lichen planus	Topical therapy: corticosteroids (as above), cyclosporine rinse 100 mg/ml, 2-3 times per day, tretinoin cream 0.1% or gel 0.01% in combination with topical corticosteroids Intralesional injection: triamcinolone 4-10 mg Systemic therapy: prednisone 40-80 mg/day for exacerbations, hydroxychloroquine 200-400 mg/day, etretinate 25-75 mg/day, azathioprine 50-100 mg/day, cyclosporine 2 mg/kg/day.
Pemphigoid and related disorders	Topical corticosteroids: clobetasol (Temovate), fluocinonide (Lidex) for mild cases Intralesional injection: triamcinolone 4-10 mg Systemic therapy: prednisone 40-80 mg/day, dapsone 50-150 mg/day, azathioprine 50-150 mg/day, cyclophosphamide 50-100 mg/day for severe cases
Pemphigus and related disorders	Topical corticosteroids: clobetasol (Temovate), halobetasol (Ultravate), betamethasone (Diprolene), fluocinonide (Lidex), triamcinolone (Aristocort) Intralesional injection: triamcinolone 4-10 mg Systemic therapy: prednisone 60-200 mg/day, azathioprine 50-200 mg/day, cyclophosphamide 50-100 mg/day, dapsone 100-200 mg/day, methotrexate 10-30 mg/wk, cyclosporine 4-6 mg/kg/day, gold sodium thiomalate 50 mg/wk IM, methylprednisolone 1 g/day IV

IM, Intramuscularly; *IV,* intravenously.

disease or recurrent aphthous stomatitis who suffer with continuous exacerbations often achieve partial or complete remission with sustained dapsone therapy. For oral diseases, daily doses of 50 to 150 mg are normally required to achieve clinical improvement. The dosage may be altered according to the severity of the disease. All patients taking dapsone require monitoring for hemolysis and methemoglobinemia, as well as for other adverse effects.

Colchicine

Colchicine, indicated for the treatment of gout, has a wide spectrum of antiinflammatory actions in disorders characterized by the accumulation of polymorphonuclear leukocytes. Its therapeutic benefit for the mucocutaneous manifestations of Behçet's disease is well known. Its efficacy in the suppression of acute attacks in patients with recurrent aphthous stomatitis has been repeatedly reported but not firmly established. Fewer than one half of patients with recurrent aphthous stomatitis can be expected to respond to colchicine. Patients with epidermolysis bullosa acquisita also respond favorably to colchicine. For oral diseases, doses of 0.6 mg may be administered two to three times a day, although gastrointestinal disturbances, most notably diarrhea, often limit its use. Prolonged administration may also result in bone marrow suppression, which necessitates hematologic monitoring.

Azathioprine

Azathioprine is an immunosuppressive antimetabolite that is one of the agents most commonly used in the treatment of the mucocutaneous blistering diseases. Its use for oral pemphigus and cicatricial pemphigoid is well established, especially when combined with systemic corticosteroids. The onset of action of azathioprine is slow, and clinical improvement may continue over months. For this reason the drug is unsuitable for acute exacerbations and should be initiated early in the course of the disease. When combined with corticosteroids, azathioprine has a significant steroid-sparing effect, reducing the steroid dose required for the induction and maintenance of remission. Patients with oral erosive lichen planus who are unresponsive to topical or other systemic agents often respond well to azathioprine. In fact, all of the oral erosive diseases, including severe cases of aphthous stomatitis, can be managed successfully with azathioprine. The drug has many potential acute and chronic toxicities, predominantly resulting from bone marrow suppression. These may be minimized by maintaining the dose under 150 mg/day and limiting its long-term use. In any event, cautious and continuous monitoring is mandatory.

Retinoids

The use of systemic retinoids for oral lichen planus is controversial. Etretinate, indicated for recalcitrant psoriasis, has demonstrated effectiveness in oral lichen planus in open and double-blind studies. Not all studies, however, support its use. Generally, daily doses of 50 to 75 mg are required to achieve clinical improvement. Erosions may take several months to heal, or they may never resolve with etretinate alone. Therefore topical corticosteroids should be applied concomitantly to obtain a more rapid and effective response. As patients improve, the dose should be lowered in an attempt to minimize toxicity. As with other therapies for lichen planus, recurrences are common after discontinuation of the medication. Because of its teratogenic potential, etretinate is contraindicated in women of childbearing potential and laboratory monitoring of all patients is required.

Miscellaneous Systemic Therapeutic Agents

Case reports and anecdotal evidence support the use of several systemic agents for a variety of oral inflammatory diseases. Hydroxychloroquine at daily doses of 200 to 400 mg administered for 6 months may improve oral lichen planus and oral lupus erythematosus. Erosions resolve slowly and patients tolerate the medication well with few adverse effects. Ophthalmologic examinations are required for patients who are maintained on chronic therapy; laboratory monitoring is also necessary.

The administration of 2 g each of tetracycline and nicotinamide may be used as alternatives to immunosuppressant therapy in patients with cicatricial pemphigoid and pemphigus vulgaris. Although this regimen has been demonstrated to be of value predominantly for cutaneous lesions, anecdotal evidence supports the use of these two drugs in the management of the oral manifestations of these diseases.

Systemic cyclosporine may be effective for many of the oral vesiculoerosive diseases. Patients with oral erosive lichen planus respond to low doses of 1 to 2 mg/kg/day, whereas patients with more severe disorders such as pemphigus, Behçet's disease, epidermolysis bullosa acquisita, and GVH disease require much higher doses, often in combination with other systemic agents. After the disease is controlled, the regimen should be substituted with a less toxic form of therapy. This drug should be administered only by practitioners familiar with its many potential side effects.

Thalidomide is available as an investigational drug in the United States. Initially marketed as a sedative, it was withdrawn after being associated with severe human fetal teratogenicity. Nevertheless, thalidomide has been demonstrated as an effective agent in suppressing painful episodes of recurrent aphthous ulcerations in patients infected with human immunodeficiency virus (HIV) and in immunocompetent patients with intractable aphthous stomatitis. Anecdotal evidence also supports its use in the treatment of oral lesions of Melkersson-Rosenthal syndrome and chronic GVH disease. Daily doses of 100 to 200 mg often achieve rapid and dramatic resolution of large and painful oral aphthae. Thalidomide use in patients with Behçet's disease also produces marked improvement in oral ulcerations. In addition to maintaining adequate contraception in women, patients receiving thalidomide require careful monitoring for neurotoxicity and other adverse effects.

Cyclophosphamide, an alkylating agent, is a potent and extremely toxic immunosuppressant. The drug is reserved for patients whose disease is refractory to other immunosuppressive therapies. Its use in pemphigus and cicatricial pemphigoid has been well demonstrated. Patients with Wegener's granulomatosis and Behçet's disease undergoing therapy for their systemic disease achieve rapid resolution of oral symptoms. Doses of 1 to 2 mg/kg/day achieve steroid-sparing effects similar to those of azathioprine. Potential side effects include cystitis, an increased risk of malignancy, and bone marrow suppression.

RETINOIDS FOR LEUKOPLAKIA

As with lichen planus, the use of retinoids as a treatment for premalignant oral leukoplakia is controversial. With the exception of beta-carotene, systemic retinoids have considerable adverse effects that limit their use. Furthermore, their benefits are transitory, with relapses occurring upon discontinuation. Nevertheless, much interest has focused on retinoids as chemopreventive agents for precancerous and cancerous lesions of the oral cavity. Several clinical studies have shown that retinoids have the capability of reversing the dysplasia found in premalignant oral lesions. Furthermore, in patients with head and neck tumors who become disease-free after therapy, systemic retinoids significantly reduce the incidence of second primary malignancies.

Of the many synthetic analogs of vitamin A, 13-cis retinoic acid or isotretinoin (Accutane) indicated for the treatment of cystic acne has been studied most extensively. Doses of 1 mg/kg/day may result in considerable reduction of lesion size after several months of therapy, but there is wide variation in its reported benefits. Laboratory monitoring is required throughout therapy, and women of childbearing potential must practice appropriate birth control methods. Patients with widespread leukoplakia involving large areas of the mouth or those who are poor surgical candidates may benefit from systemic retinoids. Some success has also been reported with topical tretinoin in the treatment of oral leukoplakia. Although intraoral use of tretinoin has minimal adverse effects, additional studies are needed to confirm its efficacy and long-term benefits. Surgical excision remains the treatment of choice for oral premalignant lesions, however, isotretinoin and newer retinoids with fewer adverse effects (e.g., 4-hydroxy phenyl retinamide) are under intense investigation as chemopreventive agents.

ANTIVIRAL THERAPY FOR HERPES INFECTIONS

The treatment of recurrent herpes simplex infections (e.g., herpes labialis) with topical acyclovir (Zovirax) in immunocompetent patients decreases viral shedding but does not diminish pain or accelerate healing. By contrast, treatment with oral acyclovir (200 mg five times a day) hastens lesion resolution and reduces pain. A dose of 400 mg twice a day can be administered prophylactically and for extended periods to patients with a history of multiple recurrences. Similar doses are effective for treatment and prophylaxis of intraoral herpes infections. Prophylactic therapy with acyclovir at doses of 600 mg four times a day has been shown to be effective in preventing the reactivation of oral herpes infections in patients undergoing bone marrow transplantation. Patients undergoing induction chemotherapy for leukemia also routinely receive acyclovir prophylactically against intraoral herpes to prevent potential viremia.

In immunocompromised patients, oral herpes infections are generally associated with extensive tissue destruction and deep ulcerations. The dosage of acyclovir should be increased or administered intravenously, and the duration of therapy should be based on healing rather than the standard 7- to 10-day regimen. The emergence of acyclovir-resistant herpes simplex has been reported primarily in HIV-infected patients and has led to the development of newer antiviral agents. The administration of the prodrug of acyclovir, valacyclovir (Valtrex), results in enhanced bioavailability and significantly greater plasma concentrations than can be achieved with oral doses of acyclovir; therefore lower and less frequent doses of valacyclovir, which may improve patient compliance, are useful in the treatment of herpetic infections. Famciclovir (Famvir), like valacyclovir, is active in vitro against herpes simplex virus types 1 and 2, accelerates healing of oral lesions, and reduces the duration of symptoms.

A newly approved topical cream, penciclovir 1% (Denavir), has been shown in double-blind, placebo-controlled, clinical trials to decrease the duration of herpes labialis lesions as well as associated pain and viral shedding when the cream is applied every 2 hours for 4 consecutive days beginning at the onset of prodromal symptoms.

ANTIFUNGAL THERAPY

The agents available for the treatment of oral candidiasis are discussed in detail in Chapter 8 and are summarized in Tables 15-4 and 15-5. In general, attention to predisposing factors in the development of candidiasis is as important as the choice of therapeutic agent. For example, dry mouths should be moistened, dentures should be routinely removed at night, underlying systemic disorders including diabetes and anemia require identification and treatment, broad-spectrum antibiotics should be substituted with more specific agents, and poor oral hygiene should be corrected.

Patients who require short-term prophylaxis against candidiasis, such as bone marrow transplant recipients, benefit more from systemic than topical antifungals because systemic agents are more effective in preventing disease. Recurrences of oral candidal infection are common in HIV-infected patients; however, continuous prophylactic use may predispose toward drug resistance. For this reason, symptomatic infections may be treated, but continuous administration of systemic antifungals is not routinely warranted. In HIV-infected patients, topical therapy may be administered for

Table 15-4   Topical Agents for Oral Candidiasis

MEDICATION	FORM	DOSAGE	COMMENTS
Nystatin (Mycostatin)	Suspension (100,000 U/ml), vaginal tablets (100,000 U), pastille (200,000 U), cream and ointment (100,000 U/g)	3-5 times daily	Suspension and pastilles contain sugar and are cariogenic Cream used to treat angular cheilitis Ointment may be placed under infected denture
Amphotericin B (Fungizone)	Suspension (100 mg/5 ml)	4 times daily	Equivalent efficacy to other polyenes
Clotrimazole (Mycelex)	Troche (10 mg)	5 times daily	Contains sugar and is cariogenic Used prophylactically in chemotherapy patients
Chlorhexidine (Peridex)	Rinse (0.12%)	2 times daily	Used as adjuvant therapy or prophylactically in immunocompromised patients

identified infections, but systemic agents are more advantageous. The emergence of drug resistance to all of the azole antifungals and the potential for numerous drug interactions should be carefully considered when selecting a therapeutic agent.

BURNING MOUTH SYNDROME

A common but frequently misunderstood condition, burning mouth syndrome, refers to abnormal burning (stomatopyrosis) or pain (stomatodynia) of the mouth in the absence of any mucosal abnormalities. The disease affects women much more frequently than men and develops most often before or shortly after menopause. Although burning may be encountered on any or all of the oral surfaces, the tongue is most frequently affected (glossopyrosis) and is often the only site of involvement. The burning may be continuous or intermittent and commonly results in taste disturbances (dysgeusia).

Certain identifiable causes of a burning mouth are correctable. For example, candidiasis and allergic and irritant reactions may elicit burning in the oral cavity. All mouthwashes and dentifrices should be discontinued, and ingested allergens should be considered as potential etiologic factors. A comprehensive clinical oral examination is necessary to detect potential etiologic factors such as poorly fitting dental prostheses and oral habits such as rubbing the tongue against the lower teeth, clenching, and bruxism. A burning sensation of the oral cavity may also be an initial manifestation of an undetected systemic abnormality. Deficiencies of iron, folate, and vitamins B_6 and B_{12}, as well as diabetes mellitus, have all been associated with intraoral burning. When these abnormalities are corrected, the burning sensation resolves.

In the absence of an identifiable cause, patients with burning mouth syndrome still require therapy for their chronic pain. In general, many patients require only reassurance that the burning mouth syndrome is a genuine disorder commonly experienced by many individuals, and that the condition is not associated with oral or systemic malignancy. Thus patient education is an integral component of any treatment and should precede its initiation.

Topical preparations that may alleviate the sensation of burning include corticosteroid mouthwashes and retinoids, although these have been found to be beneficial only for a small group of patients. Capsaicin, the active ingredient in cayenne pepper, may itself induce severe burning but, when applied in small quantities to limited oral surfaces, has been reported to alleviate burning mouth syndrome. Topical anesthetics and mouthwashes consisting of palliative agents may also be efficacious. Xerostomia frequently accompanies burning mouth syndrome, and patients may benefit from con-

Table 15-5   Systemic Agents for Oral Candidiasis

MEDICATION	FORM	DOSAGE	COMMENTS
Ketoconazole (Nizoral)	200-mg tablet	1 time daily	Highest risk for abnormal liver function tests and hepatitis
Fluconazole (Diflucan)	100-mg tablet	1 time daily	Numerous drug interactions and potential for drug resistance Agent of choice for immunosuppressed patients and prophylaxis after bone marrow transplantation
Itraconazole (Sporanox)	100-mg capsule	1 time daily	Profile similar to fluconazole

suming cold fruit juices, sugarless candy or chewing gum, and ice chips. Although the disease is most prevalent perimenopausally, resolution following estrogen replacement therapy is inconsistent. Nevertheless, empiric treatment is warranted.

As with chronic burning conditions involving the genitalia or scalp, systemic therapy with antidepressants is highly effective. Amitriptyline (Elavil) and doxepin (Sinequan) have been studied most extensively in the management of burning mouth syndrome. An initial dose of 10 mg of either agent at bedtime may be increased to 150 mg, if tolerated. If both medications fail, chlordiazepoxide (Librium) (10 mg) may be used. Antipsychotic medications including pimozide (Orap) and fluoxetine (Prozac) and anticonvulsant drugs including clonazepam (Klonopin) and carbamazepine (Tegretol) should be reserved for refractory cases and administered by practitioners familiar with the many adverse effects of these agents. The large number of medications used in the management of patients with burning mouth syndrome is indicative of the relative ineffectiveness of any one particular agent. Fortunately, many patients with burning mouth syndrome either become accustomed and accommodate to the burning sensation or undergo spontaneous remission after a period of time.

NATURAL ALTERNATIVES: GREEN TEA

The trend toward using natural ingredients for treatment of diseases has gained considerable interest in recent years. Interestingly, it has been claimed that the overall health of the oral cavity can be maintained by the consumption of green tea. After water, tea is the world's most popular beverage, with green tea accounting for approximately one fifth of all tea consumed. Green tea contains polyphenols, the active agents that are destroyed in the fermentation process of black tea production. These compounds are unique to green tea.

Highly purified polyphenols have been reported to have profound beneficial effects against a wide and diverse group of diseases including lowering blood pressure and blood cholesterol levels, stabilizing blood sugars, inhibiting bacteria that cause a variety of infections, and blocking the action of many carcinogenic agents, thereby preventing various cancers. Green tea is consumed predominantly in the Far East, where the health benefits of tea drinking have been claimed for thousands of years. Green tea polyphenols possess potent antioxidative and antiviral properties, which account for their popularity as preventive agents in maintaining oral health. In recent years, specific green tea polyphenols identified for oral cavity disorders have been zealously promoted for the prevention of dental caries and gingivitis. These agents inhibit the growth of *Streptococcus mutans,* the major etiologic bacterium in tooth decay, and *Porphyromonas gingivalis,* the etiologic bacterium in periodontal disease. In vitro and in vivo studies also support the efficacy of green tea polyphenols in the prevention of dental caries and gingivitis primarily by the inhibition of dental plaque formation. The safety of green tea consumption and its reported benefits strengthen the role of polyphenols as natural supplements in an oral health prevention program.

SUGGESTED READINGS

General

Bottomley WK, Rosenberg SW: *Clinicians guide to treatment of common oral conditions,* New York, 1983, American Academy of Oral Medicine.

Gage TW, Atherton-Pickett F: *Dental drug reference,* St Louis, 1997, Mosby.

Neidle EA, Yagiela JA: *Pharmacology and therapeutics for dentistry,* ed 3, St Louis, 1989, Mosby.

Shingler DC: *The blue book: dental prescription handbook,* Cleveland, 1996, American Academy of Oral Pharmacology.

Specific

Aufdemorte TB, De Villez RL, Parel-SM: Modified topical steroid therapy for the treatment of oral mucous membrane pemphigoid, *Oral Surg Oral Med Oral Pathol* 59:256, 1985.

Beutner KR: Valacyclovir: a review of its antiviral activity, pharmacokinetic properties and clinical efficacy, *Antiviral Res* 28:281, 1995.

Bystryn JC, Steinman NM: The adjuvant therapy of pemphigus: an update, *Arch Dermatol* 132:203, 1996.

Como JA, Dismukes WE: Oral azole drugs as systemic antifungal therapy, *N Engl J Med* 330:263, 1994.

Eisen D: The therapy of oral lichen planus, *Crit Rev Oral Biol Med* 4:141, 1993.

Eisen D et al: Effect of topical cyclosporine rinse on oral lichen planus: a double-blind analysis, *N Engl J Med* 323:290, 1990.

Epstein JB, Reece DE: Topical cyclosporin A for treatment of oral chronic graft-versus-host disease, *Bone Marrow Transplant* 13:81, 1994.

Fountzilas G: Retinoids in the management of head and neck cancer: an update, *J Chemother* 6:127, 1994.

Garber GE: Treatment of oral Candida mucositis infections, *Drugs* 47:734, 1994.

Garewal H: Antioxidants in oral cancer prevention, *Am J Clin Nutr* 62:1410, 1995.

Gorsky M, Silverman S, Chinn H: Clinical characteristics and management outcome in the burning mouth syndrome: an open study of 130 patients, *Oral Surg Oral Med Oral Pathol* 72:192, 1991.

Greenspan D: The treatment of oropharyngeal candidiasis in HIV-positive patients, *J Am Acad Dermatol* 31:51, 1994.

Hay RJ: Antifungal therapy of yeast infections, *J Am Acad Dermatol* 31:6, 1994.

Hersle K et al: Severe oral lichen planus: treatment with an aromatic retinoid (etretinate), *Br J Dermatol* 106:77, 1982.

Ho VC, Zloyty DM: Immunosuppressive agents in dermatology, *Dermatol Clin* 11:73, 1993.

Huang W, Rothe MJ, Grant-Kels JM: The burning mouth syndrome, *J Am Acad Dermatol* 34:91, 1996.

Huilgol SC, Black MM: Management of the immunobullous disorders: pemphigus, *Clin Exp Dermatol* 20:283, 1995.

Katz J et al: Prevention of recurrent aphthous stomatitis with colchicine: an open trial, *J Am Acad Dermatol* 31:459, 1994.

Kaugars GE et al: Use of antioxidant supplements in the treatment of human oral leukoplakia, *Oral Surg Oral Med Oral Pathol Oral Radiol Endod* 81:5, 1996.

Lozada-Nur F, Miranda C, Maliksi R: Double-blind clinical trial of 0.05% clobetasol propionate ointment in Orabase and 0.05% fluocinonide ointment in Orabase in the treatment of patients with oral vesiculoerosive diseases, *Oral Surg Oral Med Oral Pathol* 77:598, 1994.

Makimura M et al: Inhibitory effect of tea catechins on collagenase activity, *J Periodontol* 64:630, 1993.

Perry CM, Wagstaff AJ: Famciclovir: a review of its pharmacological properties and therapeutic efficacy in herpesvirus infections, *Drugs* 50:396, 1995.

Poskitt L, Wojnarowska F: Treatment of cicatricial pemphigoid with tetracycline and nicotinamide, *Clin Exp Dermatol* 20:258, 1995.

Rayani SA et al: Implementation and evaluation of a standardized herpes simplex virus prophylaxis protocol on a leukemia/bone marrow transplant unit, *Ann Pharmacother* 28:852, 1994.

Revuv J et al: Crossover study of thalidomide vs. placebo in severe recurrent aphthous stomatitis, *Arch Dermatol* 126:923, 1990.

Sakanaka S: Inhibitory effects of green tea polyphenols on growth and cellular adherence of an oral bacterium, *Porphyromonas gingivalis*, *Biosci Biotechnol Biochem* 60:745, 1996.

Siegel MA, Balciunas BA: Oral presentation and management of vesiculobullous disorders, *Semin Dermatol* 13:78, 1994.

Spruance SL et al: Treatment of recurrent herpes simplex labialis with oral acyclovir, *J Infect Dis* 161:185, 1990.

Spruance SL et al: Penciclovir cream for the treatment of herpes simplex labialis, *J Am Med Assoc* 277:1374, 1997.

Tourne LPM, Fricton JR: Burning mouth syndrome: critical review and proposed clinical management, *Oral Surg Oral Med Oral Pathol* 74:158, 1992.

Vincent SD, Lilly GE, Baker KA: Clinical, historic, and therapeutic features of cicatricial pemphigoid: a literature review and open therapeutic trial with corticosteroids, *Oral Surg Oral Med Oral Pathol* 76:453, 1993.

Wojnarowska F, Allen J, Collier P: Linear IgA disease: a heterogeneous disease, *Dermatology* 189:52, 1994.

Index

Page numbers followed by t indicate tables and f indicate figures.